Ovariotomy: Surgical Advances and Concerns

Ovariotomy: Surgical Advances and Concerns

Edited by Jane Edwin

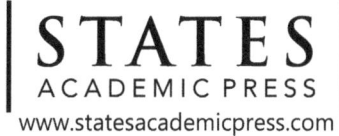

STATES
ACADEMIC PRESS
www.statesacademicpress.com

States Academic Press,
109 South 5th Street,
Brooklyn, NY 11249, USA

Visit us on the World Wide Web at:
www.statesacademicpress.com

ISBN: 978-1-63989-402-4

Cataloging-in-Publication Data

Ovariotomy : surgical advances and concerns / edited by Jane Edwin.
p. cm.
Includes bibliographical references and index.
ISBN 978-1-63989-402-4
1. Ovariotomy. 2. Ovaries--Surgery. I. Edwin, Jane.
RG481 .O83 2022
618.11--dc23

Table of Contents

Preface

The removal of ovaries through surgery is termed as ovariotomy or ovariectomy. It is also used to remove ovarian cysts and resectioning a portion of the ovaries. It plays an important part in reducing the probability of developing ovarian cancer. The surgical process in which both ovaries and both Fallopian tubes are removed is termed as bilateral salpingo-oophorectomy. Ovariotomy is recommended for people who have ovarian cancer, ovarion torsion, endometriosis or a tubo ovarian abscess. The major methods for conducting this procedure are laparotomy and minimally invasive laparoscopic surgery. The selection of the method for surgery depends on the situation. This book unfolds the innovative aspects of ovariotomy which will be crucial for the progress of this field in the future. It presents researches and studies performed by experts across the globe. The book is appropriate for students seeking detailed information in this area as well as for experts.

This book has been the outcome of endless efforts put in by authors and researchers on various issues and topics within the field. The book is a comprehensive collection of significant researches that are addressed in a variety of chapters. It will surely enhance the knowledge of the field among readers across the globe.

It gives us an immense pleasure to thank our researchers and authors for their efforts to submit their piece of writing before the deadlines. Finally in the end, I would like to thank my family and colleagues who have been a great source of inspiration and support.

Editor

1

Introduction

'It is...an interesting question to be decided as to why and wherefore a poor little Fallopian tube or withered ovary should possess the power of setting men by the ears', commented an editorial in the *Medical Press and Circular* in 1888.[1] Looking back to the nineteenth century, historians might be inclined to wonder the same thing. During this time, the ovary, as an object of physiological and pathological enquiry, and as a site of surgical intervention, engendered more debate and controversy within the profession than any other bodily organ. In the late 1830s, the removal of diseased ovaries, usually those with large non-malignant tumours, became the first surgical procedure involving major abdominal section to be performed with a degree of regularity, and in 1842, the Manchester surgeon Charles Clay began what was to become a long and unbroken series of operations where he removed the organ. During this decade, the operation was given a name that would be etched on the history of the Victorian era: 'ovariotomy', a neologism coined by the Edinburgh obstetrician James Young Simpson in 1843 to describe Clay's work.

For the next twenty-five years, the justifiability of opening the abdomen to treat ovarian disease would remain contested, causing deep schisms in the profession, through which reputations were lost and careers ruined just as often as fortunes were gained and lives were saved. It was an operation that thrilled and horrified in equal measure with its daring, as surgeons cut through the peritoneum—the membrane in which the abdominal organs were enfolded—to remove the ovaries.

Its development marked a critical juncture in the emergence of modern surgery, as the justifiability of using surgery to treat a chronic internal disease became the centre of debate. The question of whether the chance to cure a patient allowed for the substantial risk to life posed by a major surgical operation went to the heart of medical ethics and divided the profession, raising questions about the degree of power that surgeons could and should exercise over the human body. Advocates and opponents of the procedure clashed over the operation in the pages of the medical press. Robert Liston, Professor of Surgery at University College London in the 1830s and 1840s, declared those who performed ovarian surgery to be liable to charges of homicide and denounced them as 'belly-rippers', a macabre turn of phrase, which signalled the emotionally charged atmosphere surrounding the operation.[2]

In the late 1860s, mortality rates for the operation began to decline significantly, in part due to the work of two exceptionally prolific and skilful practitioners, the Edinburgh obstetrician Thomas Keith and London surgeon Thomas Spencer Wells. Keith had begun performing ovariotomy in 1862 and five years later had published the striking results of his first fifty-one cases: forty of his patients had recovered, with all but one of those individuals seemingly completely cured.[3] His recovery rate of around eighty per cent was equal to, if not better than, those of other established 'capital' operations: procedures like amputation, which came with a high risk of death.[4] By the late 1870s, ovariotomy was beginning to be depicted as one of the major surgical innovations of the past decades, gaining a status similar to that of the discovery of anaesthesia or the introduction of Listerian antisepsis.

For the rest of the century, ovariotomy would occupy a complex position within medicine. It was an operation which symbolised surgical progress, but it also remained precipitously close to the boundaries of ethical acceptability. The controversial nature of the operation did not dissipate as more patients survived the procedure. On the contrary, ovarian surgery remained a frequent catalyst for debate as the medical and cultural climate changed over the course of the nineteenth century. From the priority disputes and accusations of greed that were directed at specialists in the operation during the 1860s, to the controversies of the 1880s and 1890s when some surgeons began removing ovaries as a means of curing other bodily diseases, those who performed ovariotomy were never more than a hair's breadth from disrepute. Egos collided, and professional territories were defended by those who populated its practice; 'with its lights and its shades, its friends and its foes, its converts and its perverts, the history of ovariotomy reads like a romance', American gynaecologist William Goodell commented in 1879, capturing something of contemporary perceptions of the operation.[5]

By the end of the 1880s, many British surgeons were advancing the idea that ovarian surgery was out of control. The previous decades had seen several pioneers in the area have their careers laid waste by revelations that they had not published the full extent of their experiences with the operation, including cases which had resulted in death. The long-lasting effect of this was a peculiar paranoia among 'ovariotomists'—as those who performed the operation were increasingly known—about any hint of secrecy regarding operators' experiences with the procedure. The medical press was crammed with reports of ovariotomies well into the 1880s, as cases which saw even a slight deviation from the normal mode of operating or in outcome continued to be printed. However, some individuals expressed unhappiness that the prestige of ovariotomists still seemed to rest upon the number of ovaries that they removed. The high volume of cases—even if successful—was no longer viewed as inherently positive but rather a sign that women's reproductive organs were being removed indiscriminately.[6] The British ovariotomist George Granville Bantock reported to the British Gynaecological Society a cautionary tale from America, where surgeons were perceived as even more gung-ho than their British counterparts. It was, he claimed, 'no uncommon thing in New York to see a soup-plateful of uterine appendages presented by some of the younger surgeons to some of the societies there'.[7]

Bantock's disturbing image rivalled anything to be found in contemporary medical allegories such as Wilkie Collins' *Heart and Science* (1882–1883) or later, Bram Stoker's *Dracula* (1897), both of which, through the medium of gothic horror, addressed issues that were increasingly played out in the ovariotomy debate.[8] In the 1880s, the operation had become entwined with controversies over animal experimentation as some anti-vivisectionist campaigners claimed that 'experimental' abdominal surgery on women was analogous to vivisection, a comparison that melded all too easily with Victorian understandings of female vulnerability.[9] Cases were unearthed of women's ovaries being removed under circumstances of dubious consent and for seemingly trivial conditions. The filtering into the general press of such unpalatable aspects to ovariotomy caused anxiety among the profession. Gynaecological surgeons began acquiring an unfortunate reputation for unnecessary operating. Thus, the latter decades of the nineteenth century saw ovariotomists engaged in a battle to save their professional identity, as many tried to distance themselves from the controversies engulfing the field. Fears of excessive operating were reinforced by growing evidence that the ovaries were responsible not just for reproduction but also for the development of feminine characteristics. This made the removal of both ovaries for anything less than a serious condition, questionable, and spurred some surgeons to consider more conservative measures. By the 1890s, both radical surgery and conservative resection of the ovaries were being presented as therapeutic choices for women; thus, it was not only the *place* of ovariotomy in the surgical canon that was being called into question but, by the turn of the twentieth century, also the very *definition* of the operation that was being contested.

A GENDERED OPERATION?

Within the history of ovariotomy, one does not have to look too hard to find affirmation that the operation was used experimentally and irresponsibly and that vulnerable women were operated on in circumstances where their consent is questionable. That the procedure was used, on occasion, to 'cure' maladies like hysteria, presents troubling questions about the way invasive medical procedures were being used to control female behaviour. Historians have been rightly attentive to the connections the operation reveals between normative gender values and experimental and risky surgery. Indeed, the operation served as an important tool for women's historians in the latter half of the twentieth century, especially those intent on exposing patriarchy within the medical realm. For feminist activists Barbara Ehrenreich and Deirdre English, for example, writing in America in 1978 amid second wave feminism and an expanding women's health movement, the operation was a clear indication of the repressive sexual politics of the Victorian era. Removal of the ovaries was, as they evocatively put it, part of the 'gynecologist's exotic catalog of tortures'.[10] Ehrenreich and English set the scene for histories which viewed the operation as primarily configured upon surgical mismanagement—or at the very least over-management—of the female body. Ornella Moscucci's *The Science of Woman* (1990), Thomas Laqueur's *Making Sex* (1990) and Ann Dally's *Women Under the Knife* (1991), while less polemical than Ehrenreich and English's work, all identified the introduction of ovariotomy as a fundamental moment in the medicalisation of women, through which cultural notions of femininity were embedded into surgical practice.[11] More recent scholarship by

Deirdre Cooper Owens has nuanced understandings of the relationship between surgery, gender and race in nineteenth-century American gynaecology. Cooper Owens examines the ways in which doctors relied on gendered and racialised notions of black women, including an erroneous belief that they had a higher tolerance of pain, as a justification for their use of enslaved women's bodies as sites for experimentation with procedures centred upon the female reproductive organs, including ovariotomy.[12]

The cultural politics of ovariotomy are also explored in the works of Regina Morantz-Sanchez and Claire Brock, both of whom have drawn attention to the role female surgeons played in promoting the operation's practice on both sides of the Atlantic. Each has also highlighted the active role some female patients played in demanding ovarian surgery, showing that the position of female actors in the surgical encounter was highly variable depending on their social and economic status; patient experience did not always align to a narrative of passive patients and domineering doctors.[13] This speaks to a wider network of literature which has critiqued the 'social essentialism' that constructivist accounts of medicine may give rise to, and which can lead to a broad strokes approach to gendering medicine.[14] As the case of ovariotomy makes clear, patient agency must be taken into consideration, even if the nature of that agency was complex and, at times, compromised.

OVARIOTOMY AND INNOVATION

This book does not negate the importance of gender as a means of analysing ovariotomy. But it must be considered as one of multiple aspects at work in the introduction of the operation. In this study, it is innovation which is my conceptual focal point. Ovariotomy is one of the most significant and yet most accessible historical examples of the complexities of innovation in surgery; symbolic of the hopes and fears of the surgical profession, its performance was embedded in a network of ideas and ideals about the role of surgery in society. How was surgical innovation defined, diffused and understood? In this book, I seek to go beyond the polarisation, which has, until recently, been common in historical writing on surgery, with 'social' histories on one side, which often only pay lip service to the technical aspects of operations, and heavily technical accounts on the other, which can marginalise social and cultural considerations.[15] In this way, it speaks to recent works by historians like Thomas Schlich, Christopher Crenner, Claire Brock and Sally Wilde in attempting to recognise that the technical minutiae of operative surgery are worthy of analytical enquiry and that changes in the professional culture of surgery and in patient–practitioner relationships cannot be regarded as separate from the process of technical innovation.[16]

An approach which makes innovation its guiding framework requires some justification, or at least, clarification. 'Innovation' is a rather amorphous word and can be applied to so many different things that it can all too easily come to mean nothing as a reference point. Generally, we understand the term to convey novelty or newness. But the broadness of this definition means that 'innovation' often implies not only novelty but advancement as well. 'Innovation' is a term ascribed a great deal of value in today's cultural climate, a buzzword for businesses of all kinds. As pervasive as 'innovation' is today, the historical context to medical innovation, and particularly surgical innovation, has been less well understood. As John Pickstone noted, '"innovation" is a fashionable word, but not without reason; we are all rather weary of "progress"'.[17] As he seems to imply, innovation can become simply a more circumspect way to describe narratives of progress. Pickstone raised these concerns over twenty years ago, and yet they resonate strongly today. 'Innovation' has become the favoured term for many organisations as part of the representation of their ideas, goods and services; not least in medicine, where both private and ostensibly public initiatives have pushed the idea that the creation and diffusion of new products and processes is the only logical economic rationale for optimising and improving medical services.[18]

Emerging innovations have rarely been accepted unquestioningly. Innovation is a contested and lengthy process, not simply the invention and introduction of a 'better' product or service. In medicine especially, new procedures, technologies and theories have often triggered concerns about the risks they might bring, especially to the patient, and medical historians have been attentive to the interplay between risk, consent and innovation. Edited volumes by Pickstone, as well as Ilana Löwy and Thomas Schlich and Ulrich Tröhler, have thrown light on the diverse fates of new medicines and medical technologies.[19] More recently, Thomas Schlich and Christopher Crenner have vastly widened the scope of historical investigation of surgical innovation, with their edited volume devoted to the subject. The volume marks out the need to consider the distinct challenges and complexities of surgical innovation within the broader category of medical innovation, given its close associations with physicality and corporeality and its strong technological component.[20]

Crucially, Schlich and Crenner also stress the importance of positioning successful surgical innovations in the context of the alternative technologies and therapeutics *not* taken up by medical professionals; 'taking these alternatives into account helps understand the choices and decisions made by historical actors', they contend.[21]

Most historical work on medical innovation tends to focus upon the twentieth century, reflecting an idea that it was during this period significant doubts began to arise as to whether innovation in medicine was intrinsically a 'good' thing; 'there have been mixed feelings about medical innovations since the 1960s, and one can identify an increased interest in risk in recent times' wrote Schlich and Tröhler.[22] Disillusionment with scientific and technological innovation has become entangled with ideas of modernity.[23] This has not necessarily precluded historical analysis of medical innovations before the twentieth century: all the volumes cited above include some essays that deal with innovations from before this time.[24] Nonetheless, it has led some historians to assume that before the twentieth century medical novelties were much more readily accepted as positive changes; John Pickstone even pinpointed the nineteenth century as exemplifying this, suggesting that 'we no longer have the high Victorian confidence that change is for the best'.[25]

Just like the related concept of 'risk', because 'innovation' is fashionable *now* we might assume that projecting it onto the more distant past is presentist. But this belies a long and rich history of innovation—both as a word and concept. As historian of science Benoît Godin has observed, 'for most of its history the concept innovation, a word of Greek origin, carried pejorative connotations. As "Introducing change to the established order", innovation was seen as deviant behaviour, forbidden and punished'.[26] Often synonymic with notions of revolution—another word which would come to have important connotations for nineteenth-century surgeons—innovation had long been fraught with political and social uncertainty. Only in the nineteenth century, as the impoverished inventor was recast as the heroic Briton who fulfilled a productive role in society, did innovation begin to be understood more positively, or at least, less as a signal of radicalism or instability.[27] Surgeons were keen to apply this characterisation to themselves, and as more patients survived ovariotomy, medical men increasingly perceived the operation to be deeply symbolic, not just of Victorian progress but also of Victorian *morality*: a procedure that had saved the lives of thousands of suffering women across the social spectrum. Nonetheless, as Godin points out, 'innovation' continued to have troubling associations throughout the century. Even for those who saw ovariotomy as progress, there were ripples of unease about the extent to which surgery was being transformed by the operation; as one surgeon suggested in 1866, ovariotomy was 'perhaps the most startling innovation in surgery of late years…our old notion, that it was death to the patient to interfere with the peritoneum, has been somewhat rudely swept away by the wholesale manner in which it is now cut through, and burnt through, and mopped out with sponges'.[28] Even if innovation was not considered an outright mischief and was seen as necessary to progress, it remained shocking and, at times, brutal.

THE DISTINCTIVENESS OF SURGICAL INNOVATION

From today's viewpoint, there has been a striking continuity over the last two centuries in the way that innovation in surgery has been conceived of as distinctive. The performance of novel and experimental surgery remains contentious, continuing to be fertile ground for media speculation, feeding curiosity among the public about the closed world of surgery and the drama, emotion and medical spectacle concealed within it.[29] Recent controversies around novel procedures such as synthetic tracheal transplants and vaginal mesh implants have garnered poor press for surgeons and attest to the still very present possibility of patients undergoing risky operations in circumstances where their informed consent is debatable.[30] Moreover, the question of standardisation also concerned nineteenth-century surgeons in ways that it continues to do so today.[31] Attaining standardisation in surgery has always been checked by the aspect of performance that is central to it, which can make achieving uniformity in practice difficult. Despite the advent of minimally invasive and robotic technologies in surgery in recent years, just as in the nineteenth century, surgery today is largely the product of individual idiosyncrasies and reliant on an operating surgeon's manual dexterity. Today, this is most apparent in the difficulties of reconciling randomised controlled trials with operative surgery; 'choices about the exact size and location of the incision are individual to the surgeon and to each patient, as are the exact steps of each operation' the surgeon Peter Angelos has written; 'thus, it is often difficult to standardise procedures, which make large multicentre clinical trials of surgical procedures difficult to undertake'.[32] In his study of coronary artery bypass grafting in the 1970s, David S. Jones examined how, even in the late twentieth century, technological innovations in surgery largely remained outside the domain of the randomised controlled trial. In the shadow of trials becoming the 'gold standard' for assessing new treatments, the relative imperviousness of surgery to the method has put it increasingly at odds with other branches of medicine.[33]

Nineteenth-century surgeons likewise struggled to reach a definitive consensus as to what innovation meant to them and what was the best way to achieve it; standardisation in surgery was both desired and yet problematic to the flourishing of new procedures, which, like today, was seen to rely on a certain amount of creativity.[34] This was most obviously revealed in the well-documented tensions between 'art' and 'science' in nineteenth-century medicine. Steve Sturdy has argued that divisions between the two have been overstated by historians.[35] Certainly, such a dichotomy indicates a questionable reliance on rather essentialist concepts of 'science' and 'art' in medicine, when the two were never entirely separate entities anyway—it was perhaps more the case that an imbalance in favour of science was suspected, rather than an outward hostility to scientific surgery itself. Nonetheless, doctors *did* worry about the loss of artistic flair in the face of scientific medicine, and surgeons did imagine art and science to be two ideal constituents of surgery.[36]

These continuities are balanced out—if not outweighed—by historical contingencies. Today, clinical medicine is predicated upon levels of collective, experiential information, guidelines and managerial regulation unimagined in the nineteenth century. Thus, by reflecting on how surgical innovation was understood before the significant changes that would occur in the organisation of medicine in the twentieth century, I look to the very specific culture of the long nineteenth century and understandings of professional etiquette, patient–practitioner relationships and medical philosophies at this time. In this context, how was surgical innovation dealt with? And to what extent was surgical innovation perceived of as distinct from other types of medical innovation? The time span of this study is relatively lengthy, looking at a period from around the middle of the eighteenth century, when ovarian surgery first began to be discussed, up until the first decade of the twentieth century. But it focuses tightly on a specific technique—surgical interference with the ovaries—in what might be described as an operation-centred history, something which differentiates it considerably from previous historical work on ovariotomy and, with the notable exception of Thomas Schlich's work on osteosynthesis, most work on the history of surgery.[37]

The British experience of ovariotomy is the focus of this book. It was an experience, however, that was continually informed by international contexts. British practitioners' self-identity was in part shaped by the perception they had of themselves on the international stage and in their competitive rivalry with surgeons overseas, most noticeably those in France and America, where the operation had its roots. Within British medical culture, there were also deep divides, between general practitioners and elite consultants, obstetricians and general surgeons, and between metropolitan and provincial practitioners; all would impact upon the shaping of the operation. This book then, takes as its starting point what was ostensibly a single innovation in a single country, tracing its antecedents, diffusions and controversies. If this initial trajectory may seem linear, the outcome is anything but. This is not a story of how an innovation was developed and accepted. Rather, it shows how complex the integration of ovariotomy was into practice because its meaning and definition were continually contested.

SOURCES

The book draws upon a range of personal and institutional records. In the former category, collections containing the correspondence and papers of James Young Simpson, Robert Lee, Charles Clay and Robert Liston have helped to build a picture of practitioners' personal experiences of the operation. Archival material pertaining to lectures given by integral actors in surgery and obstetrics such as James Blundell, William Hunter and John Hunter has shed light on the ways in which senior members of the profession sought to shape students' understandings of surgical ethics.

As with many other areas of medicine, particularly those involving women's experiences, patients' first-hand accounts of ovarian surgery are lacking. For the most part, where patient experiences are cited, they are taken from archival or printed sources, and mainly derived from literature where the patient experience has been mediated through the voice of the (almost invariably male) practitioner. This should not be assumed to necessarily invalidate such accounts; in fact, many of them speak to the relationship between the patient and the networks of practitioners they encountered, where the power dynamics were not always straightforward.

Institutional records such as those for the Académie Royale de Chirurgie in Paris, the Samaritan Hospital for Women in London, the Chelsea Hospital for Women and the London Hospital have also provided significant insights. Patient records, doctors' committees, society meetings and operation registers have provided both in-depth detail about individual cases and the opportunity to find data which reveal the extent to which ovariotomies were being performed in hospital settings. These records were not always easy to analyse. At the London Hospital, for example, some cases are documented in one type of record but not in another (for instance they are listed in the Surgical Beadle's Register but not in the Surgical Index) or are indexed under different categories of operation depending on the record. An operation where both the uterus and ovaries were removed might be described as both 'ovariotomy' and 'hysterectomy', for example. Nonetheless, the records consulted were sufficiently expansive and accurate so as to make the data taken from them useful.

It might be tempting to see published sources as of secondary significance to personal correspondence and papers, which could be considered to provide a more authentic voice to historical actors because they were not intended for a public audience. In the case of ovarian surgery, however, what *was* said publicly was just as significant as what was not and none the less authentic for that. The permanence and publicity of print often made the pages of medical journals a more productive location than private correspondence for thrashing out issues of surgical morality and etiquette. Moreover, private communications were often referenced and re-published in the press anyway, blurring the boundaries between public and private. There is no question that much of the debate about ovarian surgery was very intentionally played out publicly and that this was facilitated by the emergence of medical weeklies during the first half of the nineteenth century, something which will be explored in more detail in Chapter 3. While medical societies were already well established, the introduction of titles such as the *Lancet* in 1823, the *Medical Times* in 1839, and *The Provincial Medical and Surgical Journal* in 1840 meant that a culture of print centred on medical practice was flourishing. Journals like the rabble-rousing *Lancet* seemed to encourage heated exchanges of correspondence between ovariotomists and other interested parties, while editorial pieces gave voice to strongly worded opinions about the operation that were then quickly spread among practitioners all over the country and beyond. Yet, there were significant boundaries in place which hint at the complexity to the meanings of 'public' debate; the leaking of medical discussions into the non-medical press was thought to be dangerous ground by most medical practitioners, and when reports about controversies in ovarian surgery spilled into the non-medical press, it was much to the chagrin of the profession. Popular surgical monographs have also been useful in showing the kind of pedagogical information that was being disseminated about ovariotomy on a wide scale. Surgical textbooks of the nineteenth century were by no means disinterested manuals objectively listing technical information. On the contrary, they often cited the issues of medical morality that controversial surgical innovations brought to the fore, discussing not only the technical aspects of an operation but its ethics too.

OUTLINE OF THE BOOK

While today we often associate innovation with cutting edge, radical change, the development of ovarian surgery was a drawn-out, often lumbering process, although one, crucially, that was set in motion earlier than other forms of abdominal surgery. The operation to remove diseased ovaries is most usually conceptualised as an innately Victorian invention. This is a notion that was perpetuated not only by Victorian surgeons themselves as they forged historical accounts of the operation, but also by many historians, who have viewed the procedure as reflective of Victorian ideals regarding surgical ethics and gender. Chapter 2 offers a different perspective by tracing the roots of ovarian surgery back to the eighteenth century. During this time, the diseased ovary was seen to be pathologically complex, which made it an object of curiosity in the burgeoning field of morbid anatomy. Diseased ovaries were notoriously difficult to diagnose at an early stage and considered almost impossible to treat by medical therapeutics. These difficulties led to an interest among English, Scottish, French and American medical practitioners in the possibility of finding a surgical solution to the disease. The chapter argues for the need for innovation to be understood as a process that is often temporally expansive, challenging contemporary understandings of 'innovation' which have seen it effectively become a byword for speed and efficiency.

Chapter 3 brings together two novelties of the early nineteenth century, ovariotomy and the weekly medical press, to unpack the debates around the justifiability of the operation which occurred between the 1830s and 1860s, a time during which it was given the appellation 'ovariotomy'.

The procedure polarised the medical community. For an increasingly vocal group of advocates, the operation was heralded as the beginning of a new era in surgery. For influential opponents, it was nothing more than a useless and possibly criminal procedure. How was it possible that the operation could be construed in such diametrically opposite terms? This question stimulates the key theme of the chapter: namely how representations of the operation in the public sphere were constructed, principally through the medical press. There was a thirst for knowledge about the operation. But by what means was the truth about ovariotomy's risks best conveyed? The operation was subject from both its supporters and detractors to highly emotive 'subjective' accounts, which centred upon patient narratives, as well as to 'objective' statistical deconstructions. Surgical statistics were a crucial part of conveying the risks of the operation, but, as some surgeons argued, how could mere mortality rates, stripped of details, represent the full account of a patient's pathology, or the unexpected mysteries of the internal body, and the multitude of risks in the days after an operation?

Chapter 4 looks at how the professional community assigned credit to those responsible for innovation in ovarian surgery. By the mid-1860s, the standing of ovariotomy, both within the professional sphere and beyond, was rapidly improving. As the operation's status ascended, those who had risked their reputation by performing it became more vocal about receiving credit for doing so. Claims for credit could be deconstructed into the components that formed the operation: new surgical instruments, aftercare methods and different types of incision could all be claimed as individual innovations, challenging notions of ovariotomy being a single invention. There was also a high-profile dispute, principally between Charles Clay and Thomas Spencer Wells, as to who should be credited overall with establishing ovariotomy in Britain. The quarrel between Clay and Wells attested to an instability in the definition of the operation, with both surgeons pointing to distinctions in their practices, which complicated claims to credit. Traditional legal methods of attaining intellectual property, such as patenting, were considered inapplicable to surgery for ethical and practical reasons. And yet, with reforms in patent law improving intellectual property rights for inventors in other areas of industry during the middle decades of the century, medical practitioners sought to construct alternative methods for managing and awarding credit.

Following on from some of the issues raised in the preceding chapter, Chapter 5 will explore the contentious relationship between ovariotomy and money. In the 1850s, murmurings abounded in the medical press about the lucrative nature of ovariotomy. These rumours were played upon by opponents of the operation, keen to perpetuate a characterisation of ovariotomists as money-grubbing opportunists preying upon the desperately ill. However, they contained an element of truth: a private ovariotomy could be very expensive with surgeons charging up to a hundred guineas for an operation. These powerful financial associations were revealing not only of the ascendance of surgeons' professional status but also the pecuniary gains and, potentially, losses that association with surgical innovation could bring. At a time when many other medical procedures and therapies were comparatively simple and relatively cheap, the skills and risks associated with major surgical operations, as well as the lengthy period of aftercare they required, raised questions about money distinct from the rest of medicine. In the final part of the chapter, I look more broadly at the place of ovariotomy within consumer society. In the 1880s and 1890s, as the operation became markedly safer, there were growing concerns that ovariotomy was being performed excessively, and even unnecessarily, as both surgeons and patients were swept up in a 'fashion' for ovariotomy. It led to troubling questions about the impact of consumerism upon medical authority.

Accounts of ovariotomy's history almost invariably conclude with the outcries in the 1880s and 1890s, followed by the operation's apparent decline. The reality was more complicated. In Chapter 6, I argue for a framework of surgical innovation that moves beyond simplistic dichotomies of success and failure, of straightforward beginnings and neat endings. Instead, this chapter offers something more akin to an exploration of the 'afterlife' of the operation that followed the controversies surrounding it towards the end of the century. The need to do so, I argue, is elucidated by the fractured identity of ovariotomy by the 1890s, as the methods of and reasons for operating upon the ovaries began to rapidly proliferate. As the term 'ovariotomy' became more uncertain in meaning, a range of other terms emerged to refer to new techniques in ovarian surgery that were being practiced; taxonomic and conceptual confusion was becoming readily apparent. 'Afterlife' alludes also to growing fears at the turn of the century about the long-term effects upon women's health that might come from removing their ovaries. The term speaks also to the formation of ovariotomy as an historical phenomenon during this time—even while it remained in contemporary practice—as its long history became the subject of intense reflection on the part of the profession.

NOTES

1. 'The Militant Spirit in Gynaecology Societies', *Medical Press and Circular* 45 (9 May 1888): 495.
2. The phrase was first attributed to Robert Liston by the obstetrician Robert Lee in his 1853 publication, *Clinical Reports of Ovarian and Uterine Diseases* (London: John Churchill, 1853), 83.
3. Thomas Keith, 'Fifty-One Cases of Ovariotomy', *Lancet* 90, no. 2297 (7 September 1867): 290–291.
4. James Paget, 'The Address in Surgery', *British Medical Journal* 2, no. 155 (16 August 1862): 161. In which Paget estimated that ten to fifty per cent of amputations remained fatal as did '20 or more per cent' of lithotomies.
5. William Goodell, *Lessons in Gynecology* (Philadelphia: D. G. Brinton, 1879), 299.
6. 'The British Gynaecological Society, November 11th 1885', *British Gynaecological Journal* 1, no. 4 (1886): 386.
7. 'The British Gynaecological Society, November 11th 1885', 386. 'Uterine appendages' was a term used (and still is today) to collectively describe the ovaries, Fallopian tubes and surrounding ligaments.
8. Wilkie Collins, *Heart and Science: A Story of the Present Time* (Peterborough: Broadview Press, 1996); Bram Stoker, *Dracula* (London: Penguin, 1994). First published as a serial between 1882 and 1883, *Heart and Science* was Collins' response to the vivisection debate. A vehemently anti-vivisection vehicle, the horror of doctors' experimentations were neatly characterised in Dr. Nathan Benjulia, a villainous vivisector who neglects a vulnerable young woman with brain disease in an effort to hasten death and acquire her brain for post-mortem study. Bram Stoker's *Dracula* published in 1897, when anxieties about the overuse of ovariotomy were still heightened, has equally been read as a metaphor for male medical control of female behaviour, embodied particularly in the attempts to save the vampiric and sexually charged character, Lucy Westenra. See Tabitha Sparks, *The Doctor in the Victorian Novel: Family Practices* (Farnham and Burlington: Ashgate, 2009), 118.
9. However, this was somewhat complicated by the fact that some prominent ovariotomists, most notably Robert Lawson Tait, were also strongly opposed to vivisection. For more on vivisection and gender, see

Mary Ann Elston, 'Women and Anti-vivisection in Victorian England, 1870–1900', in *Vivisection in Historical Perspective*, ed. Nicolaas A. Rupke (London and New York: Routledge, 1990), 259–294.

10. Barbara Ehrenreich and Deirdre English, *For Her Own Good: 150 Years of the Experts' Advice to Women* (London: Pluto Press, 1979), 111–112.

11. Ornella Moscucci, *The Science of Woman: Gynaecology and Gender in England 1800–1929* (Cambridge University Press, 1990), 135; Thomas Laqueur, *Making Sex: Body and Gender from the Greeks to Freud* (Cambridge, MA and London: Harvard University Press, 1990), 175; Ann Dally, *Women Under the Knife: A History of Surgery* (London: Hutchinson Radius, 1991).

12. Deirdre Cooper Owens, *Medical Bondage: Race, Gender, and the Origins of American Gynecology* (Athens: University of Georgia Press, 2017), 15–41.

13. Regina Morantz-Sanchez, *Conduct Unbecoming of a Woman: Medicine on Trial in Turn-of-the-Century Brooklyn* (Oxford: Oxford University Press, 1999); Claire Brock, *British Women Surgeons and Their Patients, 1860–1918* (Cambridge: Cambridge University Press, 2017), esp. 7–8.

14. See for example, Christina Beninghaus, 'Beyond Constructivism? Gender, Medicine and the Early History of Sperm Analysis, Germany 1870–1900', *Gender and History* 24, no. 3 (2012): 647–653.

15. Traditionally, such an approach has been associated with heavily technical, whiggish surgical histories; as Christopher Lawrence has observed: 'because it is a practice, surgery has been easily accommodated to empirical and positivist philosophies of medical progress'. Christopher Lawrence, 'Democratic, Divine and Heroic: The History and Historiography of Surgery', in *Medical Theory, Surgical Practice: Studies in the History of Surgery*, ed. Christopher Lawrence (London: Routledge, 1992), 14. Arguably surgery, more than other areas of medicine, has been disproportionately subject to 'whiggish' histories.

16. Thomas Schlich, *The Origins of Organ Transplantation: Surgery and Laboratory Science 1880–1930* (Rochester: University of Rochester Press, 2010), 9–10; Claire Brock, 'Risk, Responsibility and Surgery in the 1890s and Early 1900s', *Medical History* 57, no. 3 (2013): 325–326; Sally Wilde and Geoffrey Hirst, 'Learning from Mistakes: Early Twentieth-Century Surgical Practice', *Journal of the History of Medicine and Allied Sciences* 64, no. 1 (2009): 38–77. Wilde and Hirst, in particular, stress the practice-based nature of surgical innovation.

17. John V. Pickstone, 'Introduction', in *Medical Innovations in Historical Perspective*, ed. John V. Pickstone (Basingstoke: Macmillan, 1992), 1.

18. In 2011, the then Chief Executive of the NHS in England, Sir David Nicholson, wrote that 'innovation must become core business for the NHS'.

This was from a policy document which focused on the role of innovation in heightening the efficacy of state health care, tellingly titled 'Innovation; Health and Wealth'. Department of Health 'Innovation, Health and Wealth: Accelerating Adoption and Diffusion in the NHS' (2011), http://www.institute.nhs.uk/images//documents/Innovation/Innovation%20Health%20and%20Wealth%20-%20accelerating%20adoption%20and%20diffusion%20in%20the%20NHS.pdf, accessed 25 August 2013. Additionally, numerous companies such as 'healthcare innovation hub' Medipex focus solely on 'commercialising innovative medical products' conceived of both within the NHS and in the private sphere. http://www.medipex.co.uk/, accessed 25 August 2013.

19. Pickstone, ed., *Medical Innovations*; Ilana Löwy, ed., *Medicine and Change: Historical and Sociological Studies of Medical Innovation* (Montrouge: John Libbey Eurotext, 1993); Thomas Schlich and Ulrich Tröhler, eds., *The Risks of Medical Innovation: Risk Perception and Assessment in Historical Context* (Abingdon and New York: Routledge, 2006).

20. Thomas Schlich and Christopher Crenner, 'Technological Change in Surgery: An Introductory Essay', in *Technological Change in Modern Surgery*, ed. Thomas Schlich and Christopher Crenner (Rochester: University of Rochester Press, 2017), 1.

21. Schlich and Crenner, 'Technological Change in Surgery', 12.

22. Schlich and Tröhler (2006): Preface.

23. Thomas Schlich, 'Risk and Medical Innovation: A Historical Perspective', in *The Risks of Medical Innovation: Risk Perception and Assessment in Historical Context*, ed. Thomas Schlich and Ulrich Tröhler (Abingdon and New York: Routledge, 2006), 2. Certainly, strategies of risk analysis and methodical implementations of systems of innovation were more visible by the twentieth century. Both are perhaps best exemplified in the introduction of the randomised controlled trial into medicine in the 1950s, through which numerous dimensions of risk were built into the innovation process. See Peter Keating and Alberto Cambrosio, 'Risk on Trial: The Interaction of Innovation and Risk in Cancer Clinical Trials', in *The Risks of Medical Innovation: Risk Perception and Assessment in Historical Context*, ed. Thomas Schlich and Ulrich Tröhler (Abingdon and New York: Routledge, 2006): 225–241.

24. Ian Burney, 'Anaesthetic Death and the Evaluation of Risk in Nineteenth-Century English Surgery', in *The Risks of Medical Innovation: Risk Perception and Assessment in Historical Context*, ed. Thomas Schlich and Ulrich Tröhler (Abingdon and New York: Routledge, 2006), 38–52; Ulrich Tröhler, *Quantification in British Medicine and Surgery 1750–1830, With Special Reference to Its Introduction into Therapeutics* (PhD thesis, University College London, 1978).

25. Pickstone, 'Introduction', 1.

26. Benoît Godin, 'Social Innovation: Utopias of Innovation from c. 1830 to the Present', Project on the Intellectual History of Innovation, Working Paper No. 11 (Montreal: INRS, 2012), 8, http://www.csiic.ca/PDF/SocialInnovation_2012.pdf, accessed 25 August 2013.

27. As exemplified by James Watt and George Stephenson. See Christine MacLeod, *Heroes of Invention: Technology, Liberalism and British Identity: 1750–1914* (Cambridge: Cambridge University Press, 2007).

28. William P. Swain, 'Transactions of Branches: On Recent Improvements in Surgery', *British Medical Journal* 2, no. 298 (15 September 1866): 304.

29. For more on the relationship between surgery and the media, see Ayesha Nathoo, *Hearts Exposed: Transplants and the Media in 1960s Britain* (Basingstoke: Palgrave Macmillan, 2009). Writing on the first heart transplants in the 1960s, Nathoo contends they were 'as much media as medical events', 2.

30. In 2016, the BBC TV series *Storyville* ran a three part documentary, *Fatal Experiments: The Downfall of a Supersurgeon*, following the controversial operating practices of the Swiss-born Swedish-based surgeon Paolo Macchiarini. Macchiarini developed a synthetic trachea that he claimed could be transplanted into those suffering from congenital abnormalities of the trachea, tracheal cancer or other conditions. Six of the seven operations Macchiarini performed failed, with the patients subsequently dying after the operation. Macchiarini has since been stripped of his medical licence. In 2017, Macchiarini was found to be negligent in four cases and to have conducted fraudulent research. He narrowly escaped charges of involuntary manslaughter. The controversy over mesh implants to treat pelvic organ prolapse in women has been more wide reaching. The surgical procedure has been performed hundreds of thousands of times. However, new studies suggest the implant has been responsible for complications in large numbers of women, ranging from repeated infections to chronic pain and incontinence. At the time of writing, hundreds of women were involved in a class action lawsuit against the NHS and manufacturers of the mesh implants. Hannah Devlin and Nicola Davis, 'Vaginal Mesh Operations for Prolapse Should Be Banned, Watchdog to Say', *The Guardian* (27 November 2017), https://www.theguardian.com/society/2017/nov/27/vaginal-mesh-operations-should-be-banned-health-watchdog-to-say, accessed 5 December 2017.

31. As attested to in historical studies such as Thomas Schlich's on the introduction of osteosynthesis for bone fractures by Swiss surgeons in the 1950s. Schlich shows how the organisation responsible for innovating the technique, the AO Foundation, attempted to diffuse osteosynthesis as a standardised technique through both educational manuals and practical instruction. But Schlich also highlights the resistance of some

surgeons to the AO's brand of scientific, standardised surgery. Thomas Schlich, *Surgery, Science and Industry: A Revolution in Fracture Care, 1950s–1980s* (Basingstoke: Palgrave Macmillan, 2002), 252–253.

32. Peter Angelos, 'The Art of Medicine: The Ethical Challenges of Surgical Innovation for Patient Care', *Lancet* 376, no. 9746 (25 September 2010): 1046.

33. David S. Jones, 'Visions of a Cure: Visualization, Clinical Trials, and Controversies in Cardiac Therapeutics, 1968–1998', *Isis* 91, no. 3 (2000): 523. For more on the role of creativity, invention and innovation in twentieth-century surgery see Sally Frampton and Roger Kneebone, 'John Wickham's New Surgery: "Minimally Invasive Therapy", Innovation, and Approaches to Medical Practice in Twentieth-century Britain', *Social History of Medicine* 30, no. 3 (2017): 544–566.

34. Stefan Timmermans and Marc Berg suggest that 'the notion that predictability, accountability and objectivity will follow uniformity belongs to the Enlightenment master narratives promising progress through increased rationality and control', Stefan Timmermans and Marc Berg, *The Gold Standard: The Challenge of Evidence-Based Medicine and Standardization in Health Care* (Philadelphia: Temple University Press, 2003), 8.

35. Steve Sturdy, 'Looking for Trouble: Medical Science and Clinical Practice in the Historiography of Modern Medicine', *Social History of Medicine* 24, no. 3 (2011): 739.

36. 'Our present system of medical education is to my mind erring greatly on the side of devoting too much time to the science of our profession and too little to its art', complained the psychiatrist Lionel Weatherly in 1898. Lionel Weatherly, 'Remarks on Medical Progress', *Lancet* 152, no. 3918 (1 October 1898): 852.

37. Schlich, *Surgery, Science and Industry*. Osteosynthesis involves the implantation of metal implants to fix bone fractures. As a technique used to treat bones in various parts of the body, however, it is considerably different from ovariotomy, which is an organ-specific procedure.

2

Pathologies, Actions, Ideas

*We know what a masquerade all development is, and what effective shapes may be
disguised in helpless embryos. – In fact, the world is full of hopeful analogies and
handsome dubious eggs called possibilities.*
George Eliot, *Middlemarch*, 1874.[1]

HEROES AND VILLAINS

On a wintery day in December 1809, a forty-six-year-old woman, Jane
Todd Crawford, arrived in Danville, Kentucky, after completing an
arduous sixty-mile journey on horseback over rough terrain. Crawford
was there to meet with a surgeon, Ephraim McDowell. For some time,
Crawford had believed she was pregnant and in recent weeks had grown
so large that local doctors in her hometown of Greensburg had believed
that childbirth was imminent. Ephraim McDowell had been called in to
help deliver the child, but on examining the patient McDowell made a
surprising discovery. Crawford was not pregnant but suffering from a
rapidly growing ovarian tumour. Crawford's case immediately became
one of grave danger, 'Having never seen so large a substance extracted,
nor heard of an attempt, or success attending any operation, such as this
required, I gave the unhappy woman information of her dangerous situation' McDowell later reported.[2] Ovarian tumours were notoriously difficult to treat. Palliative procedures could bring temporary relief, but the
tumours rarely responded to any medical therapeutics that might effect

permanent change. Left untreated the growths could grow so large that they filled up the abdominal cavity, crushing the other organs. For most women, an ovarian tumour was a death sentence.

With few options available to them, McDowell and Crawford agreed to try something radical. If Crawford would make the journey to Danville, McDowell would try and remove the diseased ovary. On Christmas day, the operation took place. Despite McDowell's graphic description of the operation, at one point Crawford's intestines 'rushed out upon the table', he managed to remove her fifteen-pound tumour. The operation was, to the surprise of many, a success. Crawford recovered from the operation in a matter of days and lived for another thirty-two years. It appeared to be an unprecedented act in the history of surgery. When McDowell eventually published details of the case in 1817, along with those of two more successful procedures he had performed, the results were so extraordinary that some fellow doctors cast doubt upon their authenticity.[3]

As a consequence of his operation on Crawford, Ephraim McDowell has had a sustained grip on the title of 'father of abdominal surgery'. McDowell fitted the mould of the trailblazing surgeon, using ingenuity and self-reliance to create a new operation. Similarly, Crawford's courage has lent itself to a narrative of fortitude and bravery. Early histories of the operation reinforced this idea. Biographies of McDowell, published in 1891 and 1920, highlighted McDowell's unique role in the operation's development.[4] They emphasised the importance of his rural location, on the 'edge of civilisation' as one put it, and painted a picture of the Kentucky surgeon as the embodiment of the pioneering American spirit.[5] Indeed, McDowell's operation on Crawford would come to hold great significance for later surgeons, not only as supporting evidence of America's role in the operation, but in its identification by many in the medical profession as the effective beginning point of ovariotomy in the western world. But such narratives belie a more intricate history both to the story of Ephraim McDowell's work and of the beginnings of ovarian surgery. The idealistic portrayal of McDowell and Crawford's harmonious relationship, for example, as a 'a daring man and courageous woman coming together to settle a problem',[6] must be contextualised by McDowell's subsequent operations to extract ovaries, the next four of which were undertaken upon black women, all almost certainly enslaved, in cases in which consent for the patients to undergo surgery lay not with

the women but with their masters.[7] Moreover, the contemporary impact
of McDowell's work was hardly one of jubilant success: it would be eight
years until McDowell published a report of the case and the reception his
work received was lukewarm rather than triumphant.

The story of McDowell and Crawford, for all its drama, tells us relatively little about the genesis of the operation. Broad cultural shifts have
been suggested by several historians as precipitating interest in removing
the ovaries. But there have been few detailed explorations as to why ovarian surgery was taken up in advance of other forms of pelvic and abdominal surgery. The conceptualisation of the operation as innately Victorian
has been both the cause and effect of the scant attention paid to its
eighteenth- and early nineteenth-century roots. The analyses of Barbara
Ehrenreich and Deirdre English, Thomas Laqueur and others have largely
focused on the operation as it was in the last decades of the nineteenth
century and, in particular, the use of the operation to treat mental conditions, shaping ovarian surgery into a motif for Victorian understandings
of female pathology and sexuality and its operators into semi-villainous
characters, emblematic of the medical profession's disdainful attitude
towards women during that time. In fact, ovarian surgery had roots that
stretched far back beyond the 1800s. This chapter explores the confluence of physiological and pathological ideas which led practitioners to
believe that the removal of the ovaries was a viable operation. What made
the diseased ovary a distinctly surgical object? Was such an idea even
new? And if so, did a new idea necessarily give surgeons' licence to initiate novel practices? Or did novel practices foreground a more coherent
pathological theory? A simplistic conceptualisation of surgical innovation
might suggest that a group of authoritative practitioners encountered a
problem that needed to be solved, and that this necessarily lent itself to
action. However, any kind of linear model of innovation is complicated by
ovarian surgery where, as shall be explored, a large chasm existed between
the idea of performing the procedure and the first attempts at doing so.

LOCATING THE PATHOLOGICAL OVARY IN EARLY
MODERN MEDICINE

Towards the end of the seventeenth century, the 'testicles' of females,
previously little distinguished from their male counterparts, began to be
understood in a fundamentally different way. In 1651, the English physician William Harvey published *De Generatione Animalium* in which

he asserted his doctrine of *ex ovo omnia*: that all animals, from the low-liest creature to humankind, emerged from the *ovum*, minuscule eggs, invisible to the eye. In the 1660s and 1670s, physicians across Europe began to affirm experimentally that the female testicles were egg-producing organs and the more congruous term 'ovary' was increasingly seen fit to describe them.[8] The identification of the ovary laid the foundations for two competing theories of generation that predominated in the 1700s: preformation, which characterised the egg as the container of all future pre-formed life, merely activated by the male seed, and epigenesis, which posited that new organisms developed gradually following the sexual union of the male and female.[9] The eighteenth century saw a burgeoning research culture which centred around the female reproductive system.[10] The shift in the organ's identity from female testicle to that of the ovary, and the subsequent investigations it galvanised, was, as Thomas Laqueur has argued, a decisive moment in the shift from the 'one-sex' to 'two-sex' model, as male and female bodies became increasingly distinguished from one another during the late eighteenth and nineteenth centuries. This gave forth to understandings that women's reproductive organs were intimately connected to the production of specifically feminine bodily and behavioural characteristics. The anatomy of the male and female reproductive systems became 'the foundation of incommensurable difference' between men and women.[11]

The discovery of egg production meant it had come to be understood that the ovaries played a role in reproduction, but the intricacies of the organ's functions and its exact connection to the generative process remained unclear. The womb continued to dominate vernacular as well as medical understandings of women's reproductive functions, and its diseases were a common site of medical intervention.[12] The ovaries on the other hand were, according to Matthew Baillie, a physician and Britain's foremost morbid anatomist in the eighteenth century, 'a part of the animal oeconomy which seems to have been hitherto involved in a considerable degree of obscurity'.[13] The 'obscurity' he referred to reflected not only the mystery which still surrounded the organ's physiology but also its diseases, which were thought to occur with alarming frequency. Indeed, so often were the ovaries found to contain pathological changes following patients' deaths and the subsequent dissection of their bodies, that practitioners found it difficult to establish what exactly could be considered a

normal ovary: 'the change of condition, which these disorders produce in the ovaria, has often deceived anatomists; and made them
mistake the true structure of these parts' wrote the French physician
Jean Astruc, whose numerous textbooks were frequently translated
into English and had a considerable impact on practitioners across the
Channel.[14]

One of the most perplexing disorders of the ovary, where physiology
and pathology converged, was tumours which were found to contain
tissues like hair, teeth and bone (a condition known today as a dermoid cyst). The disease fascinated medical men. It was clear evidence of
pathological behaviour in the ovary, but how closely aligned the disease
was with embryonic development was a source of confusion and generated a multitude of theories over the years. One surgeon conjectured
that the tooth he had discovered in the ovary of one of his deceased
patients could not possibly have been formed within the organ and
instead speculated that it had been swallowed and had subsequently per-
forated the ovary.[15] Jean Astruc believed the tumours to be putrefying
embryos which had erroneously embedded themselves and then died in
the ovary.[16] Others claimed that in some cases their patients were virgins,
meaning that the condition was unlikely to be connected to pregnancy.[17]
That these strange masses defied explanation by prevailing theories of
generation did not go unnoticed by medical men. The eminent French
natural philosopher Georges Louis Leclerc, Comte de Buffon, rejected
the idea that teeth, bones and hair had even ever been found within
the organ. The Irish physician James Cleghorn claimed this to be typical of the general disregard natural philosophers had for medical facts;
'Monsieur le Comte de Buffon, finding it difficult to account for the formation of a foetus in the ovarium, like a true theorist, seems to reject
the fact altogether...thinking it of more consequence to establish his
own theory than to propagate the knowledge of truth'.[18] When in 1789
Matthew Baillie published a case of one such tumour found in the body
of a recently deceased girl, aged twelve or thirteen, and which appeared
to definitively show they were not related to pregnancy, his work demonstrated how the everyday experiences of medical practitioners could be
put to work in explaining the mysteries of the human body.[19] Andrew
Cunningham has characterised the long eighteenth century as a time
when 'the generation of humans – or certain aspects of it – became more
important for the medical or surgical practitioner than ever before'.[20] The
encroachment of male medical practitioners upon the realm of childbirth

gave further impetus to the anatomical investigation of the female reproductive system. This was borne out in the works produced by practitioners like William Smellie and William Hunter, both of whom made
their names and fortunes in London as eminent obstetricians. Hunter's
Anatomia Uteri Humani Gravidi Tabulis Illustrata (1774) especially,
provided novel knowledge about the process of embryonic development.
However, obstetrical texts were not usually written with an eye to explicitly supporting one theory of generation or another, and most obstetricians were primarily concerned with producing pedagogical texts for
fellow man-midwives or expensive illustrated volumes for their patrons.

During the eighteenth century, the ovary was considered both physiologically and pathologically complex, making it an object of curiosity
in the burgeoning field of morbid anatomy. Understandings about the
organ's generative abilities increasingly relied on the findings of medical
practitioners, whose anatomical research helped uncover its structure and
function. Anatomists like Matthew Baillie generated interest in an organ
that appeared to be frequently altered by disease. Assembling therapeutic
tools based on such anatomical findings was, however, to prove a more
challenging prospect, as practitioners looked to find a way to effectively
treat ovarian disease.

THE DROPSICAL PATIENT

Growing interest in the ovary's generative function was central to discussions of how its diseases developed. But for the patient afflicted with
ovarian disease in the eighteenth century, changing understandings of
the organ's physiology and pathology would have had little impact upon
their sufferings. Buried deep within the peritoneum, the ovary was quite
literally inaccessible. A slow and painless progression usually characterised ovarian disease in its early stages, making it difficult to determine its
existence until it had advanced to a point where it had begun to endan-
ger the patient's life. Discussions of its treatment were often suffused
with a sense of hopelessness.[21]

Despite this, most practitioners were cognisant that ovarian conditions did occur frequently among women and one disease in particular
struck with alarming regularity: dropsy.[22] Perhaps because by the mid-
nineteenth century the term 'dropsy' had become largely obsolete in
medical terminology, its role in the development of ovarian surgery has
been virtually ignored. Yet the belief among doctors that the ovary was

highly susceptible to dropsy was significant in conceptions of its pathology. Dropsy was a generic, expansive disease category, used to refer to swellings containing water, serum or air found throughout the body, usually (but not always) presenting alongside other symptoms such as retention of urine and thirst. It was generally viewed as a disease caused by some kind of constitutional imbalance.[23] The frequency with which practitioners encountered the condition in their patients meant that a detailed nosology of the disease had been in use since ancient times.[24] The disease was usually grouped into three categories: ascites (watery swelling of the belly), tympanites (windy swelling of the belly) and anasarca (swelling throughout the body).[25] During the early modern period, classification became increasingly sophisticated. Conditions like hydrocephalus (fluid in the cranium), hydrothorax (fluid in the chest) and dropsies of the womb, testicle and ovary were also referenced as different forms of the condition. Dropsy was a disease that cut across the social spectrum, affecting the young and the old, the rich and the poor. In London alone, in the late eighteenth century, it was responsible for hundreds of deaths every year.[26]

Historians Wendy Churchill and Richard Gooding have both argued that contemporary medical practitioners believed dropsy disproportionately affected women. Scottish physician Donald Monro certainly thought this was the case, writing in 1756, that 'women being more subject than men to stoppage of the natural excretions, and being also of a weaker frame, are more frequently attacked by dropsies'.[27] Reflecting the continued role of humoural theory as the explanatory mode for bodily disorders, others agreed that it was women's 'wateriness' that seemed to make them more prone to the condition. While dropsy might be thought more likely to attack women, its gendering was, however, complex. Men were by no means considered safe from the disease. The oft-made assumption that dropsy could be caused by overindulgence or excessive alcohol, which could cause an imbalance of the humours, meant it could just as easily be associated with men.[28]

Misinterpretation of the disease in both men and women was common. Dropsy was often mistaken for corpulence, something complicated by the fact that fatness was sometimes implicated as a cause of the disease too.[29] For dropsical women, misdiagnosis could have serious consequences. As would be the case with Jane Todd Crawford, patients and their practitioners very often mistook dropsy for pregnancy because of the swelling to the abdomen it caused (see Fig. 2.1).

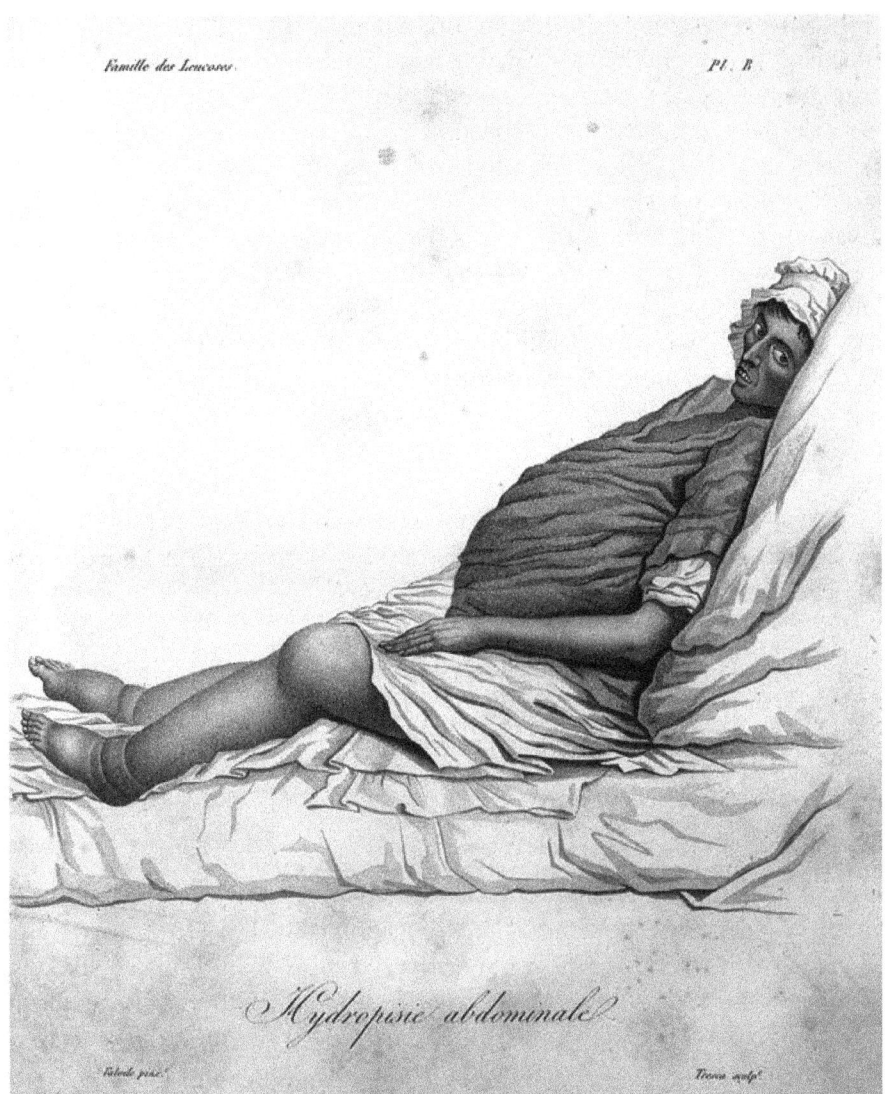

Fig. 2.1 Illustration of a woman with an abdominal dropsy taken from Jean-Louis-Marc Alibert's *Nosologie Naturelle* (1817). Her abdomen is visibly swollen with fluid, showing how the condition could easily create the illusion of pregnancy. Her swollen legs and gaunt face were other common symptoms of dropsy (*Credit* Wellcome Collection. CC BY)

Pregnancy was still shrouded in uncertainty, there being few reliable indicators as to whether a woman was pregnant or not, especially in the early months before the baby could be felt.[30] For some dropsical women, it was only when their belly continued to grow beyond the usual nine months that disease was accepted as a more likely scenario than them carrying a child.[31] The rapid growth of ovarian dropsy once it reached an advanced stage was an unnerving aspect to the disease. Dropsical ovaries could grow so big that practitioners often labelled them as 'monstrous'. The Norwich surgeon Philip Meadows Martineau reported in 1784 the case of a local woman, Sarah Kippus, whose belly had grown so large that her face had almost become obscured by it. Martineau described her appearance as 'truly deplorable, not to say shocking'.[32]

The confusion between pregnancy and dropsy left women—and especially, younger, unmarried women—vulnerable. The spectre of illegitimacy was raised by their swollen bellies which were open to scrutiny from the local community. In 1706, the Plymouth surgeon James Yonge reported one such case to the Royal Society:

> A Virgin of thirty fell into a periodical fever and afterward a total suppression of her *Menstrua*; which soon followed with a pain and tumour on the right side of her belly, which grew and encreased…till it became bigger and harder than that of a woman in her last month. When it had grown a full year, it began to soften, and then the censorious people who suspected her thought her in a dropsie.[33]

Even if the possibility of pregnancy could be disproved, the effects of the disease on one's quality of life were significant. On top of the stigma of living with a condition that observers found disturbing to look at, physically, the toll of living with a large ovarian dropsy was substantial. It could lead to breathing difficulties, trouble walking and an array of other symptoms. Practitioners noted the effect this could have on those women who had laborious and physically demanding occupations and whose livelihood depended on their health.[34]

Ovarian dropsy was set apart from other forms of dropsy in three significant ways. First, as described above, ovarian dropsy was generally symptomless until the disease reached an advanced state. Its insidious growth meant that sufferers of the condition often did not seek medical attention until their abdomen was noticeably swollen. Second, when the dropsical swelling occurred, it was often in an encysted form—when multiple sacs of fluid formed within a larger general swelling—which added complexity to the disease site, as fluid was effectively trapped in the smaller cysts. 'The ovarium dropsy being encysted, will be found to require a considerable deviation from the general mode' argued one practitioner in 1796.[35] Third, in contrast to most other dropsies, which were usually viewed as symptoms of underlying disease elsewhere in the body, it was understood to be localised, a sign of the organ's structure gone awry rather than a constitutional disorder that could be rectified by restoring humoural balance. The idiosyncrasies of the disease gave it a prominent place in discussions of potential therapeutics. The usual medical modes of treatment for dropsy, which lay in re-establishing the balance of fluids within the body, were rendered ineffective in ovarian forms of the disease.

Most practitioners came to a grim conclusion about the disease: it was simply incurable.[36] This view was endorsed in the 1785 publication *An Account of the Foxglove and some of its Medical Uses* by Birmingham physician William Withering. In what was to become a much admired text, Withering publicised his successful experimentation with the diuretic effect of *Digitalis*, commonly known as the plant foxglove, which, he argued, effectively cured many forms of dropsy. However, he excluded ovarian dropsy from the possibility of cure with this method. Failed attempts at doing so had left him convinced that 'the ovarian dropsy defies the power of medicine'.[37]

Complex in its structure, difficult to diagnose and unamenable to treatments used for other forms of the disease, a diagnosis of ovarian dropsy was a grave event for the sufferer and a hopeless case for the practitioner. A woman might labour under the disease for months, sometimes years, but few would make a full recovery. Most would eventually die from the condition. The relative powerlessness of medicine to treat the disease led some practitioners to look for more radical alternatives.

REMOVING THE OVARIES: A DISEMBODIED TECHNIQUE

The ineffectiveness of medicine meant that doctors turned to other methods for treating ovarian disease. The operation of paracentesis, commonly known as 'tapping', was one of the more common treatments for dropsies within the abdomen. It was not considered to provide a permanent cure but was held to be the only treatment which was even slightly effective in palliating ovarian disease. Paracentesis was a procedure that had been in use since ancient times and was relatively simple in its execution: after pressure had been applied to the affected area with bandages or a belt, a trocar was inserted into the abdominal cavity through which fluid was then drained off. It was a common technique, but one where the limitations were clearly perceived. Dropsical swellings would usually begin to refill soon after they had been drained and patients required multiple tappings to keep the growth at bay. The more complex and multi-cysted the swelling was, the more likely it was that a tapping would fail, a single puncture unlikely to cause effective draining in the smaller sacs of fluid. The procedure was fraught with danger, sometimes aggravating the condition and even hastening death. Most advocated performing it only when the pain had become unbearable or the vital organs were impaired. Despite the risks, many still sought repeated tappings to palliate their symptoms. Sarah Kippus, described above, was one such example. A pauper woman, her case was extraordinary for the length of time she lived with her condition; she was tapped eighty times during a period of twenty-three years, with 6631 pints of fluid altogether drawn from her dropsical ovary before she died of the disease in 1783. Evidently, the procedure became an established part of her life. Philip Meadows Martineau noted that the tapping would generally occur on a Sunday so that her neighbours could assist her. So much was it a part of her routine, he claimed, that she 'seldom regarded the operation'.[38] Throughout the late eighteenth and early nineteenth centuries, the quest to find other cures for the disease continued, with everything from douches and electricity to diuretics, mercury and iodine injections being advocated for its treatment, none of which would, however, earn the confidence of medical practitioners *en masse*.

The ineffectiveness of established treatments did not mean an inevitable path to surgery. For any disease, recourse to surgery remained undesirable. Operations were, as surgeon John Hunter, brother of William, liked to tell his students, 'the defect of surgery',[39] a necessary evil only to be performed when all else had failed. Given the common opinion that surgeons were little more than bloodthirsty and untrustworthy knife-wielders, Hunter's words of caution are not surprising.[40] Entering the abdomen was fraught with dangers to both patients' lives and practitioners' reputations.

And yet, fostered by the experimental anatomy taking hold among French and British practitioners in the eighteenth century, discussion was turning to the possibility of surgically removing internal organs. The gradual shift occurring from the traditional frameworks of humouralism and nervous pathology, which implicated the entire body, and its humoural or nervous balance, in the cause of illness, towards the idea that local tissues and organs acted as the seat of disease, was embodied within these debates. Initially, the focus was not so much upon the technical feasibility of doing so, but upon the impact of removing organs, or parts of them, upon the rest of the body. What organs was it possible for humans to live without? What would be the effect of their removal? In the early eighteenth century, attention had focused on the spleen. The exact function of the organ had long been a subject of debate among medical men. Indeed, the possibility that the spleen in fact played no functional role in the body's workings was raised. This idea was pursued by the English physician Richard Blackmore. Blackmore claimed that ancient medical authorities had, like him, viewed the spleen to lack function and to possibly even be a noxious influence on the body because of its production of black bile.[41] Joining theory with surgical experimentation, Blackmore cited the work of the seventeenth-century anatomist Marcello Malpighi who claimed to have successfully removed the spleen from a number of dogs, all of whom had survived the procedure without long-term effect.[42] As Blackmore himself acknowledged, such a view, while hardly novel, was potentially controversial, implying as it did that the organ was 'made in vain; which is to affirm, that an Intelligent and infinite wise Cause, may act without Design, and for no End'.[43] This challenged not just ingrained medical ideas of constitution and humoural balance but the Galenic idea of teleological anatomy, that every part of the body had a specific purpose, which was part of the theological concept of a designing, purposeful deity.[44]

Across the Channel, some years later, similar questions were being asked with respect to the womb. In the early 1780s, an intriguing discussion took place among members of the Académie Royale de Chirurgie in Paris. The city still led the way in surgery and obstetrics during the middle decades of the eighteenth century, and the Académie was one of a number of medical societies in operation during the Ancien Régime which cultivated a thriving culture of correspondence among its members.[45] A surgeon named Lassort appealed to his peers for responses to a question that he had become greatly interested in: namely, could a woman, once she had had children, live without her womb?

The question generated numerous replies from surgeons and *accoucheurs*, many of whom brought forward cases where extirpation of the womb had been attempted, or where in hindsight, they believed removing the organ might have saved a life. As with the spleen, the possibility of removing the womb was not an entirely new idea: the operation had once been performed by sixteenth-century surgeon Ambroise Paré who had taken a diseased mass from a woman that had later been identified as being formed from one the ovaries and the womb. Even though Paré's removal of the womb had been accidental rather than intentional, this gave the operation some historical foundation.[46] The operation Paré performed joined the other occasional reports of abdominal surgery in Europe which were scattered through medical publications in the seventeenth and eighteenth centuries.[47]

Most practitioners who joined the dialogue that Lassort had initiated believed that removal of the womb was possible, and that a woman without a womb could go on to live a healthy life. The relative expendability of the womb was emphasised, especially so after child-bearing had been completed. The womb's function was regarded as temporary; after the climacteric, the organ became useless. The discussion facilitated by the Académie provides an interesting counterpoint to arguments put forth by historians as to why the female reproductive organs became the focus of surgery. 'It is no historical accident that ovariotomy was the first major procedure in abdominal surgery to be developed and accepted' wrote Jane Eliot Sewell, 'unlike appendectomy or liver and kidney operations, which might objectively have been equally valid candidates for innovation, ovariotomy involved women's reproductive organs and these organs were bequeathed a larger-than-life status in society'.[48] Surgeons' discussions tell another story. The female reproductive organs were vital to procreation. But unlike the brain, heart or liver, most suspected they were not vital to the maintenance of life. As such, it was not so much the reproductive organs' 'larger-than-life status' that generated conversation about their possible removal, but rather their relative lack of contribution to the bodily system, particularly with the course of age. The same was thought true of men too. Male castration was not common, but it was practised as a last resort in cases of cancer.[49] This proved to practitioners that a man could survive without his generative organs, and by analogy, it seemed possible a woman could survive without hers. The crucial difference between the sexes was not so much any vital difference in their nature but that removing the female generative organs meant entering the peritoneum and thus entailed a considerably more complex and dangerous surgical operation.

It was in this context that eighteenth-century practitioners began to discuss the removal of the ovaries in those suffering from dropsy in the organ. The disease seemed to suggest itself to surgery. Visibility is at the crux of surgical encounters and the huge sizes that dropsical ovaries eventually accrued made it a striking, highly conspicuous disease that straddled the line between the internal and external and, consequently, the traditional—if not always observed—boundaries between surgery and physic. Because of this, dropsical ovaries challenged conceptual and professional boundaries. They affected an internal organ—the domain of the physician—but they were highly visible, like external tumours, and thus conceivably in the domain of the surgeon too. In 1753, a group of essays on encysted dropsies of the abdomen were published in the prestigious *Mémoires de l'Académie Royale de Chirurgie* in which the possibility of removing ovarian tumours was discussed in detail. Only five volumes of the *Mémoires* were published during the eighteenth century and those cases taken from the discussions of the Académie tended to be those 'worthy of becoming part of surgical lore'.[50] Thus, the collection of essays, entitled 'Several Accounts and Observations of the Encysted Dropsy and Schirrhus Ovary', reflected a concerted effort on the part of the Académie to focus attention upon the subject. The accounts included remarks from the eminent lithotomist Sauveur-François Morand, as well as surgeon to the Hôpital de la Charité, Henri le Dran. Like those interested in the possibility of removing the spleen and womb, Morand looked back to the ancient world for precedents. He alluded to a manuscript by the Greek author Hesychius (c. fifth century CE) in which it was suggested that women of the ancient Lydian community were surgically castrated.[51] Accounts like this provided an historical basis to any possible operation, helping to prevent it being labelled a dangerous and unnecessary novelty.

The most radical essay, however, came from a rather obscure figure, the surgeon Jean Delaporte.[52] Recounting a case of death from ovarian dropsy in his care, Delaporte was the first surgeon to publicly express his desire for a more radical operation. Delaporte affirmed his belief that the diseased ovary was not the result of a constitutional disorder but *le foyer de maladie* ('the seat of the disease').[53] The swelling took over the entire ovary until disease and organ were interchangeable. The ovary was not just the source of the disease, it *was* the disease and could only be cured, Delaporte believed, by the removal of the organ in its entirety. In his concluding comments, Morand praised Delaporte, imploring his colleagues to celebrate the surgeon's bravery in becoming the first modern practitioner to have raised the possibility of removing the diseased ovary.[54] Over the following decades, dozens of letters and reports concerning cases of ovarian dropsy were sent to the Académie, many of which conveyed the frustration of practitioners from across the country as to the ineffectiveness of current treatments. Some began to express a wish that advanced ovarian tumours be treated by major surgery and framed it as a matter of professional pride: 'surgery of our century has yet to fully triumph over this common and cruel disease' wrote one surgeon to the Académie in 1763.[55]

It was almost certainly the publication of Delaporte's essay which compelled William Hunter to bring the subject to British practitioners' attention in 1753 in an essay for the journal *Medical Observations and Inquiries*. At first, Hunter seemed to suggest the impracticality of the operation. 'It has been proposed by modern surgeons, deservedly of the first reputation, to attempt a radical cure by incision and suppuration, or by excision of the cyst' Hunter wrote, 'I am of opinion, that excision can hardly be attempted'.[56] Thus, Hunter appeared to be distancing himself from Delaporte, Le Dran and others. However, his succeeding comments left open the possibility that a radical operation might just work, if the circumstances were right:

> If it be proposed indeed to make such a wound in the belly, as will admit only two fingers or so, and then to tap the bag, and draw it out, so as to bring the root or the pedicle close to the wound of the belly, that the surgeon may cut it without introducing his hand; surely; in a case otherwise so desperate, it might be advisable to do it, could we beforehand know that the circumstances would admit such a treatment.[57]

Hunter, like Delaporte, raised the possibility of radical excision. And yet neither attempted the operation; nor did William Hunter's brother John, perhaps even more notable given John Hunter's reputation as a daring surgeon and progressive thinker. John certainly encountered the disease many times—his casebooks recorded numerous patients suspected of having the condition—and in 1785, he openly discussed the possibility of a more radical operation, decreeing that 'there was no reason why, when the disease can be ascertained in an early stage, we should not make an opening into the abdomen and extract the cyst itself'.[58] But John Hunter's conjecture similarly laid open only the theoretical possibility of surgery and he did not make any radical alterations in his own practice.

Indeed, by the end of the eighteenth century, despite the growing discussion around the subject, there had only been two cases made public in Britain involving the removal of an ovarian tumour. In 1724, the Scottish practitioner Robert Houstoun reported in the *Philosophical Transactions of the Royal Society* that in 1701 he had made an incision of about four inches into the abdomen of fifty-eight-year-old Margaret Millar, who was labouring under a 'monstrous' tumour.[59] Urged by the desperate woman to do something for her pain, Houstoun had made an incision in her belly and managed to remove large parts of a distended mass and some gelatinous substance through the incision. Millar recovered, apparently relieved of her pain. Retrospectively, a number of Victorian surgeons, most notably Robert Lawson Tait, would resurrect the case to argue Houstoun was the original pioneer of ovariotomy.[60] However, there is no evidence of either Hunter or any of the French surgeons referencing the Houstoun case, which appeared to have had relatively little contemporary impact, probably because Houstoun did not intend to remove the ovary and had not taken it away in its entirety.

The second case was reported in 1775 by St. Bartholomew's Hospital surgeon Percivall Pott. Pott had removed both ovaries from a twenty-three-year-old woman, although he only recognised them to be the ovaries upon removing them, the diseased organs having herniated and passed through the abdominal wall. Pott himself did not use the opportunity to express the significance of this incident to surgery; the case was unusual and the location of the ovaries odd. The operation had not required Pott to open the peritoneal cavity and therefore provided no guidance for treatment of the more typical presentation of ovarian disease a surgeon was likely to encounter.[61] Both Houstoun's and Pott's cases, however, would later be used to support various contentions about the justifiability of ovarian surgery, showing how older cases were often re-visited and re-positioned to suit new narratives of the operation's development.

By the end of the eighteenth century, the operation remained almost entirely hypothetical in Britain—a disembodied technique, without a surgeon willing to perform it or a patient to submit to it. In France, the situation was a little different; the surgeon Jean-Baptiste Laumonier, based at the hospital in Rouen, claimed to have successfully diagnosed and

then removed a diseased ovary from the abdomen of twenty-one-year-
old Louise Lagrange in 1782. In another case where surgical innovation
aligned dubiously with the treatment of a patient on the periphery of
society, Lagrange was a prostitute who had recently given birth, the latter an event which appeared to have precipitated her illness.[62] The significance of Laumonier's procedure to the history of ovariotomy would
be minimised by some practitioners in the nineteenth century, in an
effort to secure Ephraim McDowell's claim to having performed the
first operation. But while the British cases caused only a ripple of interest, the impact of the Laumonier case was rather more significant, in part
due to the surgeon's own attempts to press upon his professional colleagues the importance of the operation. Parisian medical societies facilitated debates on new procedures being used in surgery, acting as judge
and jury as to the justifiability of their introduction. Laumonier published
the Lagrange case in the *Histoire de la Société Royale de Médecine*, claiming that the operation, along with those cases where the womb had been
removed, meant that 'there are no organs upon which we might not
exert with advantage the various surgical operations'.[63] The Société
Royale de Médecine appeared to endorse Laumonier's proposal. A progressive organisation that had a 'brief but vigorous life history in the last
years of the Ancien Régime',[64] it praised Laumonier's work and in 1787
even awarded the surgeon a medal for his achievement with the operation.[65] But the optimism around the procedure was short-lived. In 1790,
a patient came into Laumonier's care who was initially believed to be
pregnant. With no sign of labour after the ninth month, Laumonier suspected a large tumour. Buoyed by his previous success, he proposed to
operate, only to be vehemently opposed in his plans by Jean-Antoine
Rouelle, chief physician at the hospital. Politics and practice coalesced
through their disagreement: the two appear to have been at opposing ends of the political spectrum which one might speculate influenced their opinion on radical innovation in surgery: while Laumonier
was an ardent supporter of the Revolution, Rouelle was conservative,
a believer in the Ancien Régime.[66] The matter was handed over to the
Académie Royale de Chirurgie for deliberation, who eventually backed
Rouelle, deeming the risks of the operation and difficulties of clear diagnosis too great to justify its attempt. The patient was not operated upon
and died shortly after, the autopsy revealing a large ovarian tumour.
Laumonier placed the blame for her demise squarely upon Rouelle.[67]
The Académie's decision to back Rouelle had significant consequences;

the institution publicly declared that 'the extirpation of these tumours can be neither advised nor allowed'.[68] The opposition of Europe's most powerful surgical institution to the operation clarified its identification by the surgical establishment as a dangerous and unacceptable novelty.

The relationship between theory and practice in the construction of the 'new' operation for removing diseased ovaries was complex and circular. The metropolitan, professional cultures of London and Paris planted the seed of ovarian surgery's possibility, and the case of Louise Lagrange showed the operation could be successfully performed. But there was yet to be an agreement between practitioners that the procedure should form part of regular surgical practice. Why then discordance between the idea of radical ovarian surgery and the establishment of its regular performance? Delicate negotiation was required for a procedure that signalled fundamental change, not just in technique but in surgical objective. Ovarian dropsy, as distressing a disease as it was, was one that the patient had the potential to live with for some duration. This was in stark contrast to an operation of an urgent nature like caesarean section, which was performed with relative frequency in eighteenth-century France, fostered by the country's Catholicism, which venerated the life of the child, and which in turn gave cultural impetus for the operation.[69] To open the abdomen was to put the patient at risk of exhaustion, post-operative disease and haemorrhage. Undertaking this in any case where the patient was not at the point of imminent death required a significant shift in surgical convention. For some, it was a new and exciting prospect—for others, a dangerous attack on the defined limits of surgery. Even *articulating* the possibility of the operation was thought to be a powerful and potentially dangerous move. As Anton De Haen, a leading light in eighteenth-century Viennese medicine described the operation: 'it would not do to talk about, lest some reckless surgeon should attempt to perform it'.[70]

By the of the century, the operation had become conceptualised as a procedure better suited to future rather than present-day medicine. 'I am persuaded that a time will come when this operation will be extended to more numerous cases than I have proposed, and that it will not be difficult to execute', the French surgeon Nicolas Chambon is supposed to have written in 1798.[71] Surgeons expressed the view that innovation in ovarian surgery should be neither inevitable nor random; rather it was essential that the profession waited for the right time and indeed the right case to come along—however long that may be—so that the operation began with success rather than failure. Before the operation had even materialised in physical form, complex ideas of temporality were at work. Morand's citation of ancient cases of the removal of ovaries contrasted with Chambon's contention that the operation was better suited to future generations of surgeons. Practitioners turned to both the past and the future of surgery to answer the question of the operation's justifiability in the present.

CONCLUSION

Critics and historians such as Michel Foucault and Toby Gelfand have shown that a greater focus upon anatomy and dissection led to an increasingly 'surgical' way of thinking among doctors in the late eighteenth and early nineteenth centuries.[72] Less work has been done, however, to show in what manner exactly this was expressed in the practice of surgery, or why some forms of 'new' surgery were prioritised. In this respect, ovarian surgery provides important nuance to more generalised narratives. The construction of the ovary as a surgical object was dependent on a confluence of factors. The identification of the organ's unique egg-producing function attributed to it in the seventeenth century helped make it an object of novel, physiological interest and drew attention to its pathological complexity. A visually striking, tactile disorder, dropsical ovaries were common enough for cases to be plentiful and the effects distressing enough that practitioners looked to more radical means to treat it. The claim that it was an affliction local to the ovary, rather than the result of a constitutional disorder, raised the possibility that removing the organ would cure the disease entirely. The idea of the relative dispensability of the reproductive organs in comparison with other vital, internal organs further propelled the ovary into the realm of the surgeon.

In 1817 came the claim that Ephraim McDowell had successfully removed diseased ovaries in three women, all of whom had survived.[73] McDowell was novel in that he was reporting multiple cases, in which diseased ovaries had been intentionally removed, demonstrating both a clear objective and consistency. McDowell appeared to have been motivated by practical reasons rather than by a more grandiose objective of proving empirically the theories of French surgeons and claimed to be ignorant of any other attempts to perform the operation. However, his work was not quite as independent as he implied. Many accounts have sourced McDowell's inspiration to perform the operation from his time as a medical student at the University of Edinburgh, where it is believed he studied under the anatomist John Bell, who had a special interest in diseases of the ovaries and their surgical potential. McDowell personally sent Bell a copy of his report of the cases, suggesting a degree of kinship had existed between the two.[74] However, it was only upon returning to his small practice in rural Kentucky that McDowell was remote enough from the scrutiny of his peers to be able to perform the operations with relative anonymity.[75]

McDowell had brought the operation into practice, and yet, in 1819, he echoed the fears Anton De Haen had expressed about the unregulated diffusion of the operation into the hands of any and every practitioner. McDowell openly declared his wish that the operation should not become part of regular surgical practice, implying instead that the operation needed to be carefully controlled, as its danger would be greatly increased if it fell into the hands of 'the mechanical surgeon', to whom he believed the operation should remain 'forever incomprehensible'.[76] Cognisant of the suspicion that lingered around it, McDowell took the remarkable step of cautioning against the use of an operation that he himself had helped make a reality.

By the 1820s, the operation had been discussed for over seventy years; however, its justifiability was far from established. If the technique of opening the peritoneum and cutting out the ovary was no longer completely novel, what it represented was. Far from the successes of McDowell hastening surgery into a new era, ovarian surgery was soon to be catapulted onto the pages of the medical press, where it was to become one of the most enduringly controversial topics in British medicine.

NOTES

1. George Eliot, *Middlemarch: A Study of Provincial Life* (London: Vintage, 2007), 8.
2. Ephraim McDowell, 'Three Cases of Extirpation of Diseased Ovaria', *Eclectic Repertory and Analytical Review* 7 (1817): 242–243.
3. Ezra Michener, 'Case of Diseased Ovarium', *Eclectic Repertory and Analytical Review* 8 (1818): 114–115.
4. Mary Young Ridenbaugh, *The Biography of Ephraim McDowell M.D., the Father of Ovariotomy* (New York: Charles L. Webster, 1890);

August Schachner, *Ephraim McDowell: 'Father of Ovariotomy' and Founder of Abdominal Surgery* (Philadelphia and London: J. B. Lippincott Company, 1921). Both authors had a connection to McDowell; Ridenbaugh was his granddaughter and Schachner was a fellow Kentucky surgeon who would later lead the campaign to have Ephraim McDowell's house restored and converted into a museum.

5. Schachner, *Ephraim McDowell*, 4.

6. Schachner, *Ephraim McDowell*, 61.

7. McDowell in one case refers to the woman's 'master'. Ephraim McDowell, 'Observations on Diseased Ovaria', *Eclectic Repertory and Analytical Review* 9 (1819): 551. Deirdre Cooper Owens notes that the black population of Danville was very small, making it all the more striking that McDowell's next four cases involved black patients. It suggests that McDowell actively pursued cases within the black community so as to experiment with the operation. Deirdre Cooper Owens, *Medical Bondage: Race, Gender, and the Origins of American Gynecology* (Athens: University of Georgia Press, 2017), 32.

8. Regnier De Graaf, *Regnier de Graaf on the Human Reproductive Organs: An Annotated Translation of 'Tractatus de Virorum Organis Generationi Inservientibus' (1668) and 'De Mulierum Organis Generationi Inservientibus Tractatus Novus' (1672)*, trans. H.D. Jocelyn and B.P. Setchell (Oxford: Blackwell, 1972), 135.

9. Clara Pinto-Correia, *The Ovary of Eve: Egg and Sperm and Preformation* (Chicago: University of Chicago Press, 1997), 42–44. Most preformationists believed the egg to be at the centre of generation. However, there was also a theory of 'spermist' preformation which was briefly in vogue at the end of the seventeenth century, the proponents of which suggested that it was in fact sperm that was the container of all preformed life.

10. A prominent example was John Hunter's research looking at the effect of removing one ovary upon the generative potential of pigs. Hunter was fascinated as to the physiological reasoning behind there being two ovaries, and his experimentations led him to conclude that while generation was still possible, the loss of one ovary would considerably diminish the number of young produced. John Hunter, 'An Experiment to Determine the Effect of Extirpating One Ovarium Upon the Number of Young Produced', *Philosophical Transactions of the Royal Society* 77 (1787): 239.

11. Thomas Laqueur, *Making Sex: Body and Gender from the Greeks to Freud* (Cambridge, MA and London: Harvard University Press, 1990), 149.

12. Darren Wagner, 'Visualisations of the Womb Through Tropes, Dissection and Illustration (c. 1660–1774)', in *Book Illustration in the Long Eighteenth*

Century: Reconfiguring the Visual Periphery of the Text, ed. Christina Ionescu (Newcastle: Cambridge Scholars Publishing, 2011), 542.

13. Matthew Baillie, *An Account of a Particular Change of Structure in the Human Ovarium from the Philosophical Transactions* (London: s.n., 1789), 2.

14. Jean Astruc, *A Treatise on the Diseases of Women*, vol. 3. (London: J. Nourse, 1767), 14.

15. Richard Browne Cheston, *Pathological Inquiries and Observations in Surgery, from the Dissections of Morbid Bodies. With an Appendix Containing Twelve Cases on Different Subjects* (Gloucester. R. Raikes, 1766), 47.

16. Astruc, *A Treatise on the Diseases of Women*, 60–62.

17. James Yonge, 'An Account of Balls of Hair Taken from the Uterus and Ovaria of Several Women. By Mr. James Yonge, F.R.S. Communicated to Dr. Hans Sloane, R.S. Secr.', *Philosophical Transactions of the Royal Society* 25, no. 309 (1706): 2391.

18. James Cleghorn, 'The History of an Ovarium, Wherein Were Found Teeth, Hair and Bones. By James Cleghorn M.B. Communicated by Robert Perceval M.D.', *Transactions of the Royal Irish Academy* 1 (1787): 74–75.

19. Having always accepted the dominant view that the condition was a by-product of conception, the girl's age, apparent virginity and under-developed womb led Baillie to conclude that the condition was simply an ovary that had gone pathologically awry, curiously and haphazardly imitating the process of foetal formation. In his rather fortunate position as the nephew of surgeon and anatomist John Hunter, Baillie was able to access Hunter's rich collection of anatomical specimens, unearthing further examples of the tumours which consolidated his claim. Baillie, *An Account of a Particular Change*, 6–8.

20. Andrew Cunningham, *The Anatomist Anatomis'd: An Experimental Discipline in Enlightenment Europe* (Farnham: Ashgate, 2010), 170.

21. The physician Henry Manning's extensive *Treatise of the Female Diseases*, published in 1771, devoted little more than a page to diseases of the ovaries and Fallopian tubes, Manning writing that they were 'seldom or never perceptible, even to the patient herself' until the disease had progressed to an advanced stage. Henry Manning, *A Treatise on Female Diseases* (London: R. Baldwin, 1771), 307.

22. 'Of all the parts of the female pelvis, the ovaries are most frequently diseased' wrote the Scottish surgeon Charles Bell in 1798, '...in reference to practice, the knowledge of them is unimportant, if we except that of dropsy, so frequently occurring'. Charles Bell, *A System of Dissection, Explaining the Anatomy of the Human Body, the Manner of Displaying*

the Parts, and Their Varieties in Diseases (Edinburgh: Mundell and Son, 1798), 89.

23. However, what exactly this underlying problem was would remain a subject of debate until the early nineteenth century, when it began to be understood better as a symptom of cardiac, renal and other abnormalities.

24. Physician and antiquary Richard Wilkes discussed the treatment and etymology of dropsy in ancient Greece. Richard Wilkes, *An Historical Essay on the Dropsy* (London: Law & Ray, 1781), 1–7.

25. Anonymous, *An Account of the Causes of Some Particular Rebellious Distempers* (London: s.n., 1670), 76–78.

26. Bills of mortality attest to this; the 1764 Bill for London reported 956 deaths from the disease in that year, making it the sixth most fatal of the fifty-seven diseases listed. For the year 1798, dropsy again proved the sixth most fatal of fifty-four diseases listed, the cause of 784 deaths in the city. 'General Bills of Mortality for the Year 1764', *Scots Magazine* 26 (1764): 72; 'Account of Diseases in London' *Monthly Magazine* 7, no. 41 (1799): 68–69.

27. Donald Monro, *An Essay on the Dropsy and Its Different Species* (London: D. Wilson & T. Durham, 1756), 14.

28. In 1810 for example, it was a male figure that cartoonist Thomas Rowlandson chose to represent dropsy in his caricature 'Dropsy Courting Consumption'. In the illustration, a large dropsical gentleman is courting a rake-thin, consumptive lady, using for comical effect the disparity in their weight.

29. Wilkes, *An Historical* Essay, 94–95; John Leake, *Medical Instructions Towards the Prevention, and Cure of Chronic or Slow Diseases Peculiar to Women* (London: R. Baldwin, 1777), 336–337; Thomas Short, *A Discourse Concerning the Causes and Effects of Corpulency* (London: J. Roberts, 1728).

30. Lisa W. Smith, 'Imagining Women's Fertility Before Technology', *Journal of Medical Humanities* 31, no. 1 (2010): 72. As Smith notes, an absence of menstruation was not necessarily taken as a sign of pregnancy but could be indicative of a wide range of conditions.

31. Benjamin Gooch, *Medical and Chirurgical Observations, as an Appendix to a Former Publication* (London and Norwich: G. Robinson and R. Beatniffe, 1773), 110–117.

32. Philip Meadows Martineau, 'An Extraordinary Case of a Dropsy of the Ovarium, with Some Remarks. By Mr. Philip Meadows Martineau, Surgeon to the Norfolk and Norwich Hospital; Communicated by John Hunter, Esq. F. R. S.', *Philosophical Transactions of the Royal Society* 74 (1784): 471.

33. Yonge, 'An Account of Balls of Hair', 2389.

34. Cheston, *Pathological Inquiries*, 44.
35. William Luxmoore, *An Address to Hydropic Patients* (London: W. Wilson, 1796), 18–19.
36. William Cullen, *First Lines of the Practice of Physic*, vol. 4 (Edinburgh: C. Elliot, T. Kay, & Co, 1788), 327; Benjamin Bell, *A System of Surgery*, vol. 1 (Edinburgh: Charles Elliot and G. Robinson, 1783), 415.
37. William Withering, *An Account of the Foxglove and Some of Its Medical Uses* (Birmingham: Swinney, 1785), 203.
38. Martineau, 'An Extraordinary Case', 472.
39. 'John Hunter: A Copy of Notes Taken at His Lectures on Surgery', 2 (1787), Western Manuscripts MS5598 (Wellcome Collection).
40. Lynda Payne, *With Words and Knives: Learning Medical Dispassion in Early Modern England* (Aldershot and Burlington: Ashgate, 2007), 87.
41. Richard Blackmore, *A Treatise of the Spleen and Vapours* (London: J. Pemberton, 1725), 5.
42. Richard Blackmore, *A Critical Dissertation Upon the Spleen* (London: J. Pemberton, 1725), 51–52.
43. Blackmore, *A Critical Dissertation*, 5.
44. Sarah Parker, 'Subtle Bodies: The Limits of Categories in Girolamo Cardano's *De Subtilitate*', in *Anatomy and the Organization of Knowledge, 1500–1850*, ed. Matthew Landors and Brian Muñoz (London and New York: Routledge, 2016), 79.
45. Toby Gelfand, *Professionalizing Modern Medicine: Paris Surgeons and Medical Science and Institutions in the Eighteenth Century* (Westport and London: Greenwood, 1980), 9.
46. Beauredont, 'A Monsieur le doyen de la Société de l'Ausun…', ARC 17, d. 3, no. 45 (c. 1781–1782), Archives de l'Académie Royale de Chirurgie (Académie Nationale de Médecine), 5.
47. Reports of caesarean section, for example, can be occasionally found, where a baby who had become obstructed in labour was able to be saved. The mothers almost invariably died, although in 1738 the midwife Mary Donally, in advance of any surgeon, performed a caesarean in which the mother survived after twelve days of obstructed labour in which the child had died. Donally delivered Alice O' Neal, a farmer's wife from Armagh, by cutting open her abdomen and uterus with a razor. In addition, surgical texts of the eighteenth century recommended abdominal procedures for severe injuries, and operations for hernia were also described, which involved making minor incisions in the abdomen. Lisa Forman Cody, *Birthing the Nation: Sex, Science and the Conception of Eighteenth-Century Britons* (Oxford: Oxford University Press, 2005), 40.

48. Jane Eliot Sewell, *Bountiful Bodies: Spencer Wells, Lawson Tait and the Birth of British Gynaecology* (Ph.D. thesis, Johns Hopkins University, 1990), 315.

49. Katherine A. Walker, 'Pain and Surgery in England, c. 1620–1740', *Medical History* 59, no. 2 (2015): 270.

50. Laurence Brockliss and Colin Jones, *The Medical World of Early Modern France* (Oxford: Clarendon Press, 1997), 581.

51. Sauveur-François Morand, 'Remarques sur le Observations précédentes, avec un précis de quelques autres, sur le meme sujet', in 'Plusieurs Mémoires et Observations sur l'Enkistée et le Skirre des Ovaires', *Memoires de l'Academie Royale de Chirurgie* 2 (1753): 455–460.

52. Jean Delaporte, 'Hydropsie Enkistée de l'Ovaire attaquée par incision', in 'Plusieurs Mémoires et Observations sur l'Enkistée et le Skirre des Ovaires', *Memoires de l'Academie Royale de Chirurgie* 2 (1753).

53. Delaporte, 'Hydropsie Enkistée', 455.

54. Morand, 'Remarques sur le Observations précédentes', 459.

55. Philippe, 'D'un Mémoire sur l'hydropsie de l'ovaire', as reported to the Society by Destremau, ARC 39, d.'maladies de l'ovaire', no. 74—Document (1765), Archives de l'Académie Royale de Chirurgie (Académie Nationale de Médecine), 1; 'la chirurgie de notre siècle n'a pas encor pleinement triomphée de cette commune et cruelle maladie', 9.

56. William Hunter, 'The History of Emphysema', *Medical Observations and Inquiries* 2 (1758): 17–70, 41.

57. William Hunter, 'The History of Emphysema', 44–45.

58. As quoted in Schachner, *Ephraim McDowell*, 141.

59. Robert Houstoun, 'An Account of a Dropsy in the Left Ovary of a Woman, Aged 58. Cured by a Large Incision Made in the Side of the Abdomen', *Philosophical Transactions of the Royal Society* 33, no. 381 (1724): 9.

60. Lawson Tait, 'Address on the Principle of Exploratory and Confirmatory Incisions', *Lancet* 137, no. 3519 (7 February 1891): 292–296.

61. Pott did, however, consider the implications removing the ovaries would have on the woman's physiology, reporting that after the operation her breasts had disappeared, and her body had become more muscular, challenging the predominant view that removing the ovaries would not impair the general physiology of the body. Percivall Pott, *Chirurgical Observations* (London: T. J. Carnegy, 1775), 184–186.

62. Jean-Baptiste Laumonier, 'Observations sur un Dêpot de la Trompe et sur l'Extirpation des Ovaires', *Histoire de la Société Royale de Médecine* 5 (1787): 296–300.

63. Laumonier, 'Observations sur un Dêpot de la Trompe', 300.

64. Caroline C. Hannaway, 'The Société Royale de Médecine and Epidemics in the Ancien Régime', *Bulletin of the History of Medicine* 46, no. 3 (1972): 257.

65. 'Médicine-Pratique', *Histoire de la Société Royale de Médecine* 8 (1790): 7.

66. Paul Marx, 'Un Conflit Médical à l'Hôtel-Dieu de Rouen en 1790', *Histoire des Sciences Médicales* 19, no. 4 (1985): 382.

67. Paul Marx, 'Un Conflit Médical à l'Hôtel-Dieu de Rouen en 1790', *Échanges Magazine* 19 (1992): 33.

68. Marx, 'Un Conflit Médical' (1985): 380.

69. Brockliss and Jones, *The Medical World*, 561–562.

70. As quoted in Randolph E. Peaslee, *Ovarian Tumors: Their Pathology, Diagnosis and Treatment, Especially by Ovariotomy* (New York: D. Appelton, 1872), 234.

71. Peaslee, *Ovarian Tumours*, 234–235.

72. Michel Foucault, *The Birth of the Clinic: An Archaeology of Medical Perception*, trans. A.M. Sheridan (London: Routledge, 2003), 124–148; Gelfand, *Professionalizing Modern Medicine*, 9.

73. McDowell, 'Three Cases of Extirpation', 242–245.

74. Ornella Moscucci, *The Science of Woman: Gynaecology and Gender in England 1800–1929* (Cambridge University Press, 1990), 135–136; Ann Dally, *Women Under the Knife: A History of Surgery* (London: Hutchinson Radius, 1991), 11–13. The connection between McDowell and Bell seems to have first originated with a Kentucky surgeon named John D. Jackson sometime in the nineteenth century. The role of Bell became important in asserting that while an American surgeon may have had success in performing it, the operation was, in spirit, a British one. McDowell's early biographer refuted the connection. August Schachner wrote that while McDowell may have been influenced more generally by the powerful teaching of Bell 'we are thoroughly convinced that the idea of ovariotomy originated in the fertile brain of Dr. McDowell'. Schachner, 'Ephraim McDowell', 11–12.

75. Jean Bowra, 'Making A Man A Great Man: Ephraim McDowell, Ovariotomy and History', presented at Social Change in the Twenty-First-Century (University of Queensland, October 2005), 5–6, http://eprints.qut.edu.au/3454/1/3454.pdf, accessed 13 November 2010.

76. McDowell, 'Observations on Diseased Ovaria', 548.

3

Creating a Surgical Controversy

FROM KENTUCKY TO EDINBURGH TO THE PAGES OF THE *LANCET*:
OVARIAN SURGERY IN THE EARLY NINETEENTH CENTURY

John Bell would never receive the report Ephraim McDowell sent to him about his successes with ovarian surgery in Kentucky. In May 1817, Bell left for Italy where he would remain until his death in 1820. The report instead fell into the hands of the surgeon John Lizars, who had been Bell's partner in practice. Lizars, a respected instructor in anatomy and surgery at the Edinburgh extra-mural school, had his curiosity aroused by McDowell's new operation, and the challenge of removing diseased ovaries was to become a project for him over the next several years. In 1825, he published a monograph, *Observations on Extraction of Diseased Ovaria*, in which he detailed four cases where he had attempted the procedure. Lizars' results were mixed; of his four patients, one died from peritoneal inflammation, another was discovered to have been misdiagnosed, with no tumour to be found upon opening the abdomen, and in a third, the operation had to be abandoned because of extensive adhesions. Only one case brought success, a large diseased ovary was removed from a patient who—after a tense three-month period where she suffered severe post-operative illness—had survived. But even this achievement was tempered by Lizars' revelation that the patient's other ovary had also been diseased, but which he had been unable to remove.[1]

Lizars' work received mixed reviews from the medical press. *The Medico-Chirurgical Review*, one of the more established London medical journals, edited by the surgeon James Johnson, praised Lizars' bravery in performing the operation, but his disappointing results resolved the journal's editor to continue cautioning against surgeons repeating the procedure.[2] The *Lancet*, on the other hand, gave a more enthusiastic reception to Lizars' work. Still only two years old and founded on the radical agenda of its editor Thomas Wakley, who sought to challenge the conservatism and nepotism of the medical establishment, the journal implored its readers to cut through the prejudices of the profession and judge the operation relative to others already in existence. In keeping with its growing reputation for boldness, the journal claimed to see no reason why the operation should not be performed.[3]

Lizars' publication marked the introduction of the operation into the British public sphere. It hinted also at the increasingly polarised views of the medical community with regard to it. By the 1820s, the possibility of surgically extirpating the dropsical ovary was accepted by many medical practitioners to be at least technically possible. Empirical work by the obstetrician James Blundell, published in the *Lancet* in 1828, had built a more solid foundation for the practice of abdominal surgery based on experimental physiology. Blundell's experiment, in which he had removed ovaries, uteruses, spleens, kidneys and portions of the bladder from twenty-nine rabbits—eight of whom had survived—led him to believe that it was possible for the human peritoneum to tolerate injury and interference.[4] Blundell concluded from his experiments that the ovaries, the uterus, the spleen and parts of the bladder could all be removed from the body. But it was the ovaries that remained the focus of surgeons' attention as practitioners sought to build on the work of McDowell and Lizars. Interest in removing the other organs was not pursued; innovation required greater motivation than simply technical feasibility.

Coupled with successful cases being reported in London, as well as from Germany and America, the operation hovered at the boundaries of acceptability.[5] One doctor in America in 1822 claimed already to be teaching students how to carry out the procedure.[6] Those who continued to advocate medical treatments of ovarian disease increasingly faced scepticism from their peers. When St. George's Hospital physician Edward Seymour, for example, published a lengthy tome on ovarian pathology and physiology in 1830, he faced criticism for proposing treatments that deviated little from the customary cluster of therapeutics, such as diuretics and purgatives, employed by practitioners to treat a whole host of diseases, and for not instead investigating more radical cures.[7] A more nuanced nosology of ovarian tumours was also developing, which further teased apart ovarian disease from sweeping categorisations of 'dropsy'. 'Dropsical' swellings in the ovaries could be cysts, sometimes comprising a single chamber, but more often made up of multiple small sacs of fluid; they could be hard and malignant or soft and jelly-like. Their contents ranged from watery fluid to thick, opaque substances, to matter that resembled powdery coffee-grinds; ovarian disease manifested in such disparate ways that generic treatments like tapping and diuretics simply seemed at odds with pathological understandings. The ineffectualness of such treatments for ovarian disease only reinforced the latter's distinctiveness as a category of pathological disorder; indeed, the *Edinburgh Medical and Surgical Journal* questioned the validity of using the term 'dropsy' at all when describing the ovaries, arguing the term was erroneous when used to classify their diseases.[8] The inadequacy of standard treatments was a view James Blundell communicated to his students in his lectures on midwifery at Guy's Hospital at the tail end of the 1820s. Speaking about tapping in a lecture on midwifery, he declared to his class, 'the more I have seen of this operation, the more I have felt inclined to whisper to myself, when the surgeon has taken up his instrument, "I wish he could do something better"'.[9]

A cautious optimism lingered around the new operation but its considerable hazards remained evident. Failed cases still outstripped successful ones, and experiences like that of Lizars showed the range of difficulties that might be encountered, from misdiagnosis to the presence of adhesions, which would render it impossible to remove the organ. Surgeons stood at a crossroads. Could an operation with so much potential for complication, and which required entering the unknown territory of the abdomen, ever be admitted into established practice? The debate was carried and amplified by the weekly medical press, itself a novelty of sorts. The establishment of the *Lancet* in 1823 precipitated the arrival of a multitude of other weekly and fortnightly publications in Britain over the next few decades. Together they sped up the circulation of medical knowledge, generating a culture of public correspondence through their columns and providing a space for clinical case reports, medical politics and informal dialogue which glued together the profession. It is to fundamentally misunderstand the medical press to consider it a neutral 'mirror' upon medicine. Medical journals shaped and led debates, implicitly relayed the medical and political inclinations of their editors and publishers and guided their audiences through the latest discoveries and innovations. Through this latter function, the medical press entered a reciprocal relationship with those performing the new ovarian operation, enabling surgeons to bring their experiences and results under the scrutiny of the medical community. In exchange, the operation proved a newsworthy and controversial topic, of the type that the medical press thrived upon. There was a thirst for knowledge and news of the operation within the medical profession. The question of the operation's justifiability could not, after all, be judged until its risks were adequately understood. But what methods of analysis best interpreted and conveyed the risks of what was irreducibly a *practice*-based innovation? The medical press made it possible for there to be a plethora of modes of representation. This complicated searches for the truth and reality of the procedure as British practitioners tried to make sense of the moral, technical and professional concerns that came with the growing use of a novel operation in practice.

In the rest of this chapter, I consider three different aspects to the representation of ovarian surgery in the press between the early 1830s and the 1850s when the justifiability of removing ovaries was the subject of intense debate. In the first section, by way of setting the scene, I give a brief overview of the place of ovarian surgery in British medicine in the 1830s, before going on to consider how, during this time, it could be represented as both progressive and regressive. How were these differing representations situated in a medical culture where changes in anatomy, pathology and professional politics were shaping ideas of 'progress' in surgery? I go on to consider the place of what I term 'emotive accounts' of ovarian operations that emerged in the medical press, particularly during the 1840s, as the operation began to be performed by numerous practitioners in London, bringing it closer to the metropolitan hub of English medical practice. Reports of ovarian surgery in the medical journals were distinctive in their verbosity and in their strong conveyance of the patient's narrative, constructed to elicit an emotional response from readers. This played heavily into discussions regarding responsibility in surgery and even blame. Moreover, the women who underwent the procedure were not necessarily represented as passive participants. Their active role in agreeing to the operation, as well as their behaviour before and especially after it had taken place, played an important role in the way the operative experience was presented to the rest of the medical community, both by those who advocated the operation and by those who made it their business to prevent it becoming established practice. I then turn to the role of statistics in accounts of the procedure,

considering how statistical and 'emotive' representations of the operation
complemented, challenged and complicated one other. Quantifying data,
it has often been argued, became central to medicine around the middle
of the century, and the use of statistics in settling the question of ovarian
surgery's justifiability might be assumed to be simply another reflection
of the shift towards 'scientific' medicine at this time. But, practitioners
wondered, how useful were numbers in representing surgery? Could they
provide a definitive answer to the justifiability question? And how could
they represent the moral uncertainties that hung over the operation?

Progress or Culpable Homicide?

In 1837, a paper by William Jeaffreson, a surgeon practising in the
small market town of Framlingham in Suffolk was published in the
Transactions of the Provincial Medical and Surgical Association. In
it, Jeaffreson described the case of Mrs. B, a long-time patient of his
who had laboured under suspected ovarian dropsy for some years,
the condition causing complications in two pregnancies. As was typical, Mrs. B's tumour had been slow growing at first, before beginning
to rapidly enlarge, leaving the patient in considerable pain and leading Jeaffreson to offer his distressed patient 'the one chance which I
thought remained, by operation, candidly stating its probable hazard'.[10]
With the final decision apparently left to Mrs. B—the significance of
which will be explored in more detail later in this chapter—a date for
the operation was set. A small incision of about an inch and a half in
length—much smaller than the type made by Ephraim McDowell and
John Lizars—was made between the navel and pubes. The diseased
sac, once located, was punctured and drained of twelve pints of fluid
before being seized and cut away. After a week, Mrs B was considered
cured and out of danger. Jeaffreson went on to perform four more
similarly successful procedures for ovarian disease, while colleagues of
Jeaffreson from the East Anglian medical community reported successful cases too.[11] Together with the Tonbridge practitioner William West,
who had four cases, two of which had good outcomes, provincial practitioners led the way in ovarian surgery.[12] Like McDowell before them,
Jeaffreson's and West's geographical locations arguably spurred on their
use of novel and risky procedures. Away from the more tightly bound
medical communities of London and Edinburgh, the practices of provincial doctors were less scrutinised.

Jeaffreson's operation received positive reviews from some corners of the medical press. Advocates of the operation praised Jeaffreson for his bravery, one claiming the surgeon was 'opening to us a new era in the surgery of the abdomen'.[13] But with their publication the cases were also open to critique. Two objections to the operation were put forward with increasing regularity: the first was the very real possibility of misdiagnosis, which had been visibly highlighted by John Lizars' erroneous operation upon a woman who had had no ovarian tumour at all. Performing a dangerous operation when there was a high chance of death was an ethical quandary in itself; that the pursuit might be entirely in vain was flagrantly immoral. The second criticism centred upon the propriety of performing the operation, given that it was possible for a patient to live with the condition for some time, whereas the operation 'may carry them off in a few hours'.[14] The justifiability of using surgery for what was construed as a chronic rather than an acute illness was at the heart of the controversies over the operation.

In the 1830s, there was no more outspoken opponent to the procedure than the surgeon Robert Liston. Liston, who was probably the most famous operator of his generation, had come from Edinburgh to London in 1834 when he was appointed Professor of Surgery at University College London. He was an excellent anatomist and a skilful surgeon of external diseases, including tumours. Much of his considerable fame was cultivated from his dazzling displays of operative skill, where he showcased a striking speediness in his surgical performances, and where he excelled in daring procedures such as excision of the large jaw, removal of scrotal tumours and amputations of the thigh. Liston's surgical innovations tended to spring from an audacious self-confidence in his own operating skills, a characteristic that at times led to him perpetrating grim errors in his practice.[15] He espoused simplicity above all else as the key to successful surgery.[16] In his 1837 manual, *Practical Surgery*, he communicated his 'plain, common-sense view of the most important injuries and diseases which are met with in practice', which he claimed were 'unencumbered by speculations or theories'.[17] In 1846, a year before his death, he became the first surgeon in Britain to perform an operation under anaesthetic ether, cementing his reputation as one of the nineteenth century's more influential surgeons.

Liston was not unusual at this time in troubling himself over abdominal surgery, but he was notable for the ferocity of his opposition to it, which reflected his brusque persona. In *Elements of Surgery*, first published in 1831, Liston claimed that John Lizars was 'indictable for culpable homicide' for the fatal operation he had performed. The unfortunate women who had undergone the procedure he described as 'sacrificed to a desire for false reputation'.[18] This was not the only time the operation was linked criminality by those who opposed its use. During the first half of the nineteenth century, numerous surgeons who performed the operation found themselves threatened with criminal charges. One American surgeon, Walter Burnham, recounting in 1879 his early experiences with the operation, recalled how he had 'many times been threatened with prosecution for manslaughter' and that he had 'heard one of the ablest Professors in New York denounce all ovariotomists as "deserving to be hung"'.[19] British surgeons experienced the same threats.[20] As shall be explored in detail later in this chapter, involvement in the operation came with serious risks to one's career.

For Liston and others who opposed the operation, there was nothing to suggest that opening the abdomen was the beginning of a new era, let alone a sign of progress in surgery. Rather, they used evocative language to depict it as a regression; the famous term, 'belly-rippers', which Liston coined to describe those who performed ovariotomy, suggested a throwback to baseness and butchery, while the allusion to female 'sacrifice' Liston made conjured up images of slavishness to unthinking ritual and of unnecessary death, quite contrary to any notion of progress. So powerful was sacrifice as a metaphorical trope that early proponents of the operation also used it in their representations of the procedure, instead describing the sacrifice of women to the untamed ravages of disease, left to die rather than being offered a chance of life.[21]

Liston was joined in his disavowal of the operation by William Lawrence, surgeon to St. Bartholomew's Hospital. The way Lawrence conveyed his opposition to the operation requires us to consider in more detail how 'progress' elicited complex meanings in surgery. The historian Peter Stanley has depicted the 1830s as a period when 'the only way to make a name as a surgeon...was by performing operations, and young men hoped that by performing an operation first, more daringly or more spectacularly, it would enhance their reputation'.[22] An oft-made supposition is that pre-anaesthetic surgery was a haze of speed and spectacle, and that surgeons were at liberty to innovate freely.[23] But any radical new procedure in surgery was tempered by the continued deference of surgeons to an ideal of *reducing* the number of operations performed, which, it was believed, would be increasingly possible as surgical pathology improved. It was, after all, the science of surgery rather than its manual aspects that many surgeons, concerned about their professional standing, wished to promote.[24] As Adrian Desmond has shown, during the 1820s and 1830s, British physicians and surgeons were reflecting intensely upon broader notions of progress, reform and radicalism in the organisation and philosophical underpinnings of medicine. The explosion of medical-professional politics during this time, as reformers like Thomas Wakley castigated the bloated medical corporations and hospitals for their elitism and nepotism, was closely intertwined with the transmission of radical new medical theories into British education. This included Lamarckian ideas of philosophical anatomy, which stressed commonality between organisms, rather than hierarchy, enabling radical medical men to emphasise a universal thread of progressive egalitarianism in both anatomical theory and the organisation of medicine.[25]

Conservative members of the profession worried about the unwelcome importation of French philosophies of medical practice. Some believed it explained an increase in bold and daring operations occurring in Britain, particularly gynaecological and obstetrical ones, borne of the influence of a continental culture that prided itself on risk and novelty. In 1828, the politically conservative *London Medical and Physical Journal* claimed that 'some of the operators of this island have shown an anxiety to import such operations from the continent or to invent others which vie with them in boldness'. This was no doubt in part an allusion to the French enthusiasm for caesarean sections, which were performed more often on the continent than in Britain.[26] But the journal also landed upon John Lizars' operations to remove ovaries as an example of surgical boldness.[27] In actuality, in the early 1830s, ovarian surgery was still roundly disapproved of by French surgeons. But the operation was sufficiently controversial that conservative members of the profession strove to represent it as a French idea and thus use it to support their notion that British medical men were vulnerable to the influence of dangerous foreign radicalism.

Despite the claims of the *London Medical and Physical Journal*, progressivist medical politics among surgeons did not necessarily extend to radical modes of practice, as William Lawrence exemplified. Although by the 1830s Lawrence had virtually renounced his political radicalism after being elected to the Council of the Royal College of Surgeons of

England, in the decades preceding that, no other London surgeon had
had such a profound impact on medical philosophy. Lawrence had been
an outspoken critic of the lack of democratic representation for general
practitioners, who made up the bulk of the profession, and was a close
ally of Thomas Wakley. His deep attachment to controversial French
anatomical theories also saw him adopt a materialist viewpoint that was
condemned as blasphemous. Throughout and beyond these controversies, Lawrence exercised an enormous influence as a surgical educa-
tor. A gifted orator, his lectures were warmly received by his students at
St. Bartholomew's.[28] Lawrence promoted increased unison between
physic and surgery, and in his first lecture of the winter season of 1829,
he emphasised the fluidity of the boundaries erected between the internal
and external body, deriding the capriciousness of such a division when all
diseases were so closely connected by a general physiology and pathology.
'How deep would the domain of surgery extend, according to this view?'
Lawrence pondered with more than a hint of sarcasm, 'half an inch or an
inch?'[29] Lawrence emphasised the need for internal causes to externally
recognisable ailments to be part and parcel of surgical education.

Strikingly, Lawrence's radical aspirations did not extend to any desire
for operative surgery to foray further inside the body and Lawrence continued to equate surgical practice with external disease.[30] Like Liston,
Lawrence viewed ovarian surgery as bloody, brutal and backward. He
reacted incredulously to the possibility of removing ovaries, citing the
difficulties in diagnosing what disease lay beneath, which he believed
made the operation unjustifiable. In a lecture in 1830, Lawrence subtly
married the idea of the large abdominal incision with the act of dissecting
the dead, commenting caustically that 'the operation *merely* requires an
incision to be made through the integuments of the abdomen, extending
from the pubes to the ensiform cartilage; exactly the same kind of cut
that you would make in examining a subject after death'.[31] The same idea
was later echoed by Liston, who, in a lecture published in the *Lancet*,
quoted the macabre poetry of seventeenth-century satirist Samuel Butler
to describe the ovarian operation: 'as if a man should be dissected/to see
what part is disaffected', Liston told his students.[32]

Liston and Lawrence's comments intimated repugnance at the
opening of the sealed cavities of the living body, drawing an analogy
between the violent interference which both dissection of cadavers and
surgery of the abdomen required. Represented this way, the operation
evoked all the horrors of human vivisection at a time when tension

surrounding doctors' use of cadavers was growing. Just a year before Lawrence's lecture, the labourer and cobbler William Burke had been hanged in Edinburgh for his part in a series of gruesome murders he committed with his accomplice William Hare. The bodies of those they killed had been sold as dissection material to the surgeon Robert Knox. Knox was eventually cleared of any wrongdoing in the scandal, but his reputation never quite recovered.[33] To prevent further, similar episodes, the Anatomy Act, passed in 1832, had given surgeons increased access to bodies, allowing them the unclaimed dead of the workhouses. But the Act, wrought with caveats, served only to stigmatise the bodies of the poor instead of criminals. Throughout the decade, tensions between the profession and the public remained high. The latter remained deeply suspicious of surgeons' practices with dead bodies.[34]

Certainly, some of the descriptions given by those performing abdominal surgery in the late 1830s were suggestive of an anatomical exploration of the living, fully conscious patient. Robert King, who had assisted William Jeaffreson in his first operation, reported to the *Lancet* on his numerous attempts at abdominal surgery in 1837. In 1834, King had made an eight-inch incision into the abdomen of forty-year-old Sophia Puttock, who was suffering intolerable pain caused by a suspected tumour:

> To give greater facility for examination, the wound was enlarged in the direction of the lumbar vertebrae, for about four inches. The search was repeated most carefully, not only in the perpendicular direction, but upwards, towards the liver and small extremity of the stomach. Several of the gentlemen present repeated the attempt to find the tumour, but unsuccessfully. The kidney of the same side was handled, and appeared to be more moveable than natural, as it could be raised from its position nearly two inches. After the cavity of the abdomen had been exposed for two minutes, it was determined to reclose it, which was done without difficulty, by the common interrupted sutures.[35]

Puttock's abdomen had been cut open, allowing King to handle her abdominal organs, before he then invited his colleagues to insert their hands into her body to do the same. The operation could well have proved a useful anatomy lesson to King and his colleagues; indeed, King himself presented it as an important part of the operative experience. But such accounts also allowed individuals like Lawrence and Liston to use the imagery of dissection to represent the operation as a violation of the living body.[36]

In terms of how representations were constructed, there is a crucial point to be made here: that there was discordance between notions of progress in anatomy and those in surgery. While a surgeon like Lawrence could enthusiastically promote French methods of observation and practice over textbooks and lectures, as well as embrace radical ideas of anatomy and medical politics, this did not extend to countenancing the radical newness of abdominal surgery. Undoubtedly, this was in part a response to the very real risk of patients dying, as well as the delicate public reputation of surgeons, particularly in the light of the body-snatching scandals. But it also leads to more complex questions about connections in medicine that we often take for granted. For many surgeons, the new in fact did not always represent the progressive, nor was improvement in anatomy necessarily best represented by an expansion in the remit of surgery.

At the end of the 1820s, John Lizars' advocacy of ovarian surgery was described by the *London Medical and Physical Journal* as 'exactly the opposite to ninety-nine men out of a hundred'.[37] By the end of the 1830s, little seemed to have changed. Further operations had occurred, but they remained few and far between and generally performed outside the medical metropolises of London and Edinburgh. During this time, powerful opposition to the operation was arising, which saw ovarian surgery represented by its detractors as contrary to surgical morality. Beyond the ever-present concerns regarding the hazards of the operation, competing representations of progress were at play. The operation had to be carefully situated within a medical world fraught with professional politics.

WHO'S RESPONSIBLE? PATIENTS, RISK AND EMOTIVE ACCOUNTS

Despite the powerful opposition of Liston and Lawrence, the early 1840s saw an uptake in the practice of the operation—or at least an increased reporting of cases—as it began to be performed by numerous London practitioners. Some of these operations, such as those by Charles Aston Key, Caesar Hawkins, Bransby Cooper and Benjamin Phillips, were one-offs. All but Hawkins' case had resulted in the death of the patient, and one can speculate that this may have prevented those practitioners from making further attempts. But there was also a small group of surgeons, including Samuel Lane, Daniel Walne and Frederic Bird, who had performed the operation multiple times and with greater success. Most cases were treated in private although occasionally the operation would be performed at a hospital. The most prolific operator of all, however, was Manchester obstetrician and surgeon Charles Clay, who commenced a long and unbroken series of the procedures in 1842, claiming in 1848 to have performed the operation forty times, twenty-six of which had been successful.[38] These practitioners came from a range of professional backgrounds; Bird was a young, recent graduate from Guy's, Lane was a senior surgeon at St. Mary's, Walne was a less well-known but also relatively well-established London surgeon, while Clay was part of an elite of Manchester obstetricians. It was Charles Clay who in 1843 introduced one of his cases with a new word to describe the operation: 'ovariotomy', a term he claimed had been coined for his operations by his most well-known supporter, the Scottish obstetrician James Young Simpson.[39] The term was a misnomer—technically 'ovariectomy' would have been more accurate, as the ovary was completely cut out; 'ovariotomy', as Clay used it, implied only an incision. But nonetheless the word stuck, assured by the combined clout of Simpson and Clay.

At this point, the *London Medical Gazette* and the *Medical Times* rather than the *Lancet* were where the majority of cases of ovarian surgery were published. This was possibly a bid on the part of operators to avoid the acid tongue of Thomas Wakley, for by 1844 the *Lancet*, which earlier in the century had been a cautious advocate of the operation, had come out against the procedure, publishing a strongly worded editorial condemning its use.[40] Choosing which journal to publish it was one of several factors surgeons needed to consider when opening up their cases to public scrutiny. Those who performed it were already in a precarious position, more especially if they were disclosing poor results. Crafting an account which was able to adequately convey one's experiences, the patient's journey, and which also carefully negotiated the ethics of the operation, was a delicate process.

It has been argued, not always convincingly, that it was in the nineteenth century that the patient's 'voice' began to disappear from medical accounts. The conversational, emotive style that characterised early modern narratives of illness was replaced by an altogether more dispassionate tone, dominated by the practitioner's (rather than the patient's) voice, something often closely aligned with the 'rise' of hospital medicine in the early part of the century.[41] Clinician and historian Brian Hurwitz has described the style of the nineteenth-century medical report as involving a 'ruthless curtailment of patients' accounts and the denial of their agency within case reports...accompanied by a clinical attentiveness that focuses now on the normality of body systems'.[42]

My argument here is somewhat different. It is rather that those practising ovariotomy both desired from others and were expected to provide richly subjective accounts of their own and their patients' experiences *as well as* ostensibly objective, statistical-based data. In this sense, I align more closely with the argument put forward by literary theorist Meegan Kennedy. As she contends, the case history, which had so long been a significant aspect of medical culture, was not merely ironed out or replaced by tools of 'objectivity' in the nineteenth century. Rather, the nineteenth-century case history faced 'a uniquely heterogeneous set of demands: it must produce both a fact and a story, represent both a disease and a person, display both the disinterested stance of the man of science and the physician's subjective insight'.[43] As we shall see in the next section, 'objective' statistical accounts of ovarian surgery were important. But surgeons were predominantly concerned with constructing—and journals with publishing—full, qualitative accounts that centred upon the patient narrative. These were conceived of as crucial to formulating an idea of how justifiable ovarian surgery was. They were used to convey emotional experiences that more objective accounts could not express, as well as to elicit equally emotive responses from professional colleagues. Given the ethical questions the operation raised, this style of representation was more prominent in cases of ovarian surgery than in other forms of surgery. The negotiation of responsibility between surgeons and patients was at the crux of these accounts.

Surgical responsibility has been a subject of interest to historians of late. Claire Brock's recent work on abdominal surgery in late nineteenth-century Britain elaborates upon the divisions of responsibility between surgeons and their assistants, as operations began to be performed by surgical 'teams' rather than individuals.[44] Like historians before her, including Regina Morantz-Sanchez, Brock also raises the issue of patient demand for ovarian operations in the latter part of the century, opening up the question of how far women could be deemed responsible for the outcome of operations (especially when they failed) and even in encouraging unnecessary procedures.[45] This can be connected to previous work by Morantz-Sanchez on gynaecological surgery, which has contested the notion of the patient's disappearing voice in the nineteenth century, revealing instead the pivotal role some patients were able to play in the decision-making process.[46]

As I will elaborate upon in Chapter 5, the issue of patient demand certainly became an area of increasing concern during the latter part of the century. But less is known about the patient role in ovariotomy during the middle decades. From our contemporary viewpoint, it is perhaps hard to conceive of demand for such an operation in the pre-anaesthetic era. Surgery at this time could be bloody, brutal, fearful and unimaginably painful. Moreover, a patient's power to demand certain plans of treatment would have been heavily dependent on their socio-economic status. In any event, there *was* patient demand for ovariotomy, propelled by the deep suffering and humiliation ovarian disease could cause. This factored heavily into the way surgeons presented their experiences of the operation.[47] The operations which Frederic Bird, Daniel Walne, Charles Clay and others performed were by their own admission hazardous. Yet, as they represented it, it was not they but their patients who demanded they took place.

My concern is less about the material extent to which this was occurring, which it would be hard to determine, but rather how the patient role was used and amplified in surgeons' narratives of ovarian surgery to their advantage. Take a report published in the *London Medical Gazette* in 1840, sent in by the surgeon Benjamin Phillips about his twenty-one-year-old patient, identified only as 'A.D.'. Phillips began not with the case itself but with a lengthy preamble which saw him preparing his audience for the bad result he was about to reveal: 'unquestionably it is more agreeable to detail the results of the successful than the unsuccessful practice of our profession' he stated, 'yet it is equally incumbent on the practitioner to detail the one and the other'.[48] As Phillips saw it, there was a growing prevalence among surgeons for refusing to take responsibility for a bad outcome, the consequence of 'a desire men feel to find a cause of death over which they could not have control: and that is rarely difficult: the consequence of this is, that when they estimate the results of treatment, they exclude all cases where they can find reason for death independent of the operation or the treatment'.[49]

Yet as Phillips moved on to describe the case of A.D., a striking contradiction began to emerge in his account, as the surgeon began to subtly shift the responsibility for the case's failure to the patient and her family. Phillips began by conveying A.D.'s long journey towards the operation.

A.D. had perceived an enlargement on one side of her abdomen many months before, which after a period of slow growth had begun to rapidly enlarge. With a prescribed cupping treatment proving ineffective, her case had been passed via Robert Liston on to the obstetrician Charles Locock. Whether Liston was aware of Locock's opinion of the operation is not known, but the views of the man he was sending her on to were quite the opposite of his own. Locock advised A.D. that both tapping and medicine would be useless and that there was only one hope. Phillips paraphrased Locock telling the girl that: 'within the last four years an operation had been invented by which the cyst could be extracted; that if it succeeded her disease would be cured, and he strongly advised her to undergo that operation'.[50]

Exercising a degree of consumer power, A.D. once more switched doctors, determined to find someone who would not just recommend the procedure but also perform it. Her next doctor was of a similar opinion to Locock and at once referred her on to Phillips, who at last gave her the news she wanted: that he would undertake the operation. A month later, with A.D. in 'good spirits',[51] Phillips performed the procedure with ten other medical men in attendance. The operation went well, with the ovarian sac easily removed and as Phillips had estimated, no adhesions were present. The pedicle, the small stem-like piece of tissue which contained nerves and vessels, connecting the diseased ovary to its blood supply, was cut and ligatured and the patient appeared to be recovering well. However, A.D.'s condition quickly took a downward turn. She began to experience agonising pain on the right side of her abdomen, to which morphia and opium made no difference. Blood oozed from the wound and frequent vomiting set in. A brief upturn in her health ('countenance *very* good') was followed by the ominous reporting of 'cholera-like symptoms'. She died soon after.[52] A post-mortem uncovered two potentially significant pathologies: first, that the ligature which was supposed to have secured the end of the severed pedicle had failed to contain all the vessels; second, that the intestines were grossly ulcerated, which Phillips argued showed evidence of pre-existing disease. Phillips' call for surgeons to take responsibility for their mistakes seemed to dissolve under the weight of his own desire to clear himself of blame; it was also here that the verbosity of the account and the strong presence of the patient's voice were most useful to him. Phillips went on to suggest that it was A.D.'s intestinal condition that was the cause of death rather than the operation—the issue of the ligature he proceeded to completely ignore.

Phillips revealed that subsequent conversations with A.D.'s mother had seen her admit to not informing him that her daughter was suffering serious bowel problems. When the mother had mentioned to her daughter just before the operation that she had not told Phillips of this, Phillips quoted the daughter's response to her mother as the following:

> It is lucky, mother, that you did forget it, for I have been twenty times to-day, but do not say anything to Mr. Phillips about it, or he will put off the operation.[53]

Using the patient's 'own' voice, Phillips implicated A.D. and her mother's actions in A.D.'s death.

It was not unusual for blame to be parcelled out to patients in this way. In his third published case, Charles Clay made a similar assertion of blame in the case of forty-seven-year-old Mrs. Dillon, this time in regard to the behaviour of her and her family after the operation. On opening Mrs. Dillon's abdomen, Clay and his colleagues had found a malignant tumour with significant vascularisation. Deemed inoperable, as malignant tumours usually were, the patient's abdomen had been closed without any active treatment. On the morning of the fifth day of her recovery, Mrs. Dillon's husband had requested giving his wife a mixture of gin and garlic 'as she had been accustomed to take it for the wind', a request Clay denied. When later that day he visited the patient, she had become seriously ill and Clay found it 'impossible to reflect on the progress of the case...without suspecting some interference of the most unwarrantable description in the nursing, particularly when coupled with the wish to exhibit stimulants in the morning of that day'.[54] Mrs. Dillon died six days after the operation and Clay placed the blame squarely with the family members who had been attending the patient, whom he believed had provided her with gin against his wishes.[55]

Such accounts encouraged readers to think deeply about divisions of responsibility in surgery. Where did fault lie when an operation went wrong? Was a fatal outcome always the surgeon's responsibility? Or could blame lie with the patient or those who attended them after? Surgical operations are often assumed to be discrete events in which the role of different actors is self-evident. Phillips' and Clay's reports instead pointed to the malleable nature of responsibility and blame in surgery, and the porous boundaries between the operation itself and events that occurred before and after that might influence its outcome.

As was seen in the case of A.D., it was not only a patient's consent to
the operation that was described but, often, their pursuit of it as well. In
many of these cases, the patient was depicted as the driving force and the
surgeon as the reluctant possessor of potential healing powers; an impartial adviser to the suffering woman. This was exemplified by Clay's first
case, a woman named Mrs. Wheeler in 1842:

> My patient began to express herself earnestly desirous of an operation –
> respecting which I neither persuaded her to, nor dissuaded her from, but
> faithfully detailed to her the magnitude of the means she sought, pointed
> out the particulars of every case on record, with the results, and rather if
> anything depreciated than added to the chance of recovery. Still she was
> determined I should operate.[56]

And indeed in Mrs. Dillon's case, which ultimately had ended fatally,
Clay retrospectively characterised himself as having had his own sense of
judgement overpowered by the patient's determination:

> In vain I argued that her case had not the same prospects of success as the
> others preceding hers and that if it was performed the chances were greatly
> against her; her importunities at length prevailed, and I somewhat reluc-
> tantly consented to operate.[57]

Husbands and male relatives were conspicuous in their absence in narratives of patient consent. It was stressed by surgeons that the women
made the final decision, and that their subjective understanding of their
own lived body potentially outweighed the surgeon's own feelings on the
matter. Many case reports emphasised the bodily pain that might compel women with the condition to seek help as well as the greater impact
of the disease upon their self-image. In the case of A.D., for example,
Phillips stated that her main motivation for seeking help was the stir that
her changing shape was causing among her peers, the surgeon commenting that 'the tumefaction was so far increased as to have become apparent externally, and subjected her to remarks which distressed her a great
deal'.[58] It was likely that, like countless other women, A.D. was also suspected of being pregnant. Daniel Walne's third and youngest patient,
'A.K.', was reported to have echoed similar concerns. The nineteen-year-
old girl and her family were distressed by remarks from A.K.'s teacher and
later her employer about her unusual and 'matronly' appearance; indeed,
'her size excited so much observation, and caused so many unpleasant

remarks...that she was obliged to return home'.[59] The interplay between illegitimate pregnancy and ovarian tumours and its attendant consequences—social stigma and even a detrimental effect on employability and marriageability—weighed heavily on the minds of younger patients with the condition. Even if pregnancy was not suspected, the oddity of appearance which the condition could cause—a grossly swollen belly, often coupled with a swelling of the legs or emaciation of the rest of the body—could be distressing enough, a fact that was emphasised by operators.[60] Walne's first case, fifty-eight-year-old Mrs. F., was moved to seek treatment because she had become 'unpleasantly remarkable'.[61] Surgeons constructed accounts that fleshed out patients' experiences, beyond the clinical points, and detailed the impact of the disease on their quality of life.[62]

The role of patients in initiating surgical encounters also proved useful material for those against the use of ovariotomy. Samuel Ashwell, lecturer in Midwifery at Guy's, spoke out vehemently against the operation in the 1840s. Following the publication of his monograph, *A Practical Treatise on the Diseases Peculiar to Women* (1843), Ashwell's views on the operation began to filter into both the British and American press. Journals picked up on his description of an encounter with a sixty-two-year-old woman who had travelled a long distance to visit him in London 'anxious to have extirpation performed'. The woman 'had never been tapped, although ovarian dropsy had existed for more than half her life'. Somewhat dismissively, Ashwell claimed that 'there was scarcely any suffering beyond weight and pressure, although the tumor was of immense size and partly solid' and that 'in such a case it would have been highly culpable to have operated; and yet a surgeon over-zealous about the removal of ovaries had induced the firm belief that it ought to have been done'.[63] In this case, Ashwell claimed to have made the woman sensible to the dangers of the operation and that she had changed her mind. But in another, that of a twenty-two-year-old woman who had approached him, the patient had gone on to find another surgeon to perform the operation, only for it to prove fatal. 'Many years might have been added to her existence', noted Ashwell regretfully.[64] For Ashwell, patient demand was to be quelled and not acquiesced to.

Mirroring the use of patient narrative, the small band of men who were willing to remove ovaries could also shift around ideas of responsibility when the operation was *not* performed. An article in the *Medical Times* in 1851 by Frederic Bird barely concealed the anger he felt about a young patient on whom he had wished to perform ovariotomy.

Miss F. was just twelve years old when she first perceived an abdominal swelling. After numerous encounters with a variety of physicians and surgeons, Bird met Miss F. three years later. Describing her as 'possessed of remarkable vivacity and intelligence', who complained little about her illness,[65] Bird appeared openly moved by the plight of the girl, who had by this point developed serious curvature of the spine from where the pressure of the growth was bearing down. Much to Bird's chagrin, Miss F.'s original physician, Robert Lee, was of an opinion that stood in stark contrast to his own. Lee believed an operation inadvisable and, as Bird reported it, 'with a natural desire to spare their child useless suffering, the parents were influenced by the apparent doubt based on Dr. Lee's opinion'.[66] Thus, the operation was not agreed to. A year later, Miss F.'s parents changed their mind as the state of their daughter's health became increasingly desperate and Bird was asked to perform the operation. But Miss F. had become too weak to be operated upon and she died a few months later of the disease. While Bird never directly implicated Lee in her death, it was clear that he believed it was the latter's opposition to the operation that was at fault. 'If no other lesson be taught by this case' Bird warned, 'it must at least be conceded, that, as extirpation could have been performed, so might life have been preserved'.[67] The dangers of the operation meant that its performance could be represented as a liability, morally and professionally, but so too could the absence of its performance potentially imply a lack of responsibility on the part of the doctor to alleviate a patient's pain, and to take a chance with the only operation that might save their life.

As Flurin Condrau has succinctly put it, taking a patient's medical history most often 'results in a medical construct based on information coming from the patient, while being clearly governed by perceptions, categories and the language of medicine'.[68] Even more so, one might argue, when further mediated through journals aimed at a predominantly professional medical audience. The use of the patient's narrative to reinforce the justifiability of undertaking the procedure is translucently apparent in these accounts. The voices of A.D., A.K. and other patients were deployed by surgeons as part of a damage-limitation exercise. Evocative and dramatic narratives of their encounters with patients reinforced surgeons' characterisations of themselves as following their moral conscience; the product was reports in which the ethical aspects of the operation intentionally weighed heavily upon the reader.

It would be inaccurate to assume that because the expected audience for these reports would have been a medically educated one they would have responded only to objective facts. It plays into a broader historiography that has posited objectivity and dispassion as inherent to nineteenth-century medicine, where emotion was to be exorcised from surgeons' outward representations of themselves. But recent scholarly work has sought to challenge the notion of clinical dispassion. Michael Brown has argued that pre-anaesthetic surgery must be contextualised within the broader *milieu* of the early nineteenth century, during which enlightenment values of sensibility and sympathy laid the foundation for Victorian sentimentality.[69] Historians like Peter Stanley have argued this hindered rather than helped surgeons, as they sought to repress the expression of emotion in an effort to stay true to scientific objectivity.[70] But as Brown has amply evidenced, surgeons very frequently wrote discourses of emotion into their work and used it to build a professional culture that espoused compassion.[71] Under these circumstances, it is plausible to assume that surgeons like Phillips, Ashwell and Bird wrote the accounts that they did so as to elicit emotional responses to support their cause. The medical press, no mere storehouse of clinical knowledge, but a commercially driven enterprise always looking for appealing and interesting content, authenticated and published these accounts.

The moral quality of the 'new' operation was so intertwined with its performance, that to sever the connection between the two was neither possible nor desired. Indeed, it is telling that when James Young Simpson set an examination question on ovariotomy for his students in the late 1840s, the question did not require simply an answer of technical facts, but instead asked the student to answer whether the operation was 'justifiable or not justifiable', provoking an implicit moral judgement to be made by the examinees.[72] Ovariotomy was not only a question of technical innovation, it was a question of ethics too, and both advocates and opponents sought to recognise this in the way they represented their experiences and understandings of the operation.

'An Eminently Uncertain Operation': Ovariotomy and the Trouble with Statistics

By the early 1840s, a number of British practitioners willing to perform ovariotomy, but its standing remained precarious. The *Medical Times* saw the operation as justified, describing it in 1844 as 'far too important an innovation in surgery…to be lightly given up because it has not received the favour of a journal or two'.[73] The *London Medical Gazette*, which some years before had been vocal as to the unsavoury 'French' roots of the operation, stated that they now held a neutral position on the matter.[74] But other medical journals remained resolutely opposed. The *Lancet*, as we have seen, publicly stated its position against it in 1844 and in the same year *The Medico-Chirurgical Review* also condemned it, disparagingly describing ovariotomy as '*the* surgical subject of the day. It *is* the *fashion* just now to open the abdomen and cut out the ovary. It *was* the fashion last year to lay violent hands on every squinting man, woman and child, and cut his, her or its eyes out'.[75] 'Fashion' implied limited temporality, even faddishness. Just as reckless surgeons had been unnecessarily preoccupied with new eye operations the year before,[76] so now they focused on an equally useless procedure upon the ovary. Others insinuated that it teetered dangerously close to the realm of quackery, vying with mesmerism and hydropathy in its controversy.[77] But for many critics it was not just the operation itself that was the issue, it was how to make sense of the plethora of cases now streaming into the public arena. How could a decision about the operation be made, the profession fretted, if data on it were untrustworthy, incomplete or confused? Some began to formulate statistics from the cases published in a bid to bring closure to the ovariotomy debate; 'statistics will settle the question' the obstetrician Fleetwood Churchill declared confidently in 1844.[78]

The role of statistics in medicine is a path much trodden by historians. In surgery, Ulrich Tröhler has shown that the use of statistics stretches back farther than we often assume and that they were commonly used in the eighteenth century.[79] But Ian Hacking's contention that it was during the nineteenth century that statistics began to permeate most elements of Western society through a powerful intertwining with print culture—what he describes as an 'avalanche of printed numbers'—remains convincing.[80] This is not to say that the medical profession quickly and unquestioningly accepted statistical methods. Throughout the eighteenth and nineteenth centuries, there were many in the medical profession who were not convinced by the usefulness of statistics, nor did they like what it represented about medicine—that it was, perhaps, more science than art and that it reduced their patients to mere numbers.[81] But in the mid-nineteenth century, statistics figured more prominently in medical culture than ever before—in part because the expansion of hospitals enabled the collation of greater numbers of cases.

The apparent 'rise' of statistics has sometimes been conceptualised as part of a wider history of risk, although that there might even
be a history of risk to be found in the nineteenth century is a thorny
issue. 'Risk' after all is often considered to be a twentieth-century phenomenon, associated with the increasing use of epidemiology to inves-
tigate the probabilistic aspects of illness on a mass scale, as well as with
the expansion of the life insurance industry.[82] Etymologically, too, use
of the word 'risk' increased exponentially in the mid-twentieth century. For these reasons, discussing notions of risk in the nineteenth
century has been considered presentist.[83] While one must avoid con-
flating nineteenth-century concepts of risk with modern ones, surgical risk—as in measuring the likelihood of a fatal outcome—was very
real, both as concept and as a term in nineteenth-century surgery.[84]
As Patricia Jasen has argued, historians' fears of presentism may stem
from understanding 'risk' only by what it means today, when a more
useful approach would be to understand the 'different languages of
risk' that there have been, including the way risk was understood by the
patient.[85]

How risk was represented statistically in regard to ovariotomy has
been somewhat subsumed by historians' interest in the quantification of
another surgical innovation of the 1840s: anaesthesia. Martin Pernick
cautions against assumptions that anaesthesia was the main reason for
an increase in operations in general; he nonetheless argues that in the
case of gynaecology, and particularly ovariotomies, anaesthesia 'did
indeed lead to new and more untested operations' and that before 1846
'ovariotomy had been done only as an heroic last resort'.[86] Aside from
Pernick's anachronistic depiction of ovariotomy,[87] his argument that
there was a major division between ovariotomy pre- and post-1846—
at least when applied to Britain—is debatable. While the introduction
of chloroform was welcomed by most performers of ovariotomy as an
important aide to their operations,[88] there is little evidence from the
1840s to attest to ether and chloroform either improving confidence
in the operation among its sceptics or substantially increasing the number of operations being performed. In Britain at least, as the enthusiasm
for anaesthesia began to cool soon after its introduction into practice,
fears quickly set in over its role in encouraging dangerous and unnecessary operations.[89] Its use in ovariotomy only added fuel to the fire as
critics speculated that operations would now be performed even more
recklessly.[90]

Ian Burney has argued that the introduction of anaesthesia was a prime example of the emergence of surgical risk in the nineteenth century and the use of statistics in calculating the risk of anaesthetic-related deaths as exemplifying the 'medical utilitarianism' that pervaded at the time.[91] But the use of statistics to represent ovariotomy should not be read in the shadow of anaesthesia. Not only did ovariotomy statistics precede the introduction of anaesthesia in 1846 but the innovation under scrutiny was quite different: a surgical procedure, rather than a process ancillary to the actual operation, as anaesthesia was. This impacted on the process of statistical representation, as too did the unique status many ascribed to ovariotomy in terms of both its technique and objective.

It was Charles Clay's publication of his first five operations as a stand-alone pamphlet, *Cases of Peritoneal Section*, in 1842, which seemed to first draw the medical community's attention to the statistics of ovariotomy.[92] At the end of the pamphlet, Clay had collated a list of all known large incision ovarian operations including his own (thus differentiating it from small incision procedures like that carried out by William Jeaffreson in Framlingham). As Clay calculated it, there had so far been ten successful cases and one failed case of the operation.[93] His statistics, however, were met with derision. In a vicious review of the pamphlet, the *British and Foreign Medical Review* (later re-named *The Medico-Chirurgical Review*) tore apart his methodology, the reviewer pouring scorn upon the way Clay had grouped his own fatal outcomes. Clay, it seemed, had chosen *not* to count his two fatal cases, those of Mrs. Dillon and Mrs. Hardy, because he had operated upon them only to find tumours that were not ovarian but were either uterine or of an 'anomalous' nature; thus, Clay had seen fit not to count them at all in the statistics of his operations. Clay's approach outraged the *Review*. In a testament to the power that journal editors wielded in shaping representations of the operation, the *Review* re-jigged Clay's table of statistics into two tables that they claimed provided more accurate data: one table of completed operations and another of operations where no ovarian tumour had been discovered, or where the operation had had to be abandoned because of complications. The reviewer also attacked the validity of Clay's other data regarding successful cases. His inclusion of Jean-Baptiste Laumonier's 1783 case was discounted by the *Review*, who claimed Laumonier's patient Louise Lagrange had suffered from an abscess rather than an encysted ovarian tumour (somewhat contradicting their outrage at Clay's own exclusion of cases with a different pathology).

Ephraim McDowell's successes were also, it seems, still being met with incredulity, the *Review* suggesting his operations 'stagger[ered] belief'.[94] Doubt was also cast on the validity of including John Lizars' apparently successful case, since the second ovary in the surviving patient was believed to have been diseased but not removed. The *Review* was clear in its dislike for the operation, but that these three particular operators came under so close a scrutiny spoke also to changing notions of what could be counted as valid evidence in surgery. In the eighteenth century, the boundaries between historical and contemporary data had blurred; as we have seen in Chapter 2, anecdotal evidence from the ancient world had played a role in validating the removal of the ovaries. By the 1840s, with Clay's statistics under scrutiny, older examples, unpoliced by contemporary British observers, were being discounted by critics.

Just a year later, two further statistical tables were published, one by the surgeon Benjamin Phillips in the *Medico-Chirurgical Transactions* and a second by the obstetrician Fleetwood Churchill, first published in the *Dublin Journal of Medical Science*, before being reprinted in *The Medico-Chirurgical Review*.[95] Phillips, following the fatal result in A.D.'s case, had turned his back on the operation. He had become vocal in his belief that the results of unsuccessful ovariotomies were being held back and that this was erroneously giving the impression that the operation was safer than it was.[96] Phillips inferred that multiple practitioners were choosing not to reveal cases where there had been a fatal outcome. He supported this contention by including in his table four cases (the surgeons described by the anonymous initials 'A.B.', 'C.D.' and so forth) that had never been publicly recorded in Britain but with which he was 'acquainted'. Three had resulted in death. Phillips insinuated that he knew of a number of other failed cases too, performed by surgeons who had already published on their successes but had failed to report those where the patient had died; he did not include these in his own statistics, implying instead that if these surgeons were honourable they would reveal their failed outcomes in due course.[97] By stating that he had omitted such cases, Phillips was drawing attention to the limitations of his *own* statistics in accurately conveying both the number of ovariotomies performed and the procedure's relative risk. If, as Phillips asserted, a multitude of dangerous operations were going unrecorded, this was a worrying thought indeed, for it suggested the widespread and unchecked use of a dangerous innovation.

The contemporaneous table constructed by Churchill further suggested that confusion was already present in the project to construct a 'true' statistical representation of ovariotomy's risk. Churchill's table differed considerably; it excluded several cases that Phillips had added to his, as well as including one—the contentious Laumonier case—that Phillips had not. The two men also calculated their mortality rates differently. Phillips had determined his by looking at how many times the diseased organ had been successfully removed from the patient and how many had then gone on to recover—only with both these elements in place did he believe the operation could be regarded as a success. Using this, he determined that there had been thirty-five successes out of eighty-one attempts, giving a success rate of forty-three per cent. Churchill had collated sixty-six cases and stated that there had been forty-two recoveries and twenty-four deaths, giving an overall survival rate of sixty-four per cent. In cases where the ovary had been successfully removed (he counted forty-nine cases), a success rate of sixty-seven per cent was given.[98]

How ovariotomy statistics could be related to other major operations raised further divisions. For proponents of the operation, making such a comparison was vital to their cause. If ovariotomy's risk could be shown to be similar to those of other 'capital' operations,[99] as many believed it was, then why should it be held in more disregard and fear than other procedures?[100] Opposition to the operation, Charles Clay argued, stemmed from an illiberal and conservative streak in the medical profession, happy to cut off legs at the thigh and tie major arteries because these were 'established' practices, but unable to countenance the new. Clay believed it was the excessive and unproven fears about entering the peritoneum that prevented ovariotomy's establishment, an opinion that was probably well founded given the repulsion Robert Liston and others professed at the opening of the abdomen.[101] Most questioned the validity of comparing ovariotomy with other operations; ovariotomy was a procedure based on *choice*, quite different from amputation and aneurysm, which were indispensable, emergency treatments. Supporters of ovariotomy like James Young Simpson claimed that if the meaning of a 'capital' operation was going to be scrutinised in this way, then other operations— lithotomy or tying an aneurysm—could equally be described as operations of choice for conditions that could be lived with for years.[102] But Simpson's argument largely fell on deaf ears; ovariotomy was inherently different because, as one critic put it in a letter to the *Lancet* in 1857, it was against 'surgical instinct'.[103] Opening the abdomen and entering the peritoneum was so wildly different from performing a lithotomy, amputation or other 'classic' surgical operation that it simply rendered it incomparable.

While both advocates and opponents took an interest in the quantification of ovariotomy, statistical tables—or at least published ones—were more commonly constructed by opponents. Through one man, the aforementioned obstetrician Robert Lee, statistics came to be a powerful tool for those who remained sceptical about the operation in the 1850s. Lee in fact was a fine example of how statistics were constructed when one already had a firm opinion of the operation in mind. A Scottish-born but London-based practitioner, Lee had by the late 1840s built up both a considerable private practice and a powerful reputation as an author, lecturer, anatomist and physiologist.[104] He worked relentlessly in his numerous fields of interest and was well respected, although during his career he was involved in a number of well-publicised spats, including a lengthy dispute with Thomas Snow Beck during the 1840s over which one of them had ascertained correctly the anatomy and physiology of the uterine nervous system. Lee was a known traditionalist in his approach to surgery and especially in his distaste for major operations in obstetrics and gynaecology. From the late 1840s, Lee castigated the use of caesarean section in his speciality. Equally, the increasing use of ovariotomy deeply perturbed him and he spoke out publicly against what he saw as a 'rage for cruel and bloody operations'.[105] In the case of both procedures, Lee thought the statistics to be unsatisfactory and like Benjamin Phillips believed that many unsuccessful cases were not being disclosed. The contested nature of caesarean section provides an interesting comparison to ovariotomy in this respect, as surgeons and obstetricians were similarly concerned about ascertaining its risks. In 1841, Fleetwood Churchill had produced statistical tables comparing the mortality of various obstetrical operations. Reflecting on his statistics of all caesarean sections known to him to have been performed since 1750, Churchill declared that there had been '316 operations, from which 149 mothers recovered and 129 children were saved and 53 lost, in 182 cases where the result was recorded'.[106] This suggested to Churchill that while the operation was dangerous and should still be considered a last resort, it was less dangerous than previously believed and that the risk was not dissimilar to other more established obstetric procedures like symphyseotomy, an operation where the symphysis pubis joint was divided in order to facilitate labour.[107] Churchill's statistics were swiftly questioned by *The Medico-Chirurgical Review*, who argued that his collected numbers barely scratched the surface as to the true number of caesarean sections that had been performed in Europe so far, the estimated extent of which led the *Review* to conclude that 'the real proportionate mortality can...never be accurately ascertained'.[108] Statistics were being sought as a means of attaining a definitive idea of operative risk, but like ovariotomy statistics, those for caesarean section seemed deeply uncertain. In this way, operative statistics, where data was being retrospectively collected, differed considerably from those for anaesthesia, where statistical methods had been quickly employed soon after it was introduced into practice.

Nonetheless, there were important differences between ovariotomy and caesarean section. The necessity of the latter in extreme circumstances was usually seen as justified. With caesarean section, after all, it was about comparing its risks to other serious operations for obstructed labour. With ovariotomy, the choice was between major surgery and one of the considerably less invasive treatments for ovarian tumours which were still being utilised, such as tapping, application of pressure to the tumour and iodine injections. It was perhaps for this reason that Robert Lee more ardently pursued ovariotomy. He first made his own statistics on the operation public at a meeting of the Royal Medical and Chirurgical Society at the end of the 1850, where he announced that he had collected 108 cases, by which he had calculated a thirty-five per cent mortality rate for all attempted ovariotomies.[109] The tables, like Phillips', included further cases which had never before been published, mostly constituting single cases which Lee alleged had been communicated privately to him. Two names were noticeably absent though: Daniel Walne and Frederic Bird. Lee claimed that both men had failed to furnish him with the full facts of their experience with ovariotomy and had not published all their unsuccessful cases. Lee's colleague Caesar Hawkins, who since his own failed operation had, like Phillips, become disenchanted with ovariotomy, denounced Bird for holding back details of failed cases while at the same time having 'actually put on record... his opinion of the impropriety of withholding any information from the public with regard to this very operation'.[110] Bird, who was present at the meeting, expressed shock at the demeaning public denouncement of his work and claimed that he had already sent Lee the statistics for his operations thus far: twelve cases, of which eight had been successes. But herein lay the slipperiness in defining what exactly the most desirable method of data collection was. Lee's definition of statistics was quite different from Bird's who believed his notice of twelve cases, without giving any further details, was enough to satisfy Lee in his collection of *statistical* data. But it was not. For Lee, statistics were not a matter of mere quantification and calculation when it came to operations; statistics, Lee believed, needed to be contextualised with further information about the cases, otherwise they were useless. Thus, the value of numerical data was not a given, even by those who were constructing apparently objective accounts. Rather, they were entirely contingent on narrative as well.

Things went from bad to worse for Bird during the meeting. Pushed into confirming how many attempts he had made to remove an ovarian tumour, whether successful or not, Bird admitted that on numerous other occasions, not reported, he had opened the abdomen to make an exploratory incision. Apparently weary of attempting to diagnose blindly, Bird had begun to open the belly to ensure that ovarian disease was present before he went ahead with an operation. The report of the meeting gives a palpable sense of tension in the crowded room as Bird was asked how many times he had made such an exploratory incision. Bird responded that 'probably he might startle some gentleman by stating as many as forty, or fifty; but of this number he was speaking quite at random'.[111] Bird denied that any of these exploratory incisions had been fatal, although this was contested by Lee who believed that at least one had been. Regardless, major damage had been done to both Bird's reputation and the cause of ovariotomy. Bird's public humiliation put a well-known face to the vague and nameless fear that dozens, perhaps even hundreds of ovarian procedures were being performed secretly and thus, that the true scale of the operation's mortality was not yet known.

Lee was evidently delighted with the stir his paper had caused and his role in encouraging the profession to think deeply and critically about both ovariotomy and caesarean section, '…in all of which I was victorious, or rather the truth triumphed', he wrote in his diary at the end of the year regarding his public battles.[112] Lee's use of statistics was ostensibly to attain an objective representation of the operation. But what it had really done was to provide Lee with an opportunity to rather dramatically reveal cases of clandestine abdominal surgery. Indeed, perhaps

even more important than the statistical calculations he had made—
that over a third of those being operated upon had died—was the way
in which he had made the withholding of information on ovariotomy
now seem completely unacceptable. The operation to remove diseased
ovaries had been an ostensibly private endeavour, negotiated between
patients, practitioners and eventually, a surgeon willing to undertake the
risk of doing the procedure. 'Ovariotomy' was something different; it
shifted the operation from a single act to a collective identity, in which all
occurrences were expected to be made public. Buttressed by the rapidly
expanding medical press, it was now felt the truth of the operation could
only be established if it existed publicly and in print. Surgeons who resisted
bringing their work into the public sphere were vulnerable to accusations
of misconduct. This shift in surgical practice was felt profoundly by those
personally and unfortunately involved. Daniel Walne had escaped the full
extent of Lee's wrath by sending him more complete information on his
cases, but it is telling that by the beginning of the 1850s he had given
up performing ovariotomy, as had Samuel Lane. Frederic Bird, who up to
now had done more in London than any other practitioner to promote
the cause of ovariotomy, at first appeared to escape relatively unscathed
from the debacle, responding with a letter to the *Lancet* again stating
his cases, and then publishing a series of articles on the pathology
and treatment of ovarian disease in the *Medical Times*. But in 1852,
aged just thirty-four, Bird published his last ovarian case. He retained a
respectable post lecturing at Westminster Hospital but was rarely seen in
medical society in later life. A telling glance into his world was furnished
in an obituary written upon his death in 1874. It noted with a hint of
ambiguity that Bird gave up ovariotomy as he was 'averse to the anxieties
which are naturally associated with such operations'.[113] Ironically, in a later
publication Lee included Bird's original statistics.

Despite Lee's personal victory, the controversies surrounding Bird
only clarified the unsatisfactory nature of surgical statistics. At the same
meeting where Bird was accused of concealment, William Lawrence
questioned what method was best employed to gather and represent
knowledge of the operation. Even though Lee had published as much
detail as he could on each case and, where possible, on the length of
life afterwards, Lawrence, who was still firmly against the operation,
expressed concern as to whether Lee's statistics really got to the bot-
tom of ascertaining the operation's propriety. Lawrence pondered

how much statistics could tell the profession not only about the extent to which a successful operation prolonged life but also whether that involved a decent quality of life too, a subject I will revisit in Chapter 6. The days, weeks, even months after ovariotomy had been performed were a period of considerable anxiety. Deaths on the operating table or immediately after accounted for around only half of fatal cases and it was, as one Irish surgeon described it, 'the great danger that looms in the distance'[114]—that is the expected onslaught of peritoneal inflammation—that was to be feared as much as the operation itself and which was not easily factored into statistics. Different situations, outcomes and sick bodies made it hard to imagine a typical ovariotomy, and without a sense of what was typical, it was difficult to say which operations should be included in statistics and which should not. Ostensibly, an operation is intrinsically connected to the operator; the two are indivisible: the operation is a product of the surgeon's physical actions. And yet, as Thomas Schlich has shown in his study of twentieth-century surgery, surgeons have often been troubled by how statistics blur the boundaries between the two, especially when outcomes are poor.[115] Is a fatal outcome caused by the type of operation employed or by an operator's technique? If it is the former, does this exonerate an operator from responsibility? This issue had earlier been highlighted by a Dr. Murphy, who in defending Frederic Bird's practice of the operation at a society meeting published in the *Lancet*, intriguingly described failed ovariotomies as 'the fault of the operation, not the operator'.[116] The operation had to be disembodied and made separate from the inherent subjectivities of the surgeon as a means of ascertaining its essential 'truth'.

The ovariotomy debate became a less visible presence in the medical press for several years after Lee's confrontation with Bird; certainly, fewer cases were published. Nonetheless, occasional articles regarding its justifiability cropped up and ovariotomies were still performed with regularity by Charles Clay in Manchester. A new group of London-based practitioners also began to take up the operation in the late 1850s, most notably the obstetric physician William Tyler Smith and the surgeons Thomas Spencer Wells and Isaac Baker Brown, the latter of whom had spent years cautioning against the operation, continuing to use only palliative and medical therapeutics to treat dropsical ovaries.[117] By the end of the 1850s, however, he had had a change of heart.

Now convinced that medicine and minor procedures could not effect a permanent cure, he began to advocate using the operation and eventually started performing it himself.[118] Indeed more generally, there was a significant shift in the operation's standing by the last years of that decade. Many, like Brown, were not entirely confident in the operation but by now, sufficiently unconfident in the various alternatives to do anything to treat the condition. When in 1862 Lee once more publicly derided the lack of truthful representation of ovariotomy's risks, his remarks were met more coolly.[119] In 1865, a further turning point came with Thomas Spencer Wells' publication of his monograph *Diseases of the Ovaries: their Diagnosis and Treatment*, which, despite the title, was in fact Wells' record of cases rather than a textbook. In it, Wells provided a verbose, heavily illustrated, richly informative account that he said was of every single ovarian operation he had performed, successes and failures, and where he had carefully divided the operations into completed and uncompleted, and provided noticeably detailed information on the patient's state of health, months and sometimes years after the operation. Through his vivid descriptions of patients who for years had laboured under enormous tumours, some of which were accompanied by evocative images of the suffering woman, Wells made a convincing case for early intervention (see Fig. 3.1). He also claimed a success rate of seventy-six recoveries for the 114 operations he had performed, results which two years later would be improved upon further by the Edinburgh-based obstetrician Thomas Keith, who in 1867 announced that four-fifths of his ovariotomy patients so far had survived the operation.[120] Wells' monograph, as will be discussed more thoroughly in the next chapter, was quickly regarded as influential, not least because he carefully seeded the idea among his surgical brethren that he was the surgeon responsible for 'reviving' the fortunes of ovariotomy. Wells' success was less to do with his mortality rate—which at around one-third might still have been considered high by those who depicted ovariotomy as a procedure of choice rather than necessity—but rather the way Wells *represented* his work. Honest statistics recounting a high number of cases were of the utmost importance. But it was context too that was essential in representing operative surgery, and this could only be provided by full and frank case reports which expressed both the surgeon's narrative and the patient's.

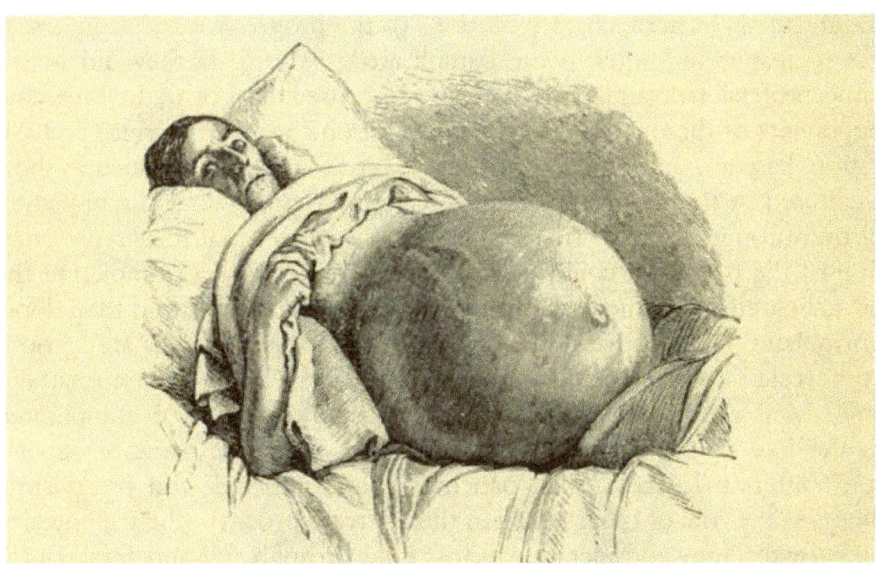

Fig. 3.1 Illustration from Thomas Spencer Wells' *Diseases of the Ovaries: their Diagnosis and Treatment* (1865) of his patient, 'C.B.', who he had first encountered in 1860. C.B. had suffered from an ovarian tumour for three years before seeking out Wells. The operation was put off for another eighteen months after C.B. was advised by another doctor to try palliative methods instead. When Wells eventually performed the operation, her abdomen was sixty inches in circumference. The patient died soon after. Wells used the case to warn of the risks of delaying ovariotomy (*Credit* Wellcome Collection/Francis A. Countway Library. CC BY)

Conclusion

During the middle decades of the nineteenth century, the justifiability of removing the ovaries or, as it was known by the 1840s, 'ovariotomy', was hotly debated in Britain by some of the most powerful surgeons in the country. Competing framings of the operation were formed, facilitated by the burgeoning medical press. On the one hand, it was depicted as a sign of advancement by a small but increasingly vocal group of advocates, on the other hand, opponents described it as a dangerous and possibly criminal procedure. Constructing an historical account of an ostensibly 'successful' innovation always runs the risk of characterising detractors along the way as conservative or even backwards looking. As I have sought to show here, characterisations of the progressive and, conversely, the regressive in surgery were complicated. Existing as they did in the same professional landscape, the language used by both advocates and opponents of the operation often mirrored one another; sacrifice and salvation, baseness and butchery: evocative terms and concepts such as these were used by the rival camps as they sought to convey an accurate picture of ovariotomy. For both sides, what was crucial was that their representation of the operation could be slotted into rather than contradicting the prevailing ethical framework of surgery. But this was easier said than done. Formulating a collective understanding of ovariotomy's risks and propriety revealed itself to be not only problematic but possibly even unattainable. Establishing the justifiability of the operation proved complicated in the face of the acknowledged messiness of lived experience—operators' differing levels of skill, patients' bodies afflicted with pre-existing illnesses, the role of other actors in the aftercare process—these all needed to be taken into consideration; thus, only through full and frank qualitative accounts of each operation could the 'real' experience of ovariotomy be represented. These accounts, punctured with emotional language and centred upon evocative narratives, allowed operators to express their reasoning for performing the operation, often by utilising the voice of the patient. This was mirrored in the similarly emotive accounts of opponents like Samuel Ashwell and Robert Lee.

This did not negate the desire, however, for clear numerical data. In the 1840s, statistics were increasingly utilised by medical men to help make sense of new and potentially hazardous innovations. They provided control and order, ostensibly permitting a definitive answer as to how risky a treatment or procedure was. The controversies surrounding operators like Frederic Bird made it more important than ever that honest, accurate numbers were provided by all who were performing new and experimental operations. While doctors' criticisms of statistics at this time are recognised by historians, particularly their concern that the individuality of cases would be stripped away, I have sought to show how surgeons negotiated these problems when faced with the urgent need to find an answer to the question of ovariotomy's justifiability. Moreover, I have argued that conceptualisations of the operation as novel and distinct also had an impact on the way its statistics were understood. Only by conveying experiences of ovariotomy through emotive, qualitative accounts *and* through statistical data, could the advantages and disadvantages of the operation be properly conveyed.

Throughout the century, the operation would continue to be painted in strikingly different ways: life-saving and life-destroying, progressive and regressive, savage and sophisticated. But it was in these middle decades that the modes used to represent the operation were most intensely scrutinised and deconstructed. The medical community was intent on settling a debate which had serious implications for the practice of surgery and where opponents often feared that the 'truth' of the operation was being obfuscated by secrecy and deception. Even as opinion began to swing in favour of the operation, the ferocity of this past opposition, when those who performed ovariotomy were castigated as 'belly-rippers', was not forgotten. Indeed, its impact would be felt for decades to come.

NOTES

1. John Lizars, *Observations on Extraction of Diseased Ovaria* (Edinburgh: Daniel Lizars, 1825), 11.
2. 'Observations on Extraction of Diseased Ovaria', *The Medico-Chirurgical Review* 3 (1825): 344.
3. 'Review: Observations on Extraction of Diseased Ovaria', *Lancet* 4, no. 103 (17 September 1825): 327.
4. James Blundell, 'On the Surgery of the Abdomen', *Lancet* 12 (27 June 1829): 355.
5. Augustus Granville, 'Case in Which an Attempt Was Made to Extirpate Ovarian Tumors', *London Medical and Physical Journal* 56, no. 330 (1826): 141–143; Alban Smith, 'Account of a Case in Which an Ovarium Was Successfully Extirpated', *North American Medical and Surgical Journal* 1 (1826): 30–38; Hopfer, 'On Extirpation of Diseased Ovaria' *London Medical Gazette* 3 (1829): 401–405.
6. Nathan Smith, 'Case of Ovarian Dropsy Successfully Removed by a Surgical Operation', *Edinburgh Medical and Surgical Journal* 18 (1822): 534.
7. Edward Seymour, *Illustrations of Some of the Principal Diseases of the Ovaria* (London: Longman, Rees, Orme, Brown and Green, 1830), 89–99; 'Review: "Illustrations of Some of the Principal Diseases of the Ovaria"', *Edinburgh Medical and Surgical Journal* 34 (1830): 139.
8. 'Review: "Illustrations of Some of the Principal Diseases of the Ovaria"', 137.
9. James Blundell, 'Lectures on the Diseases of Women and Children', *Lancet* 11, no. 290 (21 March 1829): 772.
10. William Jeaffreson, 'A Case of Ovarian Tumour Successfully Removed', *Transactions of the Provincial Medical and Surgical Association* 5 (1837): 242.

11. Robert King, 'New Operations for the Removal of Abdominal Tumours', *Lancet* 27, no. 699 (21 January 1837): 586–590; King had assisted Jeaffreson in his first operation. In 1839, Jeaffreson also reported to the *Lancet* another successful case by a practitioner in Harleston in the neighbouring county of Norfolk, named Benjamin Crisp. See William Jeaffreson, 'Ovarian Cysts', *Lancet* 33, no. 846 (16 November 1839): 287.

12. William West, 'Successful Operation for the Removal of an Ovarian Tumour', *Lancet* 29, no. 743 (25 November 1837): 307–308; John Gorham, 'Observations on the Propriety of Extirpating the Cyst in Some Cases of Ovarian Dropsy', *Lancet* 33, no. 843 (26 October 1839): 155–161.

13. John Gorham, 'Excision in Ovarian Dropsy', *Lancet* 33, no. 852 (28 December 1839): 507.

14. 'Physical Society, Guy's Hospital', *London Medical Gazette* 23 (24 November 1838): 313.

15. One of the most notorious episodes of Liston's rashness involved a small boy admitted under his care at University College Hospital who had a swelling in his neck over the carotid artery. Liston's House-Surgeon Mr. Bucknill had informed Liston that the tumour was pulsating, but Liston found it implausible that a boy so young could have an aneurysm. 'Putting his hand into his right waist-coat pocket, he took out a knife, and made a deep incision into the tumour. Out leaped the arterial blood, and the boy fell upon the floor. The wound was stitched up, and the patient put to bed, the artery being subsequently tied, but without any good result. On examination, it was found that an abscess had existed, and had ulcerated into the carotid'. J.F. Clarke, *Autobiographical Recollections of the Medical Profession* (London: J. & A. Churchill, 1874), 391.

16. For more on Liston's surgical style see Reginald Magee, 'Surgery in the Pre-anaesthetic Era: The Life and Work of Robert Liston', *Health and History* 2, no. 1 (2000): 121–133.

17. Robert Liston, *Practical Surgery* (London: John Churchill, 1837), v.

18. Robert Liston, *Elements of Surgery* (London: Longman, 1835), 54.

19. George E. Brickett, 'History of Ovariotomy in Maine', *Transactions of the Maine Medical Association* 6 (1877): 77.

20. Probably because of their libellous nature, cases where surgeons had been threatened with manslaughter charges were not openly discussed at the time. They are revealed mainly through later retrospective pieces about the history of ovariotomy. In 1895, the *British Gynaecological Journal* wrote of the Scottish obstetrician Thomas Keith in his obituary that 'it is still credibly believed that if Keith's second case had died he would have been accused of manslaughter by some of his woefully prejudiced critics'.

Although details are scant about what happened to Keith, other sources appear to corroborate the story that he narrowly escaped legal action for practising ovariotomy. In 1878, Keith himself, for example, described in an article for the *British Medical Journal* of 'being threatened by an interdict from the Court of Session'. 'Obituary: Thomas Keith', *British Gynaecological Journal* 11 (1895): 395; Thomas Keith, 'Results of Ovariotomy, Before and After Antiseptics' (1878): 590.

21. Robert King, Jeaffreson's colleague, who himself performed one (successful) extirpation, described ovarian disease as 'a morbid state which has almost invariably been left to exercise its ravages in freedom, the patient falling a sacrifice to it after a series of years of suffering, and of incapacity for useful or pleasurable exertion'. King thus evoked sacrifice too, albeit in a different context to opponents of the operation. King, 'New Operations', 586.

22. Peter Stanley, *For Fear of Pain: British Surgery, 1790–1850* (Amsterdam and New York: Rodopi, 2003), 28.

23. More recently Michael Brown has contested the idea that speed was integral to surgery in the early nineteenth century and in fact that 'many surgeons distrusted speed as a marker of skill and saw in it the spectre of self-promotion', Michael Brown, 'Redeeming Mr. Sawbone: Compassion and Care in the Cultures of Nineteenth-Century Surgery', *Journal of Compassionate Healthcare* 4, no. 13 (2017): 5.

24. Lawrence stated that it was 'the boast of modern surgery to have greatly diminished the number of operations'. William Lawrence, 'Lectures on Surgery, Medical and Operative. Lecture 1: Introduction', *Lancet* 13, no. 318 (3 October 1829): 38. See also Stephen Jacyna, *Philosophic Whigs: Medicine, Science and Citizenship in Edinburgh, 1789–1848* (London: Routledge, 1994), 115–124.

25. Adrian Desmond, *The Politics of Evolution: Morphology, Medicine and Reform in Radical London* (Chicago: University of Chicago Press, 1989), 101–110.

26. Ornella Moscucci, *The Science of Woman: Gynaecology and Gender in England 1800–1929* (Cambridge University Press, 1990), 141.

27. 'Extirpation of Ovarian Tumors', *London Medical and Physical Journal* 59 (1828): 175. The journal editor was Roderick MacLeod, a renowned conservative and rival of Thomas Wakley.

28. Keir Waddington, *Medical Education at St. Bartholomew's Hospital, 1123–1995* (Woodbridge: Boydell Press, 2003), 60.

29. Lawrence, 'Lectures on Surgery, Medical and Operative. Lecture 1', 36.

30. William Lawrence, 'Lectures on Surgery, Medical and Operative. Lecture 2: On the Nature and Seat of Diseases', *Lancet* 13, no. 319 (10 October 1829): 65.

31. William Lawrence, 'Lectures on Surgery: Lecture LXXV', *London Medical Gazette* 6 (21 August 1830): 822–828, 827.

32. Robert Liston, 'Practical Surgery: A Course of Lectures on the Operations of Surgery and Diseases and Accidents Requiring Operations', *Lancet* 45, no. 1119 (8 February 1845): 147. The couplet was taken from part two of Butler's English Civil War parody *Hudibras* (1664).

33. Helen Macdonald, *Possessing the Dead: The Artful Science of Anatomy* (Carlton: Melbourne University Press, 2010), 15.

34. For a detailed history of the body-snatching scandals and their societal impact, see Ruth Richardson, *Death, Dissection and the Destitute: The Politics of the Corpse in Pre-Victorian Britain* (London: Routledge, 1987).

35. King, 'New Operations', 587.

36. This characterisation of surgeons was most famously embodied in Charles Dickens' depiction of the bloodthirsty surgical students Bob Sawyer and Benjamin Allen in his 1837 novel *The Pickwick Papers*, in which the two young men enthusiastically relate to Mr. Pickwick the bloody operations they are witness to. Charles Dickens, *The Pickwick Papers* (London: Penguin, 1994), 483.

37. 'Extirpation of Ovarian Tumors', 175.

38. Charles Clay, *The Results of All Operations for the Extirpation of Diseased Ovaria* (Manchester: W.M. Irwin, 1848), 56.

39. Charles Clay, 'Ovariotomy', *Medical Times* 9, no. 211 (7 October 1843): 4–5.

40. 'Extirpation of Ovaria', *Lancet* 43, no. 1074 (30 March 1844): 45–47.

41. Mary Fissell, 'The Disappearance of the Patient's Narrative and the Invention of Hospital Medicine', in *British Medicine in an Age of Reform*, ed. Roger French and Andrew Wear (Abingdon: Routledge, 1991): 93.

42. Brian Hurwitz, 'Form and Representation in Clinical Reports', *Literature and Medicine* 25, no. 2 (2006): 229.

43. Meegan Kennedy, *Revising the Clinic: Vision and Representation in Victorian Medical Narrative and the Novel* (Columbus: Ohio State University Press, 2010), 23. It also speaks to work by Sarah Chaney on the history of madness. Chaney argues that, contrary to the general picture of Victorian approaches to madness as authoritarian, late nineteenth-century alienists put high value upon individual case histories and patient experience. See Sarah Chaney, '"A Hideous Torture on Himself": Madness and Self-Mutilation in Victorian Literature', *Journal of Medical Humanities* 32, no. 4 (2011): 281.

44. Claire Brock, 'Risk, Responsibility and Surgery in the 1890s and Early 1900s', *Medical History* 57, no. 3 (2013): 319–326.

45. Regina Morantz-Sanchez, *Conduct Unbecoming of a Woman: Medicine on Trial in Turn-of-the-Century Brooklyn* (Oxford: Oxford University Press, 1999), 106–107.

46. Regina Morantz-Sanchez, 'Negotiating Power at the Bedside: Historical Perspectives on Nineteenth-Century Patients and Their Gynecologists', *Feminist Studies* 26, no. 2 (2000): 287–309.

47. Stanley, *For Fear of Pain*, 198–199.

48. Benjamin Phillips, 'Extraction of an Ovarian Cyst', *London Medical Gazette* 27 (9 October 1840): 83.

49. Phillips, 'Extraction of an Ovarian Cyst', 83.

50. Phillips, 'Extraction of an Ovarian Cyst', 84.

51. Phillips, 'Extraction of an Ovarian Cyst', 85.

52. Phillips, 'Extraction of an Ovarian Cyst', 86.

53. Phillips, 'Extraction of an Ovarian Cyst', 87.

54. Charles Clay, 'Cases of Peritoneal Section', *Medical Times* 7 (26 November 1842): 141.

55. Clay, 'Cases of Peritoneal Section' (26 November 1842): 141.

56. Charles Clay, 'Cases of Peritoneal Section', *Medical Times* 7 (15 October 1842): 44.

57. Clay, 'Cases of Peritoneal Section' (26 November 1842): 140.

58. Phillips, 'Extraction of an Ovarian Cyst', 84.

59. Daniel H. Walne, *Cases of Dropsical Ovaria Removed by the Large Abdominal Section* (London: Longman, Brown, Green, and Longmans, 1843), 42. The pamphlet brought together three cases Walne had published in the *London Medical Gazette* between 1842 and 1843.

60. Joyce L. Huff has argued that within mid-nineteenth-century culture fatness potentially represented a destabilising 'otherness' to the ordered body, defying an exacting Victorian aesthetic which 'was a matter not so much of maintaining a thin body as of maintaining a "properly" shaped body'. Joyce L. Huff, 'A "Horror of Corpulence": Interrogating Bantingism and Mid-Nineteenth-Century Fat-Phobia', in *Bodies out of Bounds: Fatness and Transgression*, ed. Jana Evans Braziel and Kathleen LeBesco (Berkeley: University of California Press, 2001), 44.

61. Walne, *Cases of Dropsical Ovaria*, 8.

62. Numerous cases recorded women's anxieties over their inability to work due to their condition. See King, 'New Operations', 589; Walne, *Cases of Dropsical Ovaria*, 42. Marjorie Levine-Clarke has emphasised (albeit in a broader context than surgery) that within lower socio-economic classes, women conceptualised their own health and negotiated their health care in the context of their employability.

Marjorie Levine-Clarke, *Beyond the Reproductive Body: The Politics of Women's Health in Early Victorian England* (Columbus: Ohio State University Press, 2004), 1–11.

63. Samuel Ashwell, 'Extirpation in Ovarian Dropsy', *The Boston and Medical and Surgical Journal* 45 (4 June 1845): 357.
64. Ashwell, 'Extirpation in Ovarian Dropsy', 358.
65. Frederic Bird, 'Diagnosis, Pathology and Treatment of Ovarian Tumours', *Medical Times* 24, no. 57 (2 August 1851): 123.
66. Bird, 'Diagnosis, Pathology and Treatment', 123.
67. Bird, 'Diagnosis, Pathology and Treatment', 123.
68. Flurin Condrau, 'The Patient's View Meets the Clinical Gaze', *Social History of Medicine* 20, no. 3 (2007): 529.
69. Brown, 'Redeeming Mr. Sawbone', 3.
70. Stanley, *For Fear of Pain*, 233.
71. Brown, 'Redeeming Mr. Sawbone', 5.
72. James Young Simpson, 'Lecture Notes or Model Answers for Exams in Obstetrics and Gynaecology with a Section Discussing Ovariotomy', (c. 1848–1850) JYS/326 (Royal College of Surgeons of Edinburgh).
73. 'Ovarian Dropsy', *Medical Times* 10 (1 April 1844): 11.
74. 'Results of the Operation for the Extirpation of Diseased Ovaria: Review', *London Medical Gazette* 44 (23 November 1849): 899.
75. 'Extirpation of Ovarian Tumors', *The Medico-Chirurgical Review* 40 (1 April 1844): 557.
76. The example of surgery for squinting was not an indiscriminate choice on the part of *The Medico-Chirurgical Review*. In the early 1840s, a new operation for curing squinting by sectioning the media rectus muscle had been developed by Berlin surgeon Johann Dieffenbach and the operation had very rapidly spread across Europe.
77. Fleetwood Churchill, 'Ovariotomy', *The Medico-Chirurgical Review* 42 (1 October 1844): 528.
78. Churchill, 'Ovariotomy', 528.
79. Statistics played an integral part in eighteenth-century medicine. Tröhler cites the use of statistics, for example, to measure mortality in lithotomy and amputations. Ulrich Tröhler, *Quantification in British Medicine and Surgery 1750–1830, With Special Reference to its Introduction into Therapeutics* (PhD thesis, University College London, 1978); Ulrich Tröhler, 'Quantifying Experience and Beating Biases: A New Culture in Eighteenth-Century British Clinical Medicine', in *Body Counts: Medical Quantification in Historical and Sociological Perspective*, ed. Gérard Jorland, Annick Opinel, and George Weisz (Montreal: McGill-Queens University Press, 2005), 19–50.

80. Ian Hacking, *The Taming of Chance* (Cambridge: Cambridge University Press, 1990), 2.
81. For a useful overview on both the history and historiography of medical statistics, see Gérard Jorland and George Weisz, 'Introduction: Who Counts?', in *Body Counts: Medical Quantification in Historical and Sociological Perspectives*, ed. Gérard Jorland, Annick Opinel, and George Weisz (Montreal: McGill-Queens University Press, 2005), 3–15.
82. Thomas Schlich and Ulrich Tröhler, 'Risk and Medical Innovation: A Historical Perspective', in *The Risks of Medical Innovation*, ed. Thomas Schlich and Ulrich Tröhler (Abingdon: Routledge, 2006), 5–7.
83. For a background to this argument, see Patricia Jasen, 'Breast Cancer and the Language of Risk, 1750–1950', *Social History of Medicine* 15, no. 1 (2002): 17–43.
84. The Google Ngram Viewer (http://books.google.com/ngrams) allows one to track the use of a particular word in the 5.2 million books digitised by Google. The Ngram for 'risk' shows infrequent but growing use of the word in the nineteenth century. But a quick search of the *Lancet* during the early nineteenth century brings up a plethora of articles where operative 'risk' is described by influential surgeons. See, for example, William Lawrence, 'A Lecture Introductory to a Course of Surgery', *Lancet* 11, no. 285 (14 February 1829): 617. Lawrence warned his students: 'in any operation you have to perform, unless the knife is guided by anatomical knowledge, consider the risk of the patient, and that of yourself, as the operator', 617.
85. Jasen, 'Breast Cancer', 18.
86. Martin Pernick, *The Calculus of Suffering: Pain, Professionalism, and Anesthesia in Nineteenth Century America* (New York: Columbia University Press, 1985), 213.
87. Pernick characterises the operation in the 1840s as one where the ovaries were being removed to rectify nervous illnesses, which, as will be explored in the following two chapters, was a development that in fact came much later. Pernick, *The Calculus of Suffering*, 213.
88. Most practitioners performing ovariotomy described using chloroform in their cases soon after it was introduced. Charles Clay also wrote in private to James Young Simpson to declare himself 'converted' to chloroform. However, by 1863 Clay had begun to cast doubt on the helpfulness of chloroform in abdominal surgery, stating that if an ovariotomy patient could face the operation without it, then it would be in her favour not to have it. Letter to James Young Simpson from Charles Clay (n.d.) JYS/200 (Royal College of Surgeons of Edinburgh); 'Obstetrical Society of London', *Medical Times and Gazette* 1 (4 March 1863): 407–408.

89. Ian Burney, 'Anaesthetic and the Evaluation of Surgical Risk in Mid-Nineteenth-Century Britain', in *The Risks of Medical Innovation*, ed. Thomas Schlich and Ulrich Tröhler (Abingdon: Routledge, 2006), 38.

90. These concerns were evidently well known beyond the medical community. In 1847, the satirical magazine *Punch* published a poem entitled 'The Blessings of Chloroform' with the couplet 'Chloroform will render quite agreeable the parting with/any useless member that a patient has been smarting with'. Fears about chloroform's power to extend the realm of surgery meant that surgeons' performance of new and risky operations was more closely scrutinised than ever before. 'The Blessings of Chloroform', *Punch* 13 (18 December 1847): 232.

91. Burney, 'Anaesthetic and the Evaluation of Surgical Risk', 40.

92. Charles Clay, *Cases of Peritoneal Section* (London: Munro and Congreve, 1842). The pamphlet brought together the five cases he had published in the *Medical Times*.

93. Clay, 'Cases of Peritoneal Section', 18.

94. 'Review: "Cases of Peritoneal Section"', *British and Foreign Medical Review* 16 (1843): 394.

95. Benjamin Phillips, 'Observations on the Recorded Cases of Operations for the Extraction of Ovarian Tumours' *Medico-Chirurgical Transactions* 27 (1844): 468–492; Churchill, 'Ovariotomy', 528–531.

96. Benjamin Phillips, 'Observations on the Recorded Cases of Operations for the Extraction of Ovarian Tumours', *Medico-Chirurgical Transactions* 27 (1844): 469.

97. Phillips, 'Observations on the Recorded Cases', 475.

98. Churchill, 'Ovariotomy', 530.

99. Broadly speaking, 'capital' operations usually referred to lithotomy and lithotrity, major amputations such as at the shoulder or the thigh, operations for strangulated hernias and the ligaturing of major arteries—any operation where there was believed to be a relatively high risk of death. However, what exactly constituted a 'high' risk was never well defined.

100. This was the subject of a lecture on ovariotomy by St. Thomas' Hospital surgeon Samuel Solly in 1846. Solly, an advocate of the operation, collated numerous statistics to suggest that the mortality rate for ovariotomy was about four in ten. He compared this to the numbers for other capital operations such as amputation of the thigh, where there was a mortality rate of about three and a half out of ten, amputation of the arm (four out of ten), and Sir Astley Cooper's hernia operations, where nearly five in every ten patients had died. Samuel Solly, 'Clinical Lecture on Ovariotomy', *London Medical Gazette* 38 (3 July 1846): 54.

101. Clay, 'Cases of Peritoneal Section', 16.

102. James Young Simpson often used this argument. It formed part of a long discussion about the operation which he participated in at the Medico-Chirurgical Society of Edinburgh on 17 December 1845: 'Medico-Chirurgical Society of Edinburgh', *The Monthly Journal of Medical Science* 6, no. 4 (1846): 56–59.

103. James Matthews Duncan, 'Is Ovariotomy Justifiable?', *Lancet* 69, no. 1748 (28 February 1857): 212–214. Duncan described ovariotomy as having a 'distinct, individual character' and thus was incomparable to other operations, 213.

104. See for instance 'Biographical Sketch of Robert Lee; M.D., F.R.S.', *Lancet* 57, no. 1438 (22 March 1851): 332–337. Biographical sketches of this magnitude appeared only occasionally in the *Lancet* during the 1850s, attesting to the authority Lee wielded in the London medical world.

105. 'Royal Medical and Chirurgical Society', *Lancet* 57, no. 1432 (8 February 1851): 155.

106. Fleetwood Churchill, *Researches on Operative Midwifery* (Dublin: Martin Kenne and Son, 1841), 222.

107. Churchill estimated that about half of babies were lost when symphyseotomy was performed, compared to over two thirds when caesarean section was undertaken. He used both statistics and contextual information to claim that although more mothers survived symphyseotomy than caesarean section, many were badly injured by the former procedure, leading Churchill to declare that their risks were roughly the same. Churchill, *Researches on Operative Midwifery*, 254.

108. 'Review: "A Practical Treatise on Midwifery" by M. Chailly', *The Medico-Chirurgical Review* 41 (1 October 1844): 407.

109. 'Royal Medical and Chirurgical Society, November 13th 1850', *Lancet* 56, no. 1421 (23 November 1850): 584.

110. 'Royal Medical and Chirurgical Society', 584.

111. 'Royal Medical and Chirurgical Society', 585–586.

112. Diary of Robert Lee, Vol. 6 (1838–1872), MS3218 (Wellcome Collection).

113. 'Obituary: Frederic Bird', *Medical Times and Gazette* 1 (9 May 1874): 520.

114. Richard G. Butcher, 'On Ovariotomy, and the After-Treatment of the Patient', *Dublin Quarterly Journal of Medical Science* 40, no. 2 (1865): 283.

115. Thomas Schlich, *Surgery, Science and Industry: A Revolution in Fracture Care, 1950s–1990s* (Basingstoke: Palgrave Macmillan, 2002), 122–123.

116. 'Westminster Medical Society', *Lancet* 50, no. 1261 (30 October 1847): 467. Four years before, the surgeon John Halton similarly highlighted the distinction between surgeon and operation, suggesting that statistics

for capital operations should eschew altogether those failed cases where the performance of the operator rather than the operation itself was deemed at fault. John Halton 'On the Average Number of Deaths in Capital Operations', *London Medical Gazette* 33 (29 December 1843): 390–400.

117. Brown had also advocated a method that involved wrapping the abdomen in tight bandages so as to put pressure upon the abdomen and thus reduce swelling. Isaac Baker Brown, 'Practical Remarks on the Cure of Ovarian Dropsy Without Abdominal Section', *Lancet* 43, no. 1083 (1 June 1844): 306–307.

118. Isaac Baker Brown, *On Some Diseases of Women Admitting of Surgical Treatment* (London: John Churchill, 1854). In this publication, Brown detailed all his cases of ovariotomy so far.

119. 'Royal Medical and Chirurgical Society, Tuesday November 11th, 1862', *Lancet* 80, no. 2047 (22 November 1862): 565–569.

120. Thomas Spencer Wells, *Diseases of the Ovaries: their Diagnosis and Treatment*, vol. 1 (London: John Churchill, 1865), xiii; Thomas Keith, 'Fifty-One Cases of Ovariotomy', Lancet 90, no. 2297 (7 September 1867): 290–291.

4

Patent Concerns, Unpatentable Procedures

SITUATING SURGICAL CREDIT

In the introduction to his book *Surgical Diseases of the Ovaries and Fallopian Tubes*, published in 1891, John Bland-Sutton, gynaecological surgeon at the Chelsea Hospital for Women, commented on the publications that abounded in his specialist field: 'the literature relating to surgical diseases of the ovaries displays a notorious amount of egoism', he began, '…nearly every treatise devoted to this subject is mainly a record of personal experience'.[1] Ovariotomy, over the previous fifty years, had been one of the most enduring topics of discussion among the medical profession. The ethical issues surrounding it had meant there had long been a highly personal dimension to the debate, as practitioners risked their reputations in performing the operation. But by the 1860s, individual rivalries and disputes were in danger of becoming the defining feature of its practice.

A direct accusation of egoism, such as Bland-Sutton's, was a damning one to be cast at any sector of the medical profession. The drive for reform by practitioners in the middle decades of the nineteenth century had led to the passing of the Medical Act in 1858. Yet, for many, the Act was a disappointment, doing little to actively prevent or regulate the practice of 'quacks', and the lack of desired reform led to a heightened insecurity among doctors over their profession's status.[2] For those practitioners ostensibly operating within the parameters of orthodoxy,

immersing oneself in rhetoric that stressed altruism and the selfless acqui-
sition of knowledge was a fundamental tool in accentuating differences
between professional doctors and 'quacks'. These ideals provided a basis
upon which the morals and practices of 'orthodox' rivals could be questioned too. Any hint that practitioners might be excessively interested
in personal success was subject to intense scrutiny. Doctors inhabited a
precarious professional world where accusations of quackery and self-
interest could quickly be rolled out.

Over the mid-part of the century, those who performed ovariotomy gained an unfortunate reputation for this kind of controversy. 'Specialists' of all kinds had begun to attract negative attention
in the 1860s, as will be discussed in more detail in the next chapter,
and those identifying as specialists in gynaecological diseases were
often singled out for their predilection for bickering. An article in
The Boston Medical and Surgical Journal in 1881, reporting the news
from the London medical world, commented on a meeting of the
Royal Medical and Chirurgical Society in which the surgeon for the
Samaritan Hospital for Women, John Knowsley Thornton, had argued
for the use of antiseptic methods in gynaecological surgery: 'the subject, as usual, afforded the ladies' doctors a grand opportunity for controversy', the anonymous author commented, 'of which, as is their
wont, full advantage was taken, and in a manner too, which happily
is not usual here amongst the practitioners in other special departments'.[3] Within the speciality of the diseases of women, the unique
distinction that performers of ovariotomy were accorded, as practitioners willing to go into the abdomen, meant that they formed their own
professional subset and acquired their own peculiar reputation for controversy. Much of this was increasingly focused on one very particular
and contentious issue: the distribution of credit—that is recognition
of certain individuals' work—among those who believed themselves
responsible for the operation's innovation. That issue is the focus of
this chapter.

Historians and sociologists have long been interested in the role of
credit and priority in scientific practice. Robert K. Merton in his influential *The Sociology of Science* (1973) saw awarding credit as central to the
construction of norms within professional, scientific culture. For Merton,
it was only through credit that originality—that most prized aspect of
science—could be validated; thus, 'recognition for originality becomes
socially validated testimony that one has successfully lived up to the most

exacting requirements of one's role as a scientist'.[4] In recent years, historians of science and technology have shown revitalised interest in the subject, reflecting the growing and high-profile presence of intellectual property in the techno-sciences today.[5] With this has come a nuancing of ideas about what 'intellectual property' might have meant historically.[6] Historians of techno-science Christine MacLeod and Gregory Radick have argued that intellectual property can be understood in a narrow sense—for example as it is embodied in legal processes such as patenting—but also broadly, as it is has been expressed in priority and, perhaps more interestingly, 'productivity claims, made when a body of theoretical principles is asserted to underpin useful technologies'.[7] Such work shows historians are finding more fruitful ways of analysing claims of what credit—as we might define the concept, 'intellectual property' being rather presentist—has meant at different times and of which patenting is only one aspect.

In comparison with the history of science, the history of medicine has some way to go in examining the historical antecedents to intellectual property, although recent work suggests interest in the subject is increasing.[8] Medical practice, understood in the clinical sense, requires disentangling from the broader scope of science. The relative lack of overt engagement that 'orthodox' practitioners had with patenting in the nineteenth century has meant historians have, arguably, glossed over surgeons' anxieties about attaining credit. Histories of patenting and patent medicine, as we shall see, offer a useful contextual framework to the contemporary mores around credit and priority. But they alone do little to elucidate claims to credit in a field like operative surgery, where patenting did not occur. As medical sociologists Judith P. Swazey and Renée C. Fox have shown, however, a multiplicity of different types of credit potentially hover around surgical practice.[9] What is more, the nature of operative surgery, premised upon methods of physical intervention, has also impacted on how priority and credit have been constituted and rewarded in the field, differentiating it from other areas of medicine.

In this chapter, I consider an overlooked part of ovariotomy's history; that is, how claims to credit were constructed around what was perceived to be new surgical knowledge and practice. I purposely employ the term 'credit' to consider them. This is not only because that was the term frequently used during discussions of priority at the time, but because it also conveys the complex, somewhat obscure, relationship between honour, attribution and financial profit underpinning it. Ovariotomy was increasingly symbolic of a bold and novel way of operating. But how was this new knowledge to be owned and credited, if indeed it could be? How was it rewarded or otherwise acknowledged and why was it important that it was? How, if at all, was operative surgery to be understood as the product of intellectual labours? These issues preoccupied surgeons. Significantly, they played out in the wider context of contemporaneous debates on invention, commerce and trade. Unlike technological innovations, such as those occurring in engineering, operations were, for practical and ethical reasons, not deemed patentable. But surgeons lived in a society which increasingly sought to formalise the protection of inventors' ideas in other areas of industry; surgeons were not impervious to this development and it influenced their own internal debates. Credit claims loomed large within the medical press, which not only facilitated numerous priority disputes between medical men but often played an active role as unofficial arbitrator to them. Examining these debates expands not only our understanding of 'intellectual property' as it has been conceptualised in the medical realm, but also the nature of surgeons' professional culture. Issues of priority, patenting and credit were critical to surgeons' self-identity, at a time when their status was in ascendance.

'ATTEMPTING TO BIND THE WINDS': THE UNPATENTABILITY OF SURGERY

In the middle decades of the nineteenth century, there was increasing recognition in Britain and beyond of the contributions made to society by inventors. It resulted in growing calls for them to be better protected, legally and financially.[10] Works like *Self-Help* (1859), the journalist Samuel Smiles' hugely popular paean to self-improvement and endeavour, championed bold pioneers who had innovated in the face of adversity, including those in medicine such as Edward Jenner.[11] These changes were the manifestation of a growing cult of heroism around invention, much of which centred upon individuals from manufacturing and engineering, people like Isambard Kingdom Brunel, George Stephenson and James Watt, and the highly visible and influential products of their intellectual labours, which had so greatly transformed society. The inventor was no longer the shady eccentric or dishonest swindler but the heroic Briton, contributing to the nation's industrial might.[12]

This changing conception of inventors was most visibly embodied in public support for patenting reform; *The Times*, an early supporter of the cause, readily invoked the glories of inventors past to argue in 1850 that:

The *rights of inventors* can scarcely be spoken of as having a definite existence. It is strange that a Watt, a Hargreave, an Arkwright, should be left to present a humble petition to the crown, imploring that he may for a period of short duration be guaranteed a beneficial interest in his own discovery.[13]

With the Great Exhibition of 1851, an unprecedented platform for new industrial products and processes emerged, enabling for the first time Britons from across the social spectrum to view *en masse* the fruits of industry from all over the world. But with this platform came concerns over the ease with which inventions on display could be pirated. A hasty intermediate legal measure—the Protection of Inventions Act—gave protection to all unpatented British inventions at the exhibition.[14] More importantly, it reinvigorated and strengthened a lengthy campaign by manufacturers, inventors and other interested parties for wide-scale reform to patent law, principally to increase the short tenure of a year that patents then held and to also reduce the initial price of patents. The Patent Amendment Act, which fulfilled both these criteria, was passed in 1852.[15]

Medical practitioners were for the most part absent from these debates. When patenting was discussed within the pages of the medical journals, it was often with suspicion. For most members of the profession, there was discordance between medicine and the notion of property rights, an inherent contradiction in permitting excessive individual reward within the rhetorical framework of altruism which increasingly bound orthodox medical culture together. As Scottish physician William Gairdner put it in 1868, in a way which neatly summarised the viewpoint of the profession:

A principle now firmly established in the medical profession…that the status of its members is considered lowered by any attempt to establish property in any remedy, or other invention for the relief of disease; whether by concealment, or by patenting, or otherwise advertising the invention for the benefit of its presumed owner.[16]

In the medical world, the term 'patent' had unseemly connotations that did not reflect the changing place of patents and patentees in other fields of industry. Despite the common parlance used, most 'patent medicines' were trademarked rather than patented because the application for a trademark did not require any disclosure of the components of a medicine. Outwardly, patent medicines were treated with disdain by a profession trying hard to rid itself of old associations with useless nostrums and secret remedies. Patent medicines contravened an expectation of openness in practice, and their potential dangers were repeatedly highlighted in the medical press. A Parliamentary Bill in 1884—the Patent Medicines Bill—proposed that all purveyors of patented and trademarked medicines be forced to reveal the ingredients of their remedies, but the Bill was ultimately unsuccessful.[17] The profession's outward disdain for patent medicines belied a murkier reality; as Lori Loeb has illustrated in her exploration of patent medicines in late nineteenth and early twentieth-century Britain, in private practice, a sizeable number of practitioners prescribed patent medicines or were involved with patent medicine companies as shareholders.[18]

In surgery, the ethical dubiousness of patenting appeared to be writ large. The idea of asserting one's property over an operation was considered untenable from a moral standpoint and unworkable from a practical one. This had been clarified in the 1840s when two American practitioners, Charles T. Jackson and William T.G. Morton, attempted to patent the use of sulphuric ether following their demonstration of the substance's anaesthetic qualities in dental and surgical procedures.[19] The rapid and widespread uptake of ether among surgeons in 1846 and 1847 in light of the discovery of its astonishing pain-relieving qualities spelled a lucrative opportunity for Jackson and Morton if their claim to property could be enforced. Morton quickly enlisted a patent agent, James A. Dorr, to represent his interests in Britain. Dorr duly wrote to the *Lancet* and *Medical Times* to announce that the use of ether inhalation in England and the Colonies was now patented, and that those practitioners who used it would be liable to charges of infringement if they administered it without permission.[20] Dorr's efforts were resoundingly rebuffed by the profession. Although Morton had initially claimed the compound he used was not ether, but an original composition called 'Letheon', it was widely known that they were one and the same. Thus, the claim to novelty which the patent hinged upon was the use of ether as a *method* of procuring insensibility in surgical operations rather than the substance itself. To do so, the *Medical Times* commented, was like 'attempting to bind the winds, not less absurd but improper'.[21] The idea that practitioners would be forced to compensate Morton and Jackson financially each time they provided pain relief in an operation was considered indecent and verging on the ludicrous. It jeopardised the ability of surgeons to take on charitable and emergency cases and anyhow, would be almost impossible to enforce, given that it was widely known that the substance was ether, which was readily available. What is more, operations were performed so prolifically, and often privately, it would be impractical to try and track and manage the use of the substance. There was a slipperiness, an intangibility, in establishing ownership in a procedure. Morton tried several times in both America and Britain to enforce his patent but his attempts always failed. The patent was eventually voided.[22]

The intractability of patenting in medicine and especially surgery did not prevent intermittent criticism arising about the lack of reward for the intellectual labours of medical practitioners. Morton's patent agent James A. Dorr himself used his correspondence with the medical press to implore the profession to reconsider their disavowal of patenting, or at the very least, to look at an alternative system which made pecuniary rewards available to doctors. To Dorr's mind, the rank and honour accorded to innovative medical practitioners was hardly a replacement for financial compensation. 'What is honour without the means of subsistence?' Dorr asked.[23] Twenty-five years later, the physician and journalist Andrew Wynter put forth a similar question in an essay in the influential Whig periodical *The Edinburgh Review*. Using the successes of anaesthesia and ovariotomy as key examples, Wynter made the case for pecuniary rewards for medical and surgical innovators, arguing that 'some tangible evidence should be given that the nation appreciates the sacrifices daily and hourly made by those who devote their energies and their talents to the promotion of its physical well-being'.[24] Medical and surgical innovations were, in spirit, the same as any other type of scientific or technological innovation, and yet, when it came to awarding credit, they were treated differently. Surgery most obviously highlighted this disparity; more than other branches of medicine, it aligned with industries like engineering through its manual, practical nature, traversing divisions between medicine and technology. Wynter gloomily compared the situation in Britain to other countries in Europe where 'honours and rewards from the nation await the men who are useful to the country'.[25] In Britain, medical men were hardly ever officially recognised for their work, Edward Jenner being a rare exception.[26] In France, on the other hand, there was a long tradition of promoting and rewarding contributions to medicine and surgery with prizes, often in pecuniary form, and by the nineteenth century, both the French Academy of

Science and French Academy of Medicine offered such rewards.[27] In 1863, Eugène Koeberlé, at that point one of very few surgeons who performed ovariotomy in France—the operation was still far from established there—was awarded 2000 francs and the prestigious Prix Barbier by the French Academy of Medicine for having performed two successful ovariotomies.[28] The prize specifically rewarded the invention of instruments, surgical sundries such as new types of bandaging, and operative techniques.[29]

While patents and formal financial rewards were eschewed by the British medical establishment, invention continued to be championed ever more in the medical press. The *Lancet's* introduction in 1850 of its monthly column 'New Inventions in Aid of the Practice of Medicine and Surgery', for example, responded to doctors' clear interest in new instruments, accessories and devices being fashioned, and gave publicity to the wide range of medical and surgical aides such as siphons, trusses and respirators that were being invented by both doctors and laypeople. The medical press quickly became the main arena through which doctors attempted to claim credit and negotiate priority disputes. In 1837 the *Lancet* ran an editorial that criticised doctors' excessive interest in credit and priority and their use of journals to assert their property in discoveries and inventions. The journal complained that:

> The extent to which this evil has grown can only be fully appreciated by the conductors of the periodical press, or by those who follow with attention the debates of our medical and philosophical societies. Editors' tables are continually laden with letters from gentlemen, who would enforce their claim to 'priority' in some discovery.[30]

By the mid-nineteenth century, medical journals set out significant space for correspondence columns in their pages. The weekly frequency of the *Lancet, British Medical Journal, Medical Times* and others allowed for speedy claims to credit by doctors; in effect, medical journals became fertile ground for controversies of a personal nature. Despite the *Lancet's* protestations, the inconsistency in the profession's attitude towards priority claims can be detected. While, ostensibly, the journal proclaimed a disapproval for such disputes, it did not preclude it and other similar titles from publishing and, at times, seemingly encouraging them. Editors and publishers could not have been unaware of the tawdry appeal that personal disputations among doctors would have had among its readership. Nor were possible associations with unsavoury self-interest enough to stop practitioners airing their grievances publicly. In the absence of other channels, weekly medical journals, with their reach across both the social spectrum and geographical spread of the professional community, were the most effective tools for initiating claims. As self-declared upholders of professional ethics, journal editors and writers had a degree of authority to act as arbiters in disagreements over priority and credit.

Parallel cultures of ownership in surgery were being constructed. Claims to surgical innovation functioned through periodical correspondence, but also through other interwoven strategies of publishing and eponymy. In the next two sections, I look at two highly public disputes regarding ovariotomy, which, in different ways, attest to the methods surgeons used to attain recognition for their innovations and the difficulties they encountered.

CLAY'S ADHESION CLAM AND THE PEDICLE DISPUTE

Ovariotomy formed part of a changing landscape of knowledge management in the middle decades of the nineteenth century. As we have seen, between the 1830s and early 1860s, while controversy over ovariotomy's justifiability raged, there were still only a relatively small number of surgeons performing it, or at least admitting to performing it. As a consequence, discussion centred upon the lengthy narratives of those few men such as Frederic Bird, Charles Clay and Benjamin Phillips who spoke out publicly about their experiences with the operation; the intensely personal accounts that John Bland-Sutton would go on to admonish in the 1890s had in fact been actively encouraged earlier in the century, when claiming personal attachment to an operation had less to do with asserting a priority claim and more to do with acknowledging one's accountability when performing risky surgery. Indeed during this time, such was the polarisation of views about ovariotomy that a surgeon was just as likely to seek credit for 'disowning' the operation as he was to 'owning' it—this was evidently a concern for Robert Liston, who in a letter to the surgeon James Miller in 1835, written shortly after his move to London, expressed hopes that it would not be taken 'amiss that I have disclaimed abdominal surgery. I was first to do so'.[31]

Such was the gravity of the operation that personal responsibility was already deeply embedded in every performance of ovariotomy. But it

was only as mortality rates diminished that surgeons began to more con-
certedly use their personal experiences of the operation to make public
claims about innovations they had originated. It is no coincidence that
these began to occur in earnest in the 1860s, at the very time in which
the standing of the operation within medical circles improved considerably, making association with it by means of priority and credit desirable
rather than risky. At first, these materialised as outwardly minor, highly
technical claims, although the seriousness with which they were taken
was testament to the growing status of the operation. They also revealed
the relative ease with which ovariotomy, ostensibly a single invention,
could be deconstructed into the multiple innovations that constituted it:
the surgical instruments used, the method of aftercare, the type of incision and so forth: all had the potential to be claimed as innovative in
their own right.

One part of the operation around which multiple credit claims
emerged was the method of dividing the diseased ovary from its pedicle
and the subsequent treatment of the pedicle afterwards. This was a topic
of great interest in the 1860s as practitioners experimented with various
ways of making the division, including ligatures, clamps and cauterisa-
tion. In 1862, the professional community had had its attention drawn
to a new instrument that was being used for pedicle division by practitioners in the Midlands. The instrument, known as an 'adhesion clam',
had been devised by the Birmingham obstetrician John Clay (who was
no relation to Charles Clay).[32] John Clay had attracted attention two
years previously having translated an extensive work by Austrian obstetrician Franz Kiwisch von Rotterau on diseases of the ovaries.[33] His 'clam'
consisted of two blades which carefully secured the tissue for dividing, at
the same time forming a small groove through which either a hot or cold
cauterising iron could pass, rubbing or burning any remaining adhesions.
Clay had originally invented the instrument for complicated cases where
the ovarian tumour had formed attachments to other internal organs.[34]
However, as in principle all ovariotomies required a similar process of
tissue division, Clay envisioned that the instrument could be used more
generally in the practice of ovariotomy.[35]

John Clay's claim to innovation initially seemed secure, and he
made the details and design of the instrument accessible by publishing
both of them in the *Medical Times* in 1862. Clay and other surgeons
referred to the instrument as 'Clay's adhesion clam', marking out Clay
as its inventor. The naming of procedures, instruments, anatomical

areas and diseases after inventors was integral to the process of claiming credit and was a practice that speedily gained ground in the mid-nineteenth century, although it was far from unheard of in surgery before then.[36] Eponymy was a way of maintaining one's place within the annals of surgery as operations evolved and proliferated. If an operation was named for a surgeon, either by himself or by his supporters, and that name was accepted by peers, at least some kind of legacy was secured; for while operations might be subject to technical changes, the surgeon's name was now indelibly fixed to its development. Simpson's operation, Peaslee's operation, Tait's flap-splitting operation and Battey's operation, the latter of which will be discussed in more detail below, all became part of regular surgical taxonomy. Surgical instruments were also often named for the surgeon who had designed them. This led to a symbiotic relationship between surgeons and 'their' instruments: the most popular instruments tended to be those made by high-status surgeons, whose names suggested the trustworthiness of the tool. The popularity of their instruments then went on to further secure the surgeon's name and reputation. Instruments devised by Thomas Spencer Wells and Isaac Baker Brown, for example, proved to be some of the most fashionable in use for ovariotomy, and Wells in particular was able to enhance his visibility and professional standing with the numerous instruments he devised.[37]

John Clay's clam found favour among his fellow practitioners, and it was quickly taken up and then modified by Isaac Baker Brown as part of his routine method for dividing the pedicle. Brown carefully acknowledged that Clay had originated the instrument. But in 1866 the situation became rather more complex. That year Thomas Spencer Wells referred to Clay's priority not only in creating the instrument but also in being the first to employ the two-part method of compressing and cauterising the pedicle that the instrument enabled.[38] Published in the *British Medical Journal*, his assertion provoked a speedy and terse response from Isaac Baker Brown, who in the intervening time had claimed credit for developing this method and argued that John Clay had merely suggested the *possible* use of the instrument for dealing with the pedicle. Brown appealed to the editor of the journal, dispensing of any pretence that this was about anything other than personal credit: 'Sir, it is of little moment to me whether Mr. Spencer Wells chooses to ignore or to adopt a method of securing the pedicle which has been followed by most satisfactory results', he wrote, 'but I cannot allow him so to place the matter before my medical brethren as to lead them to infer that I had nothing whatever to do with it except as a successful operator'.[39] It was an interesting choice of words from Brown, suggesting that successful deployment of the instrument was of little compensation compared to the grander prize of originating a new technique. John Clay reluctantly involved himself in the dispute the following week, stating that he had 'a great objection to discuss personal matters in the public papers' or 'saying anything about "*due credit*"', but nonetheless did claim credit for both the instrument and the method.[40]

As was often the case, the dispute quietly died down not entirely resolved, but such was the importance of the method of managing the pedicle that it remained a frequent focal point for further innovation and high-profile priority claims.[41] Disagreements like that between Isaac Baker Brown, Thomas Spencer Wells and John Clay may seem at first to be little more than jealous medical men splitting hairs over the minor details of an invention. Indeed, the frequency with which surgeons claimed each alteration to an instrument was ridiculed by the medical press; 'we may say that if these things were expunged from any instrument maker's catalogue, that catalogue would be considerably emaciated' commented the *Lancet*, on the many instrument modifications that were advertised.[42] But they should also be read as testament to the significance even relatively minor credit claims could attain in the heated atmosphere of mid-century medicine, where the value of invention was being radically re-conceptualised. Disputes over the technical minutiae of the operation show also how credit was multifaceted. Potentially, it could be awarded for many different components of the operation, in which material inventions, their modifications, as well as operative performance, could all be, in a sense, owned.

Uneasy Pioneers: Thomas Spencer Wells and Charles Clay

By far the most controversial credit dispute involving ovariotomy was that which occurred between Thomas Spencer Wells and the more well-known Clay, Manchester obstetrician Charles Clay, in 1865 (Figs. 4.1 and 4.2). Charles Clay had, up until then, generally been considered Britain's most successful ovariotomist. No significant challenge had ever been made to his claim to have performed the first complete ovariotomy in England by major incision in 1842.[43] Since then, he had performed the operation repeatedly and by 1863 had had 104 cases, seventy-two of which were successful.[44] He was well known both in Britain and

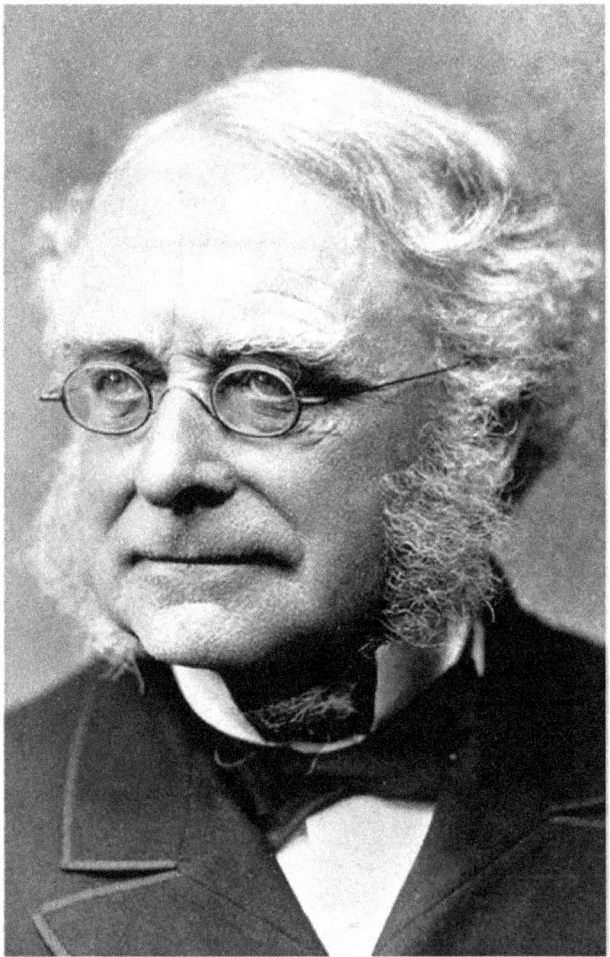

Fig. 4.1 Photograph of Thomas Spencer Wells, taken in the 1880s or early 1890s by the portrait photographer Herbert Rose Barraud. Wells was firmly ensconced within London's social elite and had received a baronetcy in 1883 (*Credit* Wellcome Collection CC BY)

abroad and attracted patients from all over the country, although he performed his operations with little fanfare. The son of a corn merchant and Edinburgh educated, up until the 1860s Charles Clay barely ever involved himself in the public debates over the justifiability of the operation, rarely appearing at society meetings and only occasionally

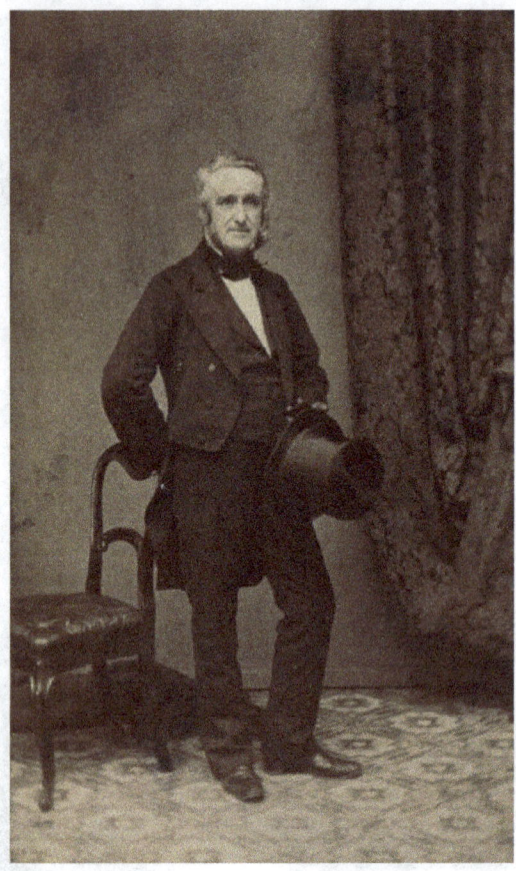

Fig. 4.2 Photograph of Charles Clay. Every inch the Victorian surgeon, the image was probably taken in 1861, by which time he was well established as a practitioner in ovariotomy (*Credit* The University of Manchester)

publishing on his cases. His only professional teaching appointment had been a brief spell as lecturer of diseases of women and in midwifery at St. Mary's Hospital in Manchester, from which he resigned after a year.[45] Indeed, he made no bones about his distaste for London medical society, remarking in private correspondence to James Young Simpson that 'the cockneys are a jealous set'.[46] Clay's publications generally received poor reviews in the predominantly London press, and this likely contributed to his dislike of the capital.

Thomas Spencer Wells, on the other hand, had chosen a very different path. Although he was at pains not to reveal it, he was from a relatively humble background. His early career consisted of a long spell in a poorly paid position as an assistant surgeon in the Royal Navy.[47] Specialism eventually enabled Wells to make a name for himself in London, initially in ophthalmology in the late 1850s, before he secured the role of surgeon at the Samaritan Hospital for Women where his interest in ovariotomy developed. In short, Wells' interest in ovariotomy might be ascribed to calculated professional risks on his part: specialism brought with it the possibility of notoriety. But if practised successfully—especially in London—it could be a ticket to both eminence and financial riches. Buttressed by his other roles as editor of the *Medical Times and Gazette* and an active and visible member of London medical society, Wells was by the early 1860s comfortably established in his practice and by the 1880s was one of the most well-respected and well-paid surgeons in London.

As discussed in Chapter 3, it was Wells' publication of *Diseases of the Ovaries: their Diagnosis and Treatment* in 1865 that sealed the permanence of his reputation. Published in response to the suspicions of opponents that failed cases were being concealed by surgeons, it was not long before the voluminous book was being depicted as a seminal publication that had definitively established ovariotomy as a 'legitimate' operation. In a rather gushing review in the *British Medical Journal*, Wells' book was readily accorded the accolade of 'the most important addition to the history of ovariotomy, which has yet been published' and was even an 'epoch in the History of Surgery, and is especially creditable to the Surgery of this Metropolis'.[48] Geographical politics was playing out here; a later review appearing in the *Edinburgh Medical Journal*, while expressing admiration for Wells' work as a 'plain and truth-like record of achievement', was somewhat more cautious and careful to recognise the contributions of non-London-based practitioners like John Lizars and Charles Clay as well as the Edinburgh-based Thomas Keith, who was achieving better results than either Wells or Clay.[49]

The book was undoubtedly influential, but Wells played an active role in encouraging the idea that his monograph was epoch-making. In the book's introduction, he neatly compartmentalised his work into a new category of literature on ovariotomy that differed considerably from that which had come before. While careful to bestow due praise on successful colleagues past and present, it was to himself that he credited the unique position of creator of what he would later term the 'revival' of ovariotomy and by doing so formed a divide both in chronology and in technique between his work and what came before. Although not claiming to have originated the operation, he argued that it was *he* who had rescued it from sliding unpopularity in the 1850s, made it trustworthy and established its re-emergence. This narrative he would continually reaffirm in later speeches, recreating what came before him as a dark phase in the operation's existence and making the new era of ovariotomy his own. Evidently this was a strong enough part of his personal and professional identity that either he or his family wished it to be his lasting legacy—in Brompton Cemetery in London lies Wells' grave, upon which a one-line epitaph is still just about visible: 'He Revived the Operation of Ovariotamy' [sic].

Wells' description of the world that ovariotomists inhabited in the 1850s, if exaggerated, contained a kernel of truth. The disgrace of Frederic Bird lay in stark contrast to Wells' very visible success and meticulous recording of cases. But in one respect his reordering of ovariotomy drew marked attention: his clear attempt to consign Charles Clay to the dubious early history of ovariotomy. Highly successful in his practice, Charles Clay had, in theory, much to his credit. Wells never directly denied Clay's claim to be the first successful ovariotomist in Britain but questioned the impact his work had had on the profession. From Wells' perspective, full credit was denied to Clay because 'his operations not being performed in an hospital before numerous professional witnesses and no connected series of cases being published, his example had but little influence'.[50] Both assertions—that Clay's claim to the operation was negated by a lack of witnesses and also by a lack of published material—went straight to the heart of contemporary notions of surgical knowledge-making. Surgical operations had, of course, long been public affairs. Surgeons observed the operations of peers as part of the pedagogical transmission of surgical knowledge, something to which Thomas Schlich has applied the Weberian idea of 'tacit knowledge' (of which surgery is arguably a prime example).[51] But witnessing was also important in terms of verifying claims about operations and could be used either to support or repudiate a surgeon's account of a performance. As Steven Shapin and Simon Schaffer argue in their now seminal work, the establishment of the experimental method in science was in part based on the witnessing of experimental observations by multiple, credible individuals, and it was no less the case in surgery.[52] Despite the often impromptu nature of operations, the necessity of having multiple witnesses was at the very least highly desirable if not rigorously policed, especially for serious or novel operations. This was not lost on Clay who, in a speedily penned and angry response to the publication of Wells' book, published in the *Lancet*, wrote of his own work:

> Every operation has been witnessed generally by *three* or *four* professional men; in many instances *seven* or *eight*; and in some instances as many as *ten* or *eleven*; I believe not less than from six to seven hundred in the whole, and nearly always very different persons from every part of Europe.[53]

Clay's personal notes and correspondence support the idea that this was so. Although filled in somewhat sporadically, Clay noted down numerous medical men who came to witness his operations, including overseas visitors.[54] But by the middle decades, the literal act of witnessing was not always sufficient in supporting an operation's veracity. Increasingly, it was the type of witness and location of the witnessing that were under scrutiny. The majority of ovariotomies continued to be performed in private dwellings. But hospitals were increasingly regarded as the ideal location for surgical spectacle, especially that which related to new methods and practices. They were places where numerous medical men could conveniently gather, and by doing so, mutually reinforce the authenticity of what was being observed. In 1847, one such spectacular event had taken place at University College Hospital when Robert Liston performed the first British operation to be conducted under ether. Liston 'posted a notice that the operation would take place and the theatre was filled with spectators'.[55] Highly public and bold performances like this projected an image of the surgical community as truthful and open, attributes which were greatly valued. This ideal permitted Wells to be dismissive of Clay's witnesses even though Clay had worked hard to ensure as many people as possible saw his operations. As Clay himself believed, Wells' allegations could only be an allusion to Clay's lack of hospital appointment. Without this role, it was easy for Wells to depict Clay as out of touch with modern practice and out of sight from his peers. With Wells in control of the wards of the Samaritan Hospital in London, but Clay residing in Manchester without any similar situation, Wells was in the stronger position in a surgical culture that was increasingly London-centric.

The second aspect to Wells' criticism of Clay was the lack of published material about Clay's cases. In a response to Clay's letter, Wells had defended his original criticism, writing:

> Half a page of tabulated matter is really all the information published of 50 of Dr. Clay's alleged cases, except some equally useless lists in one of Dr. R Lee's tables. Such meagre unauthenticated reports are absolutely worthless to the scientific inquirer; and, for all purposes of comparison with the results of other operators, Dr. Clay can only be admitted as having operated on 27 patients.[56]

Despite Clay's assertion that he had performed ovariotomy 111 times by 1865, Wells argued that only the twenty-seven operations which had been published could be counted. As we have seen, surgeons were increasingly encouraged to publish on cases to prevent accusations of concealment. But Wells' refusal to adequately credit Clay was indicative of notions once more changing as to the best way of representing surgical experience. Wells argued that cases should be connected together in a monograph form to ascertain credit—just as he had. This idea dismayed Clay; 'surely Mr. Wells cannot mean to infer that to...*ensure credit* one must publish a book (too often only a polite advertisement of the author's whereabouts?)'[57] queried Clay, who argued instead that the larger circulation and readership of journals brought cases to a wider audience and thus was a more credible means of asserting one's priority and surgical experience. Despite this seemingly logical argument, which factored in the enormous expansion of the medical press over the previous three decades, Clay had failed to acknowledge the value of the monograph in allowing practitioners to coherently bring together multiple cases, which could strengthen their authority in the field.

Clay fought back against the insinuations in Wells' book in a series of letters to the *Lancet* written between February and April 1865, in which he set out to regain a degree of ownership over the operation. For Wells, credit was intimately tied up with publication and witnessing. Clay, on the other hand, described a concept of credit that was much more closely bound to ideas of originality and priority. That he had performed the first successful ovariotomy was enough to stake his claim in the operation; 'if I had not been the pioneer for this operation in 1842, and for years after that, alone and unsupported', Clay claimed, 'neither ovariotomy as an operation, nor Mr. Wells as an ovariotomist, would most probably be heard of at this time'.[58] Clay cultivated a romantic image of himself as the isolated inventor, who had risked his reputation in the name of progress, while the profession had largely turned its back on him.

In a rather contradictory fashion, Clay encouraged readers to see both similarities and differences in his and Wells' operations. In his letters to the *Lancet* Clay, at times, represented Wells as a poor-quality imitator and spoke almost nostalgically about the days gone by when 'I had the operation to myself, when I had rather to originate than imitate plans of operation and after treatment', the insinuation being that Wells has done the latter.[59] Imitation, as the saying goes, is the highest form of flattery and could be a perfectly acceptable part of surgical practice. Emulating the methods and practices of more senior practitioners was an integral part of learning through 'tacit knowledge' and a sign of respect for one's elders. But imitation had to be acknowledged. Reproduction complicated conceptualisations of authenticity in medicine as it did in other areas of nineteenth-century industry. If the Great Exhibition marked a genuine Victorian 'moment' in its celebration of novelty and invention, it was also, as Clare Pettitt describes it, a 'moment of crisis in the history of representation', making visible, as it did the potential of new technologies to generate the mass reproduction of everything from newspapers to textiles to sculptures.[60] As wide-scale manufacturing, publishing and commercialism began their ascent, the effect was to destabilise notions of uniqueness in invention. It generated anxieties about the relative ease with which artistic and literary creations could be replicated, often to a lower quality standard, and appropriated to the detriment of authors' and inventors' intellectual property. The proliferation of ovariotomies similarly made it more difficult to pick out what was original and what was mere imitation.

Clay at other times emphasised the polarity in his and Wells' methods, arguing that their operations were 'two distinctly different modes of proceeding, if faithfully carried out', going on to detail the variations in their practice.[61] Wells, for example, completed ovariotomy by securing a clamp to the remaining pedicle, while Clay used ligatures; Wells championed an incision of about four inches to open the abdomen, while Clay made a larger one, sometimes up to twelve inches.[62] Clay was especially keen on using incision size to differentiate his style of operating from that of his competitors and used it to distinguish himself from both Wells and proponents of the 'minor' operation such as William Jeaffreson, who made incisions of only one or two inches. Both Clay and Jeaffreson insisted they practised entirely different operations from one another, to ensure they both retained a priority claim of sorts.[63]

The disagreement between Clay and Wells rapidly descended into a bitter feud that stretched beyond questions of credit and priority to matters of a more personal nature. Clay accused Wells of performing an operation on a patient with a malignant tumour knowing full well the case was incurable and would almost certainly be fatal. He insinuated that Wells had done so simply to pocket the large fee on offer. This was a step too far for Wells, who promptly took legal action against Clay, which resulted in the latter being forced to make a public apology and to retract his accusation. The *Lancet's* role in the affair was also scrutinised. The *British Medical Journal* criticised its long-standing journalistic rival for allowing Clay the space to publicly air his grievance against Wells and in encouraging the personal nature of the disagreement, a charge which stood uncomfortably at odds with the *Lancet's* professed disapproval of such disputes.[64]

The unfortunate episode between Wells and Clay did not prevent other claims arising; Clay was not the only one sceptical of Wells' depiction of ovariotomy before the 1860s as unworthy of credit. Numerous other attempts were made to draw attention to the work of early practitioners in the field. The significance of reviving older priority claims was most obviously relayed in a letter the Kent physician John Gorham sent to the *Lancet* in 1874, in which he reminded readers of the role played by the now deceased William West, one of the pioneers of the so-called minor operation. Gorham was keen to highlight West's all but forgotten role in the evolution of ovarian surgery as part of his appeal on behalf West's daughter, whom he described as living in straitened circumstances. Gorham played on the financial successes of present-day practitioners of the operation; 'I believe that some members of the profession are receiving as much as one hundred guineas for a single operation for ovariotomy', Gorham wrote, 'may it not be fair to ask these gentlemen to contribute a trifle to the daughter of one who stood foremost in introducing this operation to the metropolis of London, and so to the whole world?'.[65]

Throughout the century, numerous other claims would arise in the medical press from individuals seeking credit for practitioners now deceased and in danger of being forgotten. Most of these claims would fall on deaf ears.[66]

The dispute between Charles Clay and Thomas Spencer Wells continued until the twilight of their careers. In 1880, the public debate between the two erupted again, this time—rather ironically given its previous position—in the pages of the *British Medical Journal*. When an editorial was published which celebrated Wells' performance of his one thousandth ovariotomy, Clay responded by sending another letter reiterating once more his belief that he was the true originator of ovariotomy in Britain.[67] Fundamental to Clay's argument this time around was the fact that the term 'ovariotomy' had been coined by James Young Simpson specifically for his operation, intimately linking the procedure with his personal practice.[68] This was the last time Clay publicly involved himself in the dispute. Ultimately, the controversy strengthened Wells' grip upon the legacy of ovariotomy and for the most part the 'ovariotomy controversy', as it came to be known, did little to dent Wells' eminence. Nonetheless, his rather aggressive dismantling of Clay's legacy did not go unnoticed. In 1884, the Birmingham-based surgeon Robert Lawson Tait, who himself was making a name as a successful performer of ovariotomy, and who was a stern critic of what he saw as the highly elitist world of London surgery, took up Clay's cause. Tait wrote numerous letters condemning Wells' behaviour towards the Manchester surgeon, in one arguing that 'if it is to be contended that, from the time of McDowell till 1857, there was nothing being done in ovariotomy and that the revival took place in that year at the hands of Spencer Wells, I say it may as well be claimed for him that he revived the moon'.[69] Tait was a firebrand, always keen to dismantle the reputation of a London surgeon, but he was also astute and highly respected for his surgical work and his words stuck. Wells was accused in at least one other situation—to having been the first to perform a successful ovariotomy in Ireland—of making a false priority claim.[70] Clay's obituary in the *Lancet* suggested that Tait's defence of his work gave him some satisfaction. In what could only have been an allusion to Wells, who had been a surgeon to the Royal Household since 1863 and was created a baronet in 1883, Clay was in the habit of telling friends near the end of his life that 'some men have got baronetcies, some wealth, some positions at Court, but I have got peace of mind'.[71]

IMITATIONS AND IMPORTS: OVARIOTOMY ON THE GLOBAL STAGE

The identity and genealogy of ovariotomy were not only understood in terms of individual practitioners. Collectively, British surgeons also sought to establish ovariotomy as a definitively British invention. This was no easy task. Ostensibly, local possession of knowledge was repudiated; as historian of geography David N. Livingstone has argued, 'credible knowledge, we assume, does not bear the marks of the provincial'.[72] Moreover, by the mid-nineteenth century, the rapid diffusion of new knowledge, technologies and practices across national boundaries appeared to simply be inevitable. The French journalist and critic Edmond About, paraphrased in the popular British periodical *The New Monthly Magazine*, depicted ovariotomy as one of a number of new inventions that had quickly self-perpetuated and snaked across Europe:

> One of the characteristic features of the time we live in is the almost lightning rapidity with which progress develops itself, completes itself, spreads and bears its fruit to the extremity of the globe...in the present day, if a person makes a discovery in science in one country it is simultaneously effected in two or three others. Witness photography, ovariotomy, new planets, chloroform, new metallic bases in the spectrum, and the improvements in the sewing machine.[73]

The inevitability of imitation, and even synchronicity, which seemed to characterise modern society did not preclude resistance to narratives like About's, and on the Britishness of ovariotomy, there was for some, little question. 'Ovariotomy is an operation of British origin, and it is to the labour of British surgeons that its subsequent progress is chiefly due',[74] proclaimed Thomas Spencer Wells in 1863. Notions of the operation's British identity were consolidated by its diffusion into practice within the British colonies, where it was posited as a civilising influence. A report of the first ovariotomy in New Zealand in 1866 was received rapturously in the British medical press; the operator, Dr. McKinnon, praised for carrying 'far and wide the good deeds and the fame of British Surgery'.[75]

Retaining British identity and authorship of the operation became increasingly important in the 1860s in the face of French surgeons beginning to take up the operation. Having largely rejected ovariotomy in the early part of the century, French surgeons like Auguste Nélaton and Eugène Koeberlé had brought it into practice. It left the British with mixed feelings. Some welcomed it, seeing it as additional armour for those fighting to definitively establish the operation as respectable. But it also revealed a possessiveness on the part of the British, not only over ovariotomy but also of a general reputation for surgical authority. In a column in 1864, the *Lancet* characterised French surgeons as smug and even delusional about their own talents, contending that 'the pretensions of the French school of surgery to a distinct pre-eminence have been maintained by themselves with a self-satisfaction and an apparent confidence which have always been regarded in this country with a secret and placid amusement'.[76]

Integral to this viewpoint was the idea that the French were frequently in the habit of imitating British surgical practices without giving their counterparts over the Channel full credit. It was not long before gentle ribbing of the French turned to outright disdain, especially for their delayed uptake of ovariotomy: the *British Medical Journal* in 1864 described Koeberlé as 'merely a copyist of the English in the matter of ovariotomy'.[77] The year before, the journal had also poured scorn upon the Prix Barbier and the reward of 2000 francs Koeberlé had received as 'official' recognition for his two successful cases of the operation. The journal scoffed that 'it would be rather an expensive undertaking for the French Academy to reward our successful ovariotomists at the same rate as M. Koeberlé', reminding readers of the greater prolificacy of ovariotomists on the British side of the Channel. By the time Koeberlé wrote the first French language monograph on the operation, *L'Ovariotomie*, in 1865, it was regarded as a damp squib by the British journals. The book, aside from the accompanying raw material of the cases, was perceived to draw almost wholly on debates which had already taken place for years in Britain.[78]

The defensiveness of British surgeons was probably unfounded. Most French practitioners were happy to accept their claim to the operation, which they often described as the *mode à l'Anglaise*, even though the operation had its roots in France.[79] British doctors' hostility to their French counterparts betrayed wider concerns about the fate of British inventions on the international stage. The prospect of unprecedented competition in science and industry was looming, particularly from France, Germany and America, undermining the country's hitherto unrivalled dominance in industrial development. The *Exposition Universelle* in Paris in 1867 seemed to crystallise fears of competition and was regarded with suspicion by some British observers, concerned that successful inventions ran the risk of being copied by foreign competitors only to be then re-imported back to Britain under the guise of a different nationality.[80] These concerns infiltrated the surgical profession. That same year, the Birmingham surgeon Sampson Gamgee, who himself would later attain recognition as an important inventor of new surgical sundries, set off on a two-week holiday to Paris which took in the Exposition and was a chance for him to observe the state of surgery in the city.[81] He reported his findings to the *Lancet*: 'many are crowding to Paris, and wondering at the progress made by the French nation in a variety of manufacturing and industrial departments, in which not many years ago, we enjoyed a clear, and scarcely questioned supremacy'.[82] His investigation of French surgery was likewise infused with the language of comparison as he negotiated his way through similar and contrasting aspects of French and British surgery. Gamgee depicted French surgeons as better organised and educated—indeed perhaps too well-educated—at the cost of their technical abilities. British surgeons, on the other hand, he viewed as practically minded doers, who, consequently, were more fearless as operators. Gamgee stretched out this analogy to British industry as a whole:

> The engine-driver on a French railway is often a good pupil of the École des Arts et Métiers, knows a great deal about physics, and every now and then is nearly as good a mathematician as he is a mechanic; but he would be sorely puzzled to match one of our men in piloting the Holyhead mail at fifty miles an hour through a November fog.[83]

It was these uniquely British characteristics of courage, practicality, persistence and boldness that for Gamgee defined both British surgeons and engineers and enabled them to retain their standing even in the face of national competition. And yet, while it became increasingly acceptable for engineers to patent their inventions, relatively free of accusations of impropriety, surgeons were bereft of official channels through which to make similar claims.

The relationship between British and American surgeons was of a rather different nature. The kinship British surgeons felt towards their American counterparts was strong and based on an assumption of shared surgical style; 'the bent of the mind of the American surgeon is, like ours, practical rather than scientific', reflected the University College Hospital surgeon John Erichsen after a trip to America in 1874.[84] While there were a small number of surgeons practising ovariotomy in America in the middle decades, in general American societies and journals were content to let the British lead on the topic; most articles on ovariotomy published in the American medical press simply recounted discussions of the operation's justifiability from the other side of the Atlantic.[85] John Burnham has argued that it was not really until the latter part of the century that American practitioners began to forge their own sense of professional culture distinct from British medicine.[86] But as American surgeons began to find their voice, some expressed concern about the lack of contribution their country had made to ovariotomy's development, lamenting that British surgeons had been quicker to accept the operation than their American counterparts.[87] America had been able to maintain its claim to the 'first' ovariotomy, in the form of Ephraim McDowell's operation, but its surgeons were perceived to have not built upon this with further innovation in the field. Moreover, McDowell's contribution was easily slotted into the operation's 'British' identity, because McDowell had been educated in Edinburgh, allowing the operation to still be conceived of as borne of British medical education.[88]

For British surgeons, what happened in America regarding the operation initially made little impact on their own discussions. But in the 1870s things started to change. The work of James Marion Sims had put American gynaecology on the map. Sims was a well-known figure on both sides of the Atlantic, having spent periods working in London and Paris performing his operation for vesico-vaginal fistula, a condition often brought on by childbirth, where a tract formed between the vagina and bladder, usually leading to urinary incontinence. Sims has become notorious in the history of medicine and beyond. In recent years, scholars have called attention anew to Sims' use of enslaved women in his formulation of new surgical operations. Sims' early procedures for fistula were exclusively practised on a small group of captive women; at least three of them, Anarcha, Betsey and Lucy, were subject to multiple surgeries by Sims; Anarcha was operated upon at least thirty times.[89] Sims operated on the women without an anaesthetic agent, despite its coming into use around the time he began performing the operation, based on a common assumption that black people did not feel pain to the extent that white people did. His protestation that he was merely alleviating their upsetting condition on behalf of their benevolent owners belies a darker reality.[90] As Deleso Alford Washington has argued, the treatment the women faced '"othered" their skin based upon a construction of "race," yet "samed" their bodies for purposes of extracting reproductive knowledge, surgical inventions, and innovation to benefit all women'.[91]

It is perhaps not surprising then that it was Sims who at the end of 1877 introduced to Britain another procedure that was to become notorious, 'Battey's operation', named after its claimed originator, the surgeon Robert Battey. Born in 1828 in Georgia and trained in Philadelphia, Battey returned from his duties as a Confederate Army surgeon in 1865, settling into practice in Rome, Georgia. He began to perform ovariotomy in 1869, his interest in the operation having been piqued in the late 1850s when a tour of Europe had led him to meet many practitioners of the operation, including Thomas Spencer Wells. Battey had begun to hypothesise the use of ovarian surgery for conditions other than tumours soon after his return to practice. Perturbed by the numerous physical and psychological problems suffered by his patients with menstrual irregularities, Battey ascribed to the ovular theory: that ovulation was directly connected to menstruation. He theorised that if both ovaries were removed, menopause would ensue, thus effecting a cure. He put theory into practice in 1872 when he removed both ovaries from his thirty-year-old patient Julia Olmberg, who was suffering from a range of gastric, rectal and epileptic symptoms. Battey and others following in his footsteps would go on to perform the operation for a wide range of conditions, including, most controversially, upon women whose menstrual disorders were believed to be causing mental afflictions such as hysteria and nymphomania. The indications for the operation appeared strikingly vague and led to immediate scepticism about the pathological basis of the operation.[92] It was an unseemly cross-pollination of alienism and surgery, of the type that had recently laid waste to the career of the ovariotomist Isaac Baker Brown. Brown had become embroiled in one of nineteenth-century London's greatest medical scandals when, in the late 1860s, he began to perform clitoridectomies (the removal of the clitoris) to treat hysteria, epilepsy and a range of other ailments in women. The operations were performed at his specialist institution, the London Surgical Home, without the clear consent of his patients and, in the opinion of many London medical men, with little sound physiological reasoning; Brown was subsequently expelled from the Obstetrical Society.[93] Operations which traversed into the mental sciences tended to be treated with a degree of suspicion.

In the beginning, Battey referred to the operation as 'normal ovariotomy', a reference to his belief that 'normal' ovaries, without any obvious signs of disease, were the cause of maladies elsewhere in the body.

He had chosen it also because he believed his method to be a 'truer' ovariotomy than that which was usually performed, which he described as 'irregular ovariotomy', because it involved grossly diseased ovaries. As he rather audaciously described it, 'it was *I* who had really and truly done an ovariotomy rather than Dr. Ephraim McDowell, as I understand the *rule*, or *law*, or principle, which governs medical nomenclature in such cases', assigning himself credit for his purportedly new operation.[94] Battey's peers were critical of his use of the word 'ovariotomy'. The inference that perfectly normal ovaries were being removed was likely to raise eyebrows and was far from ideal given that the propriety of ovariotomy had so often been questioned already. It was partly for this reason that the operation was renamed by Battey and Sims in the late 1870s. But it was also a convenient opportunity to try and rebrand the operation. In 1877, Sims urged European surgeons to 'unite with us in America in giving it the name of the man who originated the operation'.[95] The renaming served a number of functions. First, it formed a connection between Battey and the procedure. In what was a calculated risk, Battey's professional reputation was now intertwined with the fate of the operation. Second, it was used to more firmly differentiate the procedure from ovariotomy, expunging the confusion that 'normal' ovariotomy had brought. But most importantly, it was meant to signal the distinctly American nature of the operation, a way of reintroducing American ingenuity back into the ovariotomy narrative. Battey and Sims were moderately successful in their endeavour. The American identity of Battey's operation was generally accepted by British practitioners and filtered into patients' perceptions too. Writing in the *British Medical Journal* in 1879, the obstetrician Alexander Russell Simpson recounted a patient with chronic menstrual pain who had implored Russell to perform Battey's operation upon her after he had mentioned the developments occurring in American surgery. According to Russell, the patient claimed to have been 'reading all about' the new operation, asking Russell 'can't you do here what the doctors in America can do?'.[96] However, the renaming of the operation did not catch on entirely. In 1872, the American surgeon Edmund Peaslee had drawn attention to the failure of 'ovariotomy' as an explanatory term and had suggested 'oöphorectomy' as a more accurate description (the suffix '-ectomy' denoting removal, whereas 'otomy' implied only incision). British practitioners began to use the latter term interchangeably with 'Battey's operation' to describe procedures that involved the removal of both ovaries to treat conditions other than ovarian tumours. And by the late 1880s, it was 'oöphorectomy' that was more commonly used to describe the procedure Battey claimed as his own. The complex nomenclature around ovarian surgery will be discussed in more detail in Chapter 6.

The uniqueness of Battey's operation was also contested across the international stage. Recalling Edmond About's pronouncement of the rapid and widespread diffusion of modern innovations, it quickly became apparent that German gynaecologist Alfred Hegar had begun performing similar operations to Battey at around the same time.[97] In Britain, Robert Lawson Tait also had his own procedure, 'Tait's operation', involving the removal of the ovaries and Fallopian tubes to cure inflammatory disease. Tait always denied using ovarian surgery to treat mental afflictions, but his operation was similar enough to Battey's that he repeatedly felt the need to emphasise their difference: 'what Dr. Battey has advocated and practised, I, for one, practically have never performed' he wrote to the *British Medical Journal*.[98]

Battey's operation received mixed reviews from the British medical press. The revelation that it was being used experimentally to treat forms of insanity startled many, even those who were themselves ovariotomists. Thomas Spencer Wells spoke out forcibly against the new operation. In an essay published in the *American Journal of the Medical Sciences* in 1886, and later reprinted as a pamphlet, he described the procedure as an 'unnecessary mutilation of young women'.[99] For Wells, this unwelcome development could only be understood through the framework of nationality, its roots in the 'fanaticism' of American surgeons.[100] But, he warned, its implications were global; 'the danger is now increasing as the operation is becoming world-wide' Wells wrote, 'the oöphorectomists of civilization touch hands with the aboriginal spayers of New Zealand'.[101] Wells picked his words carefully, crafting an image of oöphorectomy that suggested savagery, in stark contrast to ovariotomy, which he depicted as a model of colonial advance, likening it to 'the discovery of the Californian diggings or the African diamond mines'.[102] Wells entitled the essay 'On the Castration of Women', provocatively ignoring the more respectable nomenclature, to use instead a word which carried stigma and which suggested a violent, animalistic procedure rather than a progressive one. Battey's operation was never able to achieve full acceptance in Britain. Battey had gambled his name in the hope that personal association with his innovation would bring fame and prestige. Instead, it has brought enduring notoriety.

Was the nationality of an operation determined by its country of origin or the country where it had been most successful? Through what ways could a country make a claim of ownership to an operation? And why was there a need to do so? Broadly speaking, ovariotomy was identified as a British innovation; British practitioners succeeded in making it so through consistently espousing their contributions, but perhaps more so by calling into question the contributions of other countries. Defensive and possessive in equal parts, British surgeons were suspicious of the alleged imitations of the French and the deviations of the Americans, both of which potentially threatened the carefully cultivated identity of ovariotomy within Britain. On the international stage, retaining the Britishness of the operation was essential in the face of growing professional and industrial competition from other nations.

CONCLUSION

This chapter has tried to make explicit how surgeons managed and claimed the vast proliferation of knowledge that was being generated around ovariotomy. At first glance, there may seem little to connect the operation with notions of intellectual property beyond the personal disputes that doctors were notorious for. After all, medicine and surgery played a lesser role within wider societal debates on patenting and credit occurring at the time, and no patenting existed in relation to the operation. Yet on closer inspection, the apportioning of the knowledge and practice that constituted 'ovariotomy' reveals cultural and political concerns. The chronology of these disputes also signals the ostensible establishment of the operation; it was only in the 1860s as ovariotomy came to be viewed as justifiable by most of the profession that credit claims around it proliferated. In an atmosphere of heightened awareness about the role of the inventor in society, ovariotomists found methods for crediting those who innovated in the field. Being the first to perform an operation—even being the first to *consistently* perform an operation—did not necessarily secure one's legacy. Nor was credit an inevitable consequence of innovation. Rather, to ensure credit one had to maintain it, remaining visible through publishing, inviting high-profile practitioners to witness operations, inventing instruments and using eponyms. The ability to maintain a claim was also as much to do with a surgeon's social status and location, as Charles Clay would have been only too painfully aware.

Settling priority disputes was not only about personal reputations. It brought order to the operation and it allowed surgeons to reshape the narrative of ovariotomy, imbuing it with a desired sense of teleology, a national identity and its own assemblage of heroes. The need for definition and classification was fundamental to bringing respectability to the operation—both while it was being established and later in the century when new forms of ovarian surgery began to flourish. To do so was no mean feat. Debates over the nuances of the operation highlighted that the procedure was the sum of multiple innovations; the size of the incision made, the method of treating the pedicle, the type of instrument used—all could potentially hold value to those who had originated them. Moreover, it was not always easy to reconcile individual practices of the operation with a concrete definition of ovariotomy; operations tended to be highly individualistic, moulded by the idiosyncrasies of the operator and patient. In ovariotomy especially, where there was so often disagreement about what the best mode of performance was, the operation's identity was malleable.

Intellectual property in medical practice has generally been integrated into broader narratives of science and technology, but knowledge production in surgery frequently defied 'scientific' organisation and management. The idea of surgery as both an art and a science was evoked as a positive characteristic of the profession, yet the dual components existed in tension with one another. 'People...forget that operative surgery is an art', wrote the surgeon and lithotomist Sir Henry Thompson to Ernest Hart, editor of the *British Medical Journal* in 1886, 'the personality of the artist should be largely taken into account'.[103] Practitioners of ovariotomy wished desperately to have their personal contributions to the field recognised, but always present was a fine line between attaining sufficient credit and potential accusations of egoism. Social credit—with the hope of future financial reward—was hard won but easily lost by surgeons. The process of securing credit could be lengthy, delayed and complex or even fail completely. Nonetheless, if one was successful, the rewards could be bountiful; these accolades made the risks of innovation worthwhile.

Notes

1. John Bland-Sutton, *Surgical Diseases of the Ovaries and Fallopian Tubes* (Philadelphia: Lea Bros, 1891), v.
2. M.W. Weatherall, 'Making Medicine Scientific: Empiricism, Rationality, and Quackery in Mid-Victorian Britain', *Social History of Medicine* 9, no. 2 (1996): 175–194. More recent scholarship has emphasised that the 1858 Act was a process of negotiation between MPs and medical

men, in which the former limited the powers of the act for the sake of patient choice. See M.J.D. Roberts, 'The Politics of Professionalization: MPs, Medical Men, and the 1858 Medical Act', *Medical History* 52, no. 1 (2009): 37–56.

3. Anonymous, 'Letter from London', *The Boston Medical and Surgical Journal* 104, no. 6 (10 February 1881):142–143.

4. Robert K. Merton, *The Sociology of Science* (Chicago: Chicago University Press, 1973), 293.

5. To take one example, the increasing pervasiveness of 'technology transfer' in the UK, that is, the securing of intellectual property for scientific research at educational institutes, and its subsequent commercial exploitation.

6. The term 'intellectual property' did not emerge as part of regular legal vernacular until the end of the nineteenth century. However, it can be used to broadly desrcibe the range of issues surrounding the ownership of intellectual labours, from patenting to trade marking, to non-legal methods of managing and recognising credit such as publication, peer recognition and pecuniary reward.

7. Christine Macleod and Gregory Radick, 'Claiming Ownership in the Technosciences: Patents, Priority and Productivity', *Studies in History and Philosophy of Science Part A* 44, no. 2 (2013): 181.

8. See, for example, James F. Stark, 'Introduction: Plurality in Patenting: Medical Technology and Cultures of Protection', *British Journal of the History of Science* 49, no. 4 (2016): 533–540.

9. Judith P. Swazey and Renée C. Fox, 'The Clinical Moratorium', in *Essays in Medical Sociology: Journeys into the Field*, ed. Renée C. Fox (New York: Transaction Publishers, 1988), 337 incl. n. 32.

10. Christine MacLeod, *Heroes of Invention: Technology, Liberalism and British Identity: 1750–1914* (Cambridge: Cambridge University Press, 2007), 2–3.

11. Samuel Smiles, *Self-Help: With Illustrations of Conduct and Perseverance* (Rockville: Serenity, 2008). Smiles cites Edward Jenner (1747–1823) as an example, 102–103.

12. MacLeod, *Heroes of Invention*, 33–34. This reputation came in part from the fact that, in the early modern period, patentees were often favourites of the Royal Court who had been issued monopolising patents that ruined other 'honest' tradesmen, and who often charged the public extortionate prices.

13. Anonymous, 'Editorial', *The Times* 20665 (6 December 1850), 4.

14. Clare Pettitt, *Patent Inventions: Intellectual Property and the Victorian Novel* (Oxford and New York: Oxford University Press, 2004), 123–124.

15. There were numerous attempts earlier in the century to reform the patenting system, and minor changes were made with the Patent Act of 1835, which allowed the extension of some patents. But overall the Act made relatively little difference. For an overview, see H.I. Dutton, *The Patent System and Inventive Activity During the Industrial Revolution, 1750–1852* (Manchester: Manchester University Press, 1984), 34–56.

16. Anonymous, 'The Theory of Professional Remuneration', *British Medical Journal* 1, no. 371 (8 February 1868): 122.

17. *House of Commons Debate, Hansard 286 ser.3* (26 March 1884), 801–811, http://hansard.millbanksystems.com/sittings/1884/mar/26, accessed 8 August 2013. The Bill never made it to a second reading, most likely because the profession's disdain for the industry in patent medicines did not reflect the opinion of the public, who had an increasing appetite for such products throughout the second half of the century; additionally, the continued revenue patent medicines generated was probably enough to dissuade parliament from their regulation. See T.A.B. Corley, 'Interactions Between the British and American Patent Medicine Industries, 1708–1914' (pamphlet reprint from *Business and Economic History*, Series 2, 16, 1987), 112.

18. Lori Loeb, 'Doctors and Patent Medicine in Modern Britain: Professionalism and Consumerism', *Albion: A Quarterly Journal of British Studies* 33, no. 3 (2001): 416–418. For more on 'orthodox' practitioners' financial and professional interests in patented devices, see Takahiro Ueyama, *Health in the Marketplace: Professionalism, Therapeutic Desires, and Medical Commodification in Late-Victorian London* (Palo Alto: The Society for the Promotion of Science and Scholarship, 2010).

19. Sally Frampton, '"Honour and Subsistence": Invention, Credit and Surgery in the Nineteenth Century', *British Journal of the History of Science* 49, no. 4 (2016): 562.

20. Frampton, 'Honour and Subsistence', 566.

21. 'To Correspondents', *Medical Times* 15, no. 381 (16 January 1847): 307.

22. S. S. Fisher, *Reports of Cases Arising Upon Letters Patent for Inventions Determined in the Circuit Courts of the United States*, vol. 2 (Cincinnati: Robert Clarke & Co., 1871), 320–330.

23. J.A. Dorr, 'Are Improvements in Medicine and Surgery Proper Subjects of Patents?' *Lancet* 49, no. 1237 (15 May 1847): 524.

24. Andrew Wynter, 'Review Essay', *Edinburgh Review, or Critical Journal* 136, no. 278 (1872): 515.

25. Wynter, 'Review Essay', 514.

26. Edward Jenner received £30,000 from Parliament for his pioneering work on vaccination. Anonymous, 'The Theory of Professional Remuneration', (8 February 1868): 122.

27. George Weisz, *The Medical Mandarins: The French Academy of Medicine in the Nineteenth and Early Twentieth Centuries* (Oxford: Oxford University Press, 1995), 98–103.

28. L.F. Hollender, 'Eugène Koeberlé (1828–1915): Père de la Chirurgie Moderne', *Annales de Chirurgie* 126, no. 6 (2001): 574.

29. Anon. 'Le Prix Barbier ses Métamorphoses', *Revue de Thérapeutique Medico-Chirurgicale* 2, no. 21 (1861): 562.

30. 'Editorial', *Lancet* 28, no. 726 (29 July 1837): 670.

31. Letter from Robert Liston to James Miller (26 May 1835) MS6085 (Wellcome Collection).

32. Even though John Clay was no relation to Charles Clay, their similar names were a cause for confusion. In fact, John Clay first publicly addressed the issue of the clam's priority because of a lecture Brown had given describing the instrument as originated by a 'Dr. Clay', leading John Clay to raise concerns that this would suggest the instrument had been created by Charles Clay. John Clay, 'Ovariotomy: Clay's Adhesion Clam', *British Medical Journal* 1, no. 225 (22 April 1865): 418–419.

33. John Clay, *Chapters on Diseases of the Ovaries Translated, by Permission, from Kiwisch's Clinical Lectures* (London: Churchill, 1860).

34. Diseased ovaries were commonly found to be adhering to other organs and tissues such as the liver, stomach and omentum.

35. John Clay, 'Adhesion Clam; A New Instrument for Aiding the Removal of Ovarian Tumours etc', *Medical Times and Gazette* 1 (21 June 1862): 640–641.

36. In 1720, for example, the surgeon John Douglas claimed to have introduced the supra-pubic lithotomy (or 'high' operation) into British surgical practice in a pamphlet that was rather proprietarily entitled *Lithotomia Douglassiana* (London: Thomas Woodward, 1720).

37. 'Wells' artery forceps, originally used to prevent bleeding in ovariotomy cases, remain a staple of the operating theatre even today.

38. Thomas Spencer Wells, 'Clinical Remarks on Different Modes of Dealing with the Pedicle in Ovariotomy', *British Medical Journal* 2, no. 301 (6 October 1866): 378.

39. Isaac Baker Brown, 'Management of the Pedicle in Ovariotomy', *British Medical Journal* 2, no. 302 (13 October 1866): 421.

40. John Clay, 'On Management of the Pedicle in Ovariotomy', *British Medical Journal* 2, no. 303 (20 October 1866): 449.

41. This included American surgeon James Marion Sims as well as the Birmingham-based surgeon Robert Lawson Tait. Sims pioneered the use of silver wire ligatures for those ovariotomists who preferred to secure the pedicle stump within the peritoneal cavity, while Lawson Tait in the 1890s further innovated on Brown and Clay's inventions by

introducing a cautery-clamp which ran an electric current through the cautery, sufficiently ensuring the pedicle was 'cooked' and thus reducing the chance of haemorrhage. See James Marion Sims, 'Ovariotomy: Pedicle Secured by Silver-Wire Ligatures: Cure', *British Medical Journal* 1, no. 432 (10 April 1869): 326; Robert Lawson Tait, 'The Evolution of the Surgical Treatment of the Broad Ligament Pedicle', *Lancet* 147, no. 3794 (16 May 1896): 1338–1841.

42. 'Reviews and Notices of Books: The Story of My Life by J. Marion Sims', *Lancet* 126, no. 3232 (8 August 1885): 247.

43. Some ascribed the first successful ovariotomy in *Britain* to John Lizars who, as we have seen, had successfully removed a diseased ovary in 1825 but probably not cured the patient, whose other ovary was also diseased. Clay acknowledged Lizars and credited himself only as the first to have performed ovariotomy in *England*. See Charles Clay, 'Dr. Clay's Reply to Dr. Granville on Ovarian Extirpation', *Medical Times* 8, no. 204 (19 August 1843): 327.

44. 'Obstetrical Society of London: Wednesday March 4', *Lancet* 81, no. 2067 (11 April 1863): 417. This appears to have been a rare visit made by Charles Clay to the Obstetrical Society of London.

45. Peter D. Mohr, 'Clay, Charles (1801–1893)', in *Oxford Dictionary of National Biography* (Oxford University Press, September 2004); online edn, October 2006, http://www.oxforddnb.com/view/article/5558, accessed 4 May 2010. Mohr suggests this was due to 'the pressure from his private practice'.

46. Letter from Charles Clay to James Young Simpson (March 25 c. 1848) GB 779 RCSEd JYS/37 (Royal College of Surgeons of Edinburgh).

47. Jane Eliot Sewell, 'Wells, Sir Thomas Spencer, First Baronet (1818–1897)', in *Oxford Dictionary of National Biography* (Oxford University Press, 2004); online edn, October 2008, http://www.oxforddnb.com/view/article/29018, accessed 9 August 2013.

48. 'Review: Diseases of the Ovaries: their Diagnosis and Treatment', *British Medical Journal* 1, no. 214 (4 February 1865): 117.

49. 'Review: Diseases of the Ovaries: their Diagnosis and Treatment', *Edinburgh Medical Journal* 13, no. 1 (1867): 565–566.

50. Thomas Spencer Wells, *Diseases of the Ovaries: their Diagnosis and Treatment*, vol. 1 (London: John Churchill & Sons, 1865), x.

51. Thomas Schlich, *Surgery, Science and Industry: A Revolution in Fracture Care, 1950s–1990s* (Basingstoke: Palgrave Macmillan, 2002), 65.

52. Steven Shapin and Simon Schaffer, *Leviathan and the Air-Pump: Hobbes, Boyle, and the Experimental Life* (Princeton: Princeton University Press, 2011), 56–60.

53. Charles Clay, 'On Ovariotomy and Ovariotomists', *Lancet* 85, no. 2165 (25 February 1865): 201.

54. Charles Clay's case book, M/C Medical Collection—cat.9.11.54 MNB (Manchester Medical Collection, University of Manchester). Furthermore, Clay's remaining archives indicate that at least one prominent foreign medical man—the American physician and later inventor William Francis Channing—visited Clay to observe his work; letter from William Channing to Charles Clay (14 August 1855) no class mark (Manchester Medical Collection, University of Manchester).

55. D'Arcy Power, 'Liston, Robert (1794–1847)', rev. Jean Loudon, *Oxford Dictionary of National Biography* (Oxford University Press, 2004), http://www.oxforddnb.com/view/article/16772, accessed 29 July 2013.

56. Spencer Wells, 'Results of Ovariotomy', *Lancet* 85, no. 2167 (11 March 1865): 272.

57. Clay, 'On Ovariotomy and Ovariotomists' (25 February 1865): 201.

58. Clay, 'On Ovariotomy and Ovariotomists' (25 February 1865): 201.

59. Charles Clay, 'The Ovariotomy Controversy', *Lancet* 85, no. 2171 (8 April 1865): 380.

60. Pettitt, *Patent Inventions*, 85.

61. Charles Clay, 'On Ovariotomy and Ovariotomists', *Lancet* 85, no. 2166 (4 March 1865): 227.

62. Charles Clay, 'On Ovariotomy and Ovariotomists' (4 March 1865): 227.

63. The division between the two styles was certainly encouraged by Jeaffreson who, in the wake of others beginning to practise the 'major' operation, described himself in a letter in 1843 to the *Lancet* as 'the *originator* of the *minor* operation'. William Jeaffreson, 'Mr Jeaffreson's Operation for Ovarian Dropsy', *Lancet* 41, no. 1055 (18 November 1843): 217.

64. 'Freedom V License', *British Medical Journal* 2, no. 259 (16 December 1865): 637–638.

65. John Gorham, 'On the Revival of Ovariotomy', *Lancet* 103, no. 2639 (28 March 1874): 441.

66. In the 1870s, there was an attempt to resurrect the name of Frederic Bird, the memories of whose earlier work in the field had been marred by the controversy surrounding his use of exploratory incisions, described in Chapter 3. Samuel Lane's nephew also wrote to the *British Medical Journal* in 1884 to remind readers that his uncle performed the first successful ovariotomy in London, while the physician Heywood Smith wrote to the *Lancet* to claim that his father, Protheroe Smith, had performed a successful ovariotomy even before Charles Clay. Jonathan Potter, 'The History of Ovariotomy', *British Medical Journal* 2, no. 678 (27 December 1873): 770–771; James R. Lane, 'The Revival of Ovariotomy', *British Medical Journal* 2, no. 1250 (13 December 1884): 1212; Heywood Smith, 'The Early History of Ovariotomy', *The Lancet* 142, no. 3658 (7 October 1893): 898.

67. 'Ovariotomy', *British Medical Journal* 1, no. 1016 (19 June 1880): 931–932.

68. Clay claimed that Simpson had written to him 'my dear Dr. Clay, the operation is your own; none can rob you of your claim. Call it ovariotomy, not peritoneal section'. Charles Clay, 'History of Ovariotomy', *British Medical Journal* 2, no. 1020 (17 July 1880): 110.

69. Lawson Tait, 'The Revival of Ovariotomy', *British Medical Journal* 2, no. 1249 (6 December 1884): 1165.

70. 'Dublin', *Lancet* 82, no. 2098 (14 November 1863): 578–579.

71. 'Obituary: Charles Clay', *Lancet* 142, no. 3657 (30 September 1893): 846.

72. David N. Livingstone, *Putting Science in Its Place: Geographies of Scientific Knowledge* (Chicago: The University of Chicago Press, 2003), 1.

73. 'Progress in a French Point of View', *New Monthly Magazine* 131, no. 523 (1864): 255.

74. Thomas Spencer Wells, 'On the History and Progress of Ovariotomy in Great Britain', *Medico-Chirurgical Transactions* 46 (1863): 36.

75. 'Ovariotomy in New Zealand', *Medical Times and Gazette* (16 June 1866): 640.

76. 'Medical Annotations: A Laurel for English Surgeons', *Lancet* 79, no. 2001 (4 January 1862): 12.

77. 'The Week', *British Medical Journal* 2, no. 201 (5 November 1864): 528.

78. 'Reviews and Notices of Books', *British Medical Journal* 2, no. 239 (29 July 1865): 121.

79. Jean Delaporte, 'Hydropsie Enkistée de l'Ovarie Attaquée Par Incision', *Mémoires de l'Académie Royale de Chirurgie* 2 (1753): 455.

80. Graeme Gooday, 'Lies, Damned Lies and Declinism: Lyon Playfair, the Paris 1867 Exhibition and the Contested Rhetorics of Scientific Education and Industrial Performance', in *The Golden Age: Essays in British Social and Economic History, 1850–1870*, ed. Ian Inkster (Aldershot: Ashgate, 2000), 105–120, 116. English patent law would be unable to protect against this.

81. His most famous invention was 'Gamgee tissue', a new type of dry, absorbent surgical dressing which contained cotton wool.

82. Sampson Gamgee, 'The Present State of Surgery in Paris', *Lancet* 90, no. 2296 (31 August 1867): 273.

83. Sampson Gamgee, 'The Present State of Surgery in Paris', *Lancet* 90, no. 2313 (28 December 1867): 802.

84. John Erichsen, 'Impressions of American Surgery', *Lancet* 104, no. 2673 (21 November 1874): 717.

85. Randolph E. Peaslee, *Ovarian Tumors: Their Pathology, Diagnosis and Treatment, Especially by Ovariotomy* (New York: D. Appleton, 1872), 247.

In a situation akin to that of Charles Clay, Philadelphia surgeon Washington Atlee was the only surgeon performing the operation with consistency in America during the 1850s and 1860s, but with little publicity of his operations.

86. John Burnham, 'The *British Medical Journal* in America', in *Medical Journals and Medical Knowledge: Historical Essays*, ed. William F. Bynum, Stephen Lock, and Roy Porter (London and New York: Routledge, 1992), 166.

87. Peaslee, *Ovarian Tumors*, 250.

88. However, even McDowell's legacy was threatened. As Jean Bowra has noted, the partial excision of an ovary by Scottish surgeon Robert Houstoun in 1701 was, by the late nineteenth century, being claimed by some British surgeons to have been the first ovariotomy rather than Ephraim McDowell's procedure in 1809. Lawson Tait, in particular, championed this version of ovariotomy's history. Jean Bowra, 'Making a Man a Great Man: Ephraim McDowell, Ovariotomy and History', http://eprints.qut.edu.au/3454/1/3454.pdf (Paper Presented to the Social Change in the 21st Century Conference, Centre for Social Change Research, Queensland University of Technology, 28 October 2005): 4.

89. Deleso Alford Washington, 'Critical Race Feminist Bioethics: Telling Stories in Law School and Medical School in Pursuit of "Cultural Competency"', *Albany Law Review* 72, no. 4 (2009): 972.

90. James Marion Sims, *The Story of My Life* (New York: D. Appleton, 1884), 228.

91. Washington, 'Critical Race Feminist Bioethics', 964.

92. Lawrence D. Longo, 'The Rise and Fall of Battey's Operation: A Fashion in Surgery', *Bulletin of the History of Medicine* 53, no. 2 (1979): 249.

93. 'Obstetrical Society of London', *Lancet* 89, no. 2275 (1867): 429–441. The Obstetrical Society called a special meeting to consider the fate of Brown and for members to vote as to whether he should be expelled from the organisation. The debate, published in the *Lancet*, makes for fascinating reading. Society members packed into the crowded hall to hear the case for and against Brown, although his fate was likely sealed before he had even entered the room, for Brown's supporters were few and far between by this point. The surgeon was barely able to speak before jeers broke out. He was expelled with 194 votes for and 38 against.

94. Robert Battey, *Normal Ovariotomy* (Atlanta: Herald Publishing Company, 1873), 5. As quoted in Longo, 'The Rise and Fall of Battey's Operation', 249.

95. James Marion Sims, 'Remarks on Battey's Operation', *British Medical Journal* 2, no. 877 (29 December 1877): 918.

96. Alexander Russell Simpson, 'History of a Case of Double Oophorectomy, or Battey's Operation: With Remarks', *British Medical Journal* 1, no. 960 (24 May 1879): 763.

97. Alfred Hegar, Robert Battey and Thomas Spencer Wells, 'Castration for Nervous and Mental Diseases: A Symposium', *American Journal of Medical Sciences* 184 (1886): 455–490.

98. Lawson Tait, 'Removal of the Uterine Appendages', *British Medical Journal* 2, no. 1125 (22 July 1882): 153. For more on Tait's operation, see Regina Morantz-Sanchez, *Conduct Unbecoming A Woman: Medicine on Trial in Turn-of-the-Century Brooklyn* (Oxford: Oxford University Press, 1999), 100.

99. Thomas Spencer Wells, *Modern Abdominal Surgery: The Bradshaw Lecture Delivered at the Royal College of Surgeons of England. With an Appendix on the Castration of Women* (London: J. A. Churchill, 1891), 35.

100. Wells, *Modern Abdominal Surgery*, 42.

101. Wells, *Modern Abdominal Surgery*, 43.

102. Wells, *Modern Abdominal Surgery*, 36.

103. Letter from Sir Henry Thompson to Ernest Hart (29 August 1886) MS 5424/13; emphasis in original (Wellcome Collection).

5

The Business of Surgery

MEDICINE, MONEY AND MORALITY

Ovariotomy was the product of a medical culture that had a convoluted relationship with money. Two differing ideas regarding doctors' financial interests had long been present within the profession. One was that doctors should be impartial providers of the best possible care for their patients, motivated primarily by humane and altruistic concerns. The other was that they were men of trade, profiting financially from attending the sick. It was a dichotomy that had first been explicitly clarified in Britain by the Scottish physician John Gregory in his popular guide to ethical doctoring, *Observations on the Duties and Offices of a Physician* (1770). Gregory did not necessarily see these two identities as incompatible.[1] But that such a distinction could be made was to factor into one of the most complex quandaries nineteenth-century doctors faced: how to make money while retaining a moral foundation to one's practice. As Gregory's work suggests, this concern was not new to the Victorian era. But by the middle decades of the nineteenth century, rhetorical strategies were increasingly being employed by doctors to prise medicine away from any notion of it being motivated by personal gain. This was part of a wider move towards driving out medical corruption in all its forms, and establishing a more regulated profession.[2] Increasingly, as the ethics around money-making in medicine began to be realigned, medical practitioners were drawn into a torturous relationship with their finances, as growing constraint was put upon discussion of money. And yet, every individual doctor remained deeply in the thrall of economic circumstance.[3]

With the 'rise' of social history in the late twentieth century and that discipline's prevailing concern with class and material wealth, historians of medicine have been attentive to the relationship between medicine and money with its complexities, confusions and occlusions. In relation to surgery, historian Sally Wilde has rightly concluded that it is unsatisfactory to consider the economics of surgery as 'driven exclusively by the logic of market forces', and argues that the influence of the moral economy must be examined too.[4] Yet aside from Wilde, economic work on the history of surgery, especially in its nineteenth-century context, has been scant. The historiographic trend towards scrutinising divisions (or lack thereof) between 'orthodox' and 'unorthodox' practitioners, and in thinking about the commercialisation of medicine through the prism of patent medicines, has generated significant work.[5] But as a trend it also suggests historians have been embedded in—perhaps even confused by—the Victorian profession's guarded attitude towards money matters. To focus upon patent medicines, devices, advertising and other of medical men's forays into explicitly commercial medicine is to draw away from explorations of the implicit role money played in all areas of medicine—including operative surgery. It reinforces an arbitrary division between commercial and non-commercial forms of medicine when, in reality, all modes of medical practice had some kind of relationship to commerce. Dig a little deeper, and the question of pecuniary gain permeates professional discourse; money was everywhere, even where its presence was not immediately obvious.[6]

Ovariotomy was closely embedded in this moral-economic nexus and its financial implications were of particular importance in the last twenty-five years of the century when the operation came to be definitively recognised as a successful and perhaps even revolutionary procedure. It was a time when a great deal else was happening in the field; the introduction of antiseptics had an influential effect on surgery, although as we shall see, its use in ovariotomy was greatly contested. There was also increasing concern about the overuse of the operation, something which has been well addressed by historians, but which requires a more critical examination of the financial implications entangled within it. Thus, the intention of this chapter is to offer a new approach to the period by setting the expansion of the operation within a discourse of trade and business, rather than reading it solely through changing notions of

female pathology—although the two concerns were by no means separate. Increasingly, ovariotomy was understood as an innovation of specialist and private practice, as those who performed the operation began
to be identified (and identified themselves) as specialist 'ovariotomists'.
It could also be an expensive operation and its price was determined by
a multitude of factors, some of which were closely connected to its status as an innovative procedure. Its value was also entwined with broader
debates that were occurring in the profession as to the need for more
regulation and guidance in relation to professional income. In the 1880s
and 1890s, in Europe and America, ovariotomy was derided by some as
a 'fashion', as growing concerns were voiced regarding the frequency
with which ovarian operations were being performed. This led to troubling questions regarding the impact of ovariotomy's remunerative
nature upon medical authority. 'Ovariotomies are a source of income;
many have grown rich on them and you strike at the root of a very thriving industry', wrote one correspondent to the *Journal of the American
Medical Association* in 1896, responding to a critique of the operation.[7]
Was it possible, as commentators inferred, that ovariotomy had become
nothing more than a business? By the end of the century, this question
was coming to dominate discourse around the operation, as its respectability and justifiability were once more called into question.

THE OPERATOR BECOMES THE OVARIOTOMIST: SPECIALISM AND PRIVATE PRACTICE

The mid-to-late nineteenth century is usually characterised as a period
that saw the 'rise' of hospital medicine; that is, that medical theory, practice and innovation became centred within the walls of the large general hospitals.[8] Surgical advance in particular has been closely linked to
the changes brought about by the establishment of antiseptic and aseptic
techniques in the 1870s and 1880s, and especially the germ theory and
wound management system of Joseph Lister, which in itself informed
late nineteenth-century visions of the hospital space as a locale of cleanliness and social order.[9] Lister himself saw the decline in hospital fever
(hospital-acquired infection) as his most important achievement.[10]

The idea, once pervasive, that Lister's theory and practice constituted
a rapid and uncontested 'revolution' in surgery has been dispelled by historians. It is clear that not only did Lister himself frequently modify his

system, but many surgeons were either sceptical of his theories or, as was more often the case, his practice.[11] Many failed to see what was novel or innovative about his system, when the majority of surgeons already employed scrupulous aseptic techniques in their practice.[12] Ovariotomy frequently featured in these debates. While many ovariotomists used and even championed Lister's techniques, in no other field of surgery was the usefulness of the antiseptic system more fiercely contested. Some practitioners expressed doubts about the effectiveness of the system when used within the abdomen. The peritoneum—the membranous covering of the abdominal cavity—was known to have rapid absorbing qualities, and if the peritoneum was found to be in a healthy state upon opening the abdomen, the combination of a drainage tube and the tissue's natural absorption mechanism was seen as sufficient in preventing any build-ups of fluid that could lead to putrefaction, a view even Lister himself appeared to have endorsed.[13] Even more persuasive to opponents of Listerian antisepsis was the fact that operators like Thomas Keith in Edinburgh had had great success with ovariotomy some time before the introduction of carbolic acid for the treatment of surgical wounds. Keith was a quiet, guarded man who rarely involved himself in the controversies of the day, not least one that involved his friend and contemporary Joseph Lister. But in a letter to the *British Medical Journal* in 1878, Keith set out his position. While believing that antiseptics, overall, had improved his results, he argued that technical developments like the use of drainage tubes, the wide-scale application of the cautery (rather than the clamp) when treating the pedicle, and the introduction of compression forceps had been of equal importance in precipitating a declining mortality rate for ovariotomy.[14] Other prominent practitioners of the operation were, however, more damning in their assessment of antiseptics. Robert Lawson Tait, for example, was an avowed opponent of the Listerian system of surgery.

Debates about technical developments in antiseptics only barely masked the fact that claims to the professional landscape—and its pecuniary rewards—were at stake. A source of particular tension was the relationship between ovariotomy, innovation and hospital medicine. Ovariotomies were increasingly performed in general hospitals towards the end of the century. But up until the 1890s, the majority of ovarian operations still continued to take place in private lodgings (including patients' homes) or in smaller specialist hospitals for women, the latter of which included both charitable and private institutions.[15]

This was reflected in the professional positions of those who had become pre-eminent in the field: both Thomas Spencer Wells at the Samaritan Free Hospital and Robert Lawson Tait at the Birmingham and Midland Hospital for Women retained their high status without ever having an appointment at one of the large teaching hospitals. Charles Clay had resigned his position at St. Mary's Hospital in Manchester in 1858 after just one year, due, he claimed, to the burden of his private practice, and never had a hospital affiliation again, even a specialist one. Although his lack of institutional work would lead to his respectability later being questioned by Wells, as described in Chapter 4, it did little harm to his local reputation and practice, the latter of which remained sizeable.[16] Many specialists in ovarian disease, including George Granville Bantock, Wells' successor at the Samaritan, Thomas Keith and Lawson Tait also set up private nursing homes for their ovariotomy patients.[17]

As the Manchester practitioner David Lloyd Roberts—who made a fortune out of his practice in ovariotomy—once quipped, it seemed that 'a hospital was useful to a man during the first ten years on the staff; during the second ten years, honours were about equal; during the third ten years the man was useful to the hospital'.[18] Charitable hospitals, which paid their medical staff nothing more than an honorarium, were only ever one arrow in the quiver of the successful doctor, providing prestige, honour and clinical material to complement the private work through which they made their money. As the careers of practitioners progressed, they often became increasingly immersed in private practice. Wells was a case in point: he retired from the Samaritan in 1877 aged fifty-nine, but his private practice flourished for another decade, his reputation both as a charitable and skilful operator established enough that he could focus on private cases. The career trajectories of the top ovariotomists support the observation made by Marguerite Dupree and Anne Crowther that during this time 'specialists' in diseases of women and in obstetrics were especially notable for their tendency to remain attached to smaller hospitals throughout their career and, in general, were less dependent on appointments at larger, charitable institutions for the provision of social cachet.[19]

The understanding that ovariotomists were specialists had important currency in medical politics, as debates raged in the profession as to the value of specialist practice in general. Medical specialists of all kinds, particularly those who set up their own institutions, had long faced hostility from within the profession. Many practitioners continued to ascribe to

the idea that hospitals which catered to specific types of disease were little more than money-making ploys, ostensibly charitable, but in fact set
up only to gain the patronage and support of the rich, who could then
be used to gain a precious foothold in the market for private practice.
Those who described themselves as specialists in diseases of women were
often considered the most avaricious of all.[20] A pamphlet which appeared
in 1877, wittily entitled *Contradiction! Or English Medical Men and
Manners*, authored by a practitioner named James O'Flanagan, reserved
particular venom for specialists in female disease. O'Flanagan played on
the word 'speculum', the instrument used to make vaginal examinations,
to insinuate the unsavoury financial aspects to this particular specialist's
relationships with their patients:

> If named after his occupation he would have – as in some other trades he
> has – the amiable title of "ladies' man". I propose however, to call this
> gentleman the speculum specialist......from nervousness or indigestion or
> hysteria, and certain deranged functions, a woman gets it into her head
> that she is a subject for the speculum. She sets out, is "speculated" upon,
> and re-returns to the operation with periodicity in recurrence equal to a
> complete repetend in circulating decimal fractions.[21]

Despite these connotations of impropriety, as ovariotomy became more
successful, those who performed it became confident in—and increasingly protective of—the operation's status as a specialist procedure.
Indeed, in the eyes of those practitioners who saw the development of
specialism in medicine as a sign of growing maturity in the profession,
ovariotomy was a prime example of a genuine innovation that had ema-
nated from private and specialist practice and not from the larger hospitals, whose emphasis on the systematic management of large numbers of
patients was viewed as a hindrance to innovation rather than a catalyst.
'Are the triumphs of ovariotomy and abdominal section to be reckoned
among "the great advancements" which have come from general hospitals?' wrote the laryngologist and ardent advocate of specialism, Morell
Mackenzie in 1885, 'the fact is that a general hospital is about the last
place from which one would naturally expect any striking innovation to
come. Such institutions are from the conditions of their existence schools
of routine'.[22]

Many ovariotomists wished to see the procedure retain a distinctive
identity, performed only by those with 'special' skill in the area. This was

in part a response to technical concerns: the alleged incompatibility of ovariotomy with Listerian antisepsis, claimed by some surgeons, seemed to clarify continued, fundamental differences between surgery that ventured into the abdomen and that which did not. But layered upon this were deep-seated professional and financial implications. Much to the chagrin of some specialists, general hospital surgeons were increasingly asserting their right to perform the operation, arguing that antiseptics and the general move towards scrupulous cleanliness had had a democratising effect on ovariotomy, opening the abdomen to all who practised clean, safe surgery. As Ornella Moscucci has highlighted, the economic implications of this were clear: if general hospital surgeons took up the operation with regularity, they would eventually gain a foothold in the market for private ovariotomies too.[23]

It was perhaps for these reasons that the term 'ovariotomist' was one increasingly used in the medical press during the 1880s.[24] Along with 'lithotomist' it was one of the few titles used to denote an operator's special skill at one particular operation. The way the term was used was varied and not always clear-cut. Occasionally it meant anyone who performed ovariotomy; after all, surgeons were, by this point, generally expected to be trained in and ready to perform the operation if necessary in an emergency situation, an operation as essential to the young surgeon's repertoire as amputation, lithotomy or ligation. It was also on occasion a label thrust upon others with derogatory connotations, particularly in the early days of the operation. But for the most part 'ovariotomist' was a term of self-identification used with pride by those who performed ovariotomies frequently. It referred to a particular *identity*: those who considered themselves and were considered by others as especially skilled and experienced in the operation. By sculpting a reputation for specialist surgical skill, successful ovariotomists were also able to manoeuvre themselves into the surgical elite, in spite of their professional rivalries with general surgeons. This was especially the case for ovariotomists practising in London, many of whom played important roles in the city's surgical societies.[25] Thus, as British medicine began to remould itself into a bifurcate model of 'consultants' (those who were in the elite of 'pure' physicians and surgeons) and general practitioners, ovariotomists slipped easily into the former group. As Dupree and Crowther have argued, this division between general practitioner and consultant was not necessarily one with any definitive demarcations of practice; a reputation as a surgical 'consultant' was cultivated rather than acquired with any inevitability. Nor was a definition of surgical skill set in stone; rather understandings of skill were heavily dependent on their context and often re-imagined depending on the individual characteristics and motivations of prominent surgeons of the day.[26] Asserting surgical skill, it is fair to say, was often in part a rhetorical device and not always an exact reflection of technical proficiency. It was not unusual for obituaries and biographical recollections of elite surgeons in the late nineteenth century to note a relative lack of technical ability on the subject's part, suggesting the importance of other qualities like sociability, personality and a carefully cultivated reputation for intellectualism that could equally play a role in propelling one to the higher echelons of the profession.[27] Thomas Spencer Wells' assistant at the Samaritan Hospital, Alban Doran, for example, despite being a successful ovariotomist, was described in one obituary as 'having no surgical hands' but was remembered as a 'learned and accurate litterateur'.[28] And yet to attain a position as a consultant-level practitioner had significant financial implications. Elite surgeons could build lucrative practices, trading on their reputation and standing. This was perhaps nowhere more so the case than in the practice of ovariotomy, where the financial rewards could be significant.

Surgical Fees: Determining the Cost of Ovariotomy

The suggestion that ovarian surgery was especially remunerative was present from its beginnings and in the earlier days of the operation it was an association that was almost invariably negative. No one had emphasised the operation's connection with money more so than its staunchest critic, Robert Lee. In 1862, when Lee was still actively denouncing the operation, and at one of the many meetings around this time where practitioners argued over its justifiability, the obstetrician had declared that 'the question now under discussion was a money question, and not one of science and humanity'. Lee defended this claim by producing anecdotal evidence that at least one English ovariotomist had charged the rather extraordinary sum of three hundred guineas for an operation performed in Ireland, and had expected a hundred guineas each day afterwards that he was to be in attendance. Lee reported that the operation had resulted in the death of the patient just eighteen hours later.[29]

While Lee could well have been exaggerating the fees demanded in this particular case, they were by no means figures pulled out of the air. Although a private ovariotomy could be purchased for as little as five guineas, if you were lucky enough to find a surgeon willing to perform on poorer cases, fees for private ovariotomies in London and in the major metropolitan cities could easily stretch to a hundred guineas.[30] Indeed, this appears to have been the accepted price for an ovariotomy from around the 1860s until at least the mid-1880s.[31] Given the oblique manner in which doctors discussed money, few ovariotomists directly addressed the question of how much they earned. But this did not prevent the subject being speculated upon in the medical press, although noticeably more so in the pages of the American journals than the British, as in the former, doctors' finances were more openly discussed. As *The American Practitioner* put it in 1877, rumour had it that Thomas Spencer Wells did 'not lift a knife for less than one hundred guineas'—a claim that Wells never directly denied.[32] As Ornella Moscucci has shown, such a fee was about equal to the annual income of a doctor in the early years of their practice, thus underscoring the appeal the operation might have held for a young practitioner.[33]

Extending this comparison with wages into the broader economic context of nineteenth-century income, one gains an understanding of just how expensive a private ovariotomy was. One study of nineteenth-century wages has posited the average annual income in 1871 for an engineer at around £579, that of a Government employee at around £281 and that of a schoolmaster at just £97.[34] It seems likely, then, that most sufferers of ovarian disease seeking surgery would have been priced out of the private market and that for all but the reasonably well-off, the services of a charitable institution would need to be sought instead, be it one of the larger hospitals or, as was more likely, through the charity of a specialist institution like the Samaritan Hospital. A supplement that appeared in the *Lancet* in 1886 as part of a Hospital Sunday Fund appeal, and likely aimed towards the wider public, seems to confirm this. The appeal claimed that every hospital-based ovariotomy cost the institution a sizeable £10, mainly because of the amount and intensity of nursing that was required after an ovariotomy was completed.[35] Keen to draw attention to the amount of surgical work that was dependent on charity, the appeal noted that in the case of ovariotomy, 'except with well-to-do people, the doctors mostly recommend the hospital'.[36]

Thus, while the private ovariotomy market was lucrative it was also small; to pursue a career as an ovariotomist was a high-risk strategy in terms of regular income generation. Practitioners were nonetheless cognisant of the appeal that brilliant operations could retain among their younger brethren, especially in comparison with the more routine work of minor operations and obstetrical deliveries. Besides which, the operation was now safer than it had ever been. So much so that Thomas Keith was moved to remark in 1878 that 'it almost makes one envy the younger ovariotomist to whom the way in these days is made easy', calling into question the assertion of specialists that ovariotomy still required a specific skill set.[37] The appeal of ovariotomy rested on its dramatic history and the operation continued to engender a sense of daring, of singularity, of being something *special*. It was a combination of factors that gave performers of the operation a visible authority. Major operative surgery, with its sense of urgency and drama, had an electric impact.[38] It could offer a potential one-off quick fix for chronic conditions that made patients miserable and socially isolated. It was precisely in these terms that surgeon and ovariotomist Isaac Baker Brown framed a successful surgical case in 1865 that had taken place at the London Surgical Home for Women, an institution set up by Brown in 1858, where patients paid fees according to what they could afford. Conveying a sense of desperation on the woman's part, Brown recounted how she had:

> Spent her substance in obtaining medical aid, but God had not seen fit to give her relief. She was a patient sufferer truly, and a great invalid when she came into this Home. I said to her "I think I can cure you, but the operation is new; it is almost experimental" she replied – "Do what you like;" and I think her expression was "Cut me to pieces, if you can cure me." [39]

Nowhere more so was this drama apparent than with ovariotomy, where the change in condition—the removal of a large tumour—was immediately noticeable to the patient and her friends and family. This had numerous economic implications. Specifically, it meant ovariotomists could imply that their services, despite their high prices, were actually a more financially sensible option than continually resorting to medical palliatives. More broadly one can speculate upon the appeal that specialising in ovariotomy would have had in what was a rather gloomy economic climate in Britain in the 1870s and 1880s. Most economic historians agree that if there was not a depression per se, the 1870s did see a tailing off of the economic boom that had characterised the mid-century, when new technological industries had rapidly expanded.[40] As a result, the 1870s and 1880s were times of comparatively slow growth. Doctors were aware of this and worried about the consequences of commercial depression upon their profession. This showed itself in renewed anxieties about overcrowding, much of which centred upon the idea that medical schools were overfilled with unsuitable students, men who in brighter economic circumstances would have gone into business and industry, but who were instead entering into an already overcrowded profession, selecting medicine because of a dearth of other opportunities.[41] Medicine, it was feared, was increasingly viewed in stark economic terms by young men as the profession which would give the quickest financial return.[42] With the passing of the 1876 Medical Act, which allowed women to qualify as doctors in Britain, fears were further stoked about increased crowding and competition from women, particularly for female patients, which might lead to male doctors' income being reduced.[43]

How much substance there was to claims about overcrowding is debatable, but the spectre of it touched a raw nerve in doctors. Economic questions began to place high on the agenda of the weekly medical press.[44] Many felt that, disproportionately to other occupations, those in the medical profession were not sufficiently rewarded for their services, and that their fees were incompatible with their status as men of culture and refinement.[45] It compelled medical men to address an issue that it could be difficult to talk about openly without risking accusations of impropriety: making money. Of particular concern was the damage inflicted by the tradition of the annual billing system that most practitioners worked under and which, as Anne Digby has shown, often resulted in large patient debts remaining unpaid for long periods of time, if not permanently.[46] This frequently left doctors having to chase down their debtors in a manner considered undignified to the learned practitioner. The crudeness of the financial exchange was a perennial concern in the profession. What marked out the debates emerging in the 1870s was concern over correctly identifying the *value* of medical and surgical services.[47] The *British Medical Journal* became the central focus point for this campaign and the journal pushed for the British Medical Association to produce a thoroughly investigated, standardised scale of fees to counteract the generic prices for medical services usually charged, which did little to connect specific financial values to different services. In 1878, the *British Medical Journal* wrote that:

> It is somewhat disgusting for the professional mind to have to discuss fees at all. This sentiment is materially expressed by the piece of paper in which the fee is habitually wrapped, and the tacit manner in which it is paid. But advantage should not be taken of this attempt to bind professional men to the uniform acceptance of an insufficient payment for services of very various value.[48]

Practitioners wrote in to express gratitude to the journal for vocalising a taboo subject. As one grateful correspondent put it, 'I feel sure you have struck off once and for all the galling fetter of the uniform guinea-fee'.[49]

The British Medical Association itself never produced a definitive scale of fees. But various other medical societies did, some of them affiliated branches of the Association. These scales were often limited in their coverage and especially so in relation to surgery. In their tariff of medical fees issued in 1879 for example, the Manchester Medico-Ethical Association refused to make a judgment regarding the costs of surgery, including suggested fees only for general practitioners and consulting physicians' visits and advice. 'The Association cannot undertake to define individual skill or reputation in this respect', it decreed. This remained the case throughout the editions of the tariff produced in the following decades.[50] The reluctance to judge the financial value of operations perpetuated the idea of surgical skill as esoteric, its value beyond the judgment of those outside the surgical profession. It also left a nebulous gap in the pricing of major operations, in which the value of different procedures was left to be self-defined by surgeons, suggesting how much more lucrative surgery could potentially be compared to medicine.

But why, some observers reasoned, construct scales of fees only for surgery to be left out? There was a vague understanding among practitioners that all operations which imposed a serious risk to life—ovariotomy, lithotomy and major amputations—should cost at least a hundred guineas, and many felt that leaving prices to individual judgement was not desirable.[51] In 1874 there appeared the first tariff in Britain that addressed the issue. The pamphlet, titled *The Medico-Chirurgical Tariffs* (Fig. 5.1), was authored by Jukes de Styrap, a general practitioner who would later solidify his reputation as an authority upon issues of medical morality with his well-known work *A Code of Medical Ethics* (1878).[52] Written on behalf of the Shropshire branch of the British Medical Association and with four further editions produced, *The Medico-Chirurgical Tariffs* was the first of its kind to include a suggested scale of operative fees.[53] Prices were given for over sixty surgical operations and the pamphlet was envisioned as a guide to general practitioners as well as younger physicians and surgeons starting out in their career. Thus, the prices given were considerably lower than those that London consultants were charging. Indeed, to the disappointment of some reviewers, de Styrap, like others, had avoided

General Surgical Practitioners.	Minimum.			Medium Fees.	Maximum.		
	£	s.	d.	£ s. d.	£	s.	d.
For the Talicotian Operation	5	5	o	to	21	0	o
For the operation for the removal of a Nævus or Aneurism by Anastomosis	1	1	o		5	5	o
For the operation for the removal of Cicatrices	1	1	o		5	5	o
For the operation of Dermic-Grafting ...		10	6		3	3	o
For the operation for Cleft-Palate ...	5	5	o		15	15	o
For the operation for Hare-Lip	2	2	o		10	10	o
For the removal of Polypus Nasi... ...		10	6		5	5	o
For the removal of Foreign bodies from the Ear, Eye, Nose, Pharynx, or Œsophagus		10	6		2	2	o
For the operation of Tracheotomy ...	3	3	o		10	10	o
For the introduction of the Stomach Pump	1	1	o		3	3	o
For the operation of Trocar-Suction-or 'Aspiration'	1	1	o		5	5	o
For Paracentesis Thoracis	2	2	o		5	5	o
For Paracentesis Abdominis	1	1	o		5	5	o
For the reduction of Hernia by Taxis ...	1	1	o		5	5	o
For the operation for Strangulated Hernia	5	5	o		15	15	o
For the operation of Cholecystotomy ...	5	5	o		21	0	o
For the operation of Colotomy	5	5	o		15	15	o
For the operation of Duodenostomy ...	5	5	o		21	0	o
For the operation of Enterostomy ...	5	5	o		15	15	o
For the operation of Gastrostomy ...	5	5	o		15	15	o
For the operation of Hysterectomy ...	10	10	o		21	0	o
For the operation of Laparotomy... ...	5	5	o		21	0	o
For the operation of Laryngotomy ...	3	3	o		10	10	o
For the operation of Lithotomy	10	10	o		26	5	o
For the operation of Lithotrity	5	5	o		26	5	o
For the operation of Nephrotomy ...	10	10	o		21	0	o
For the operation of Œsophagotomy ...	3	3	o		10	10	o
For the operation of Ovariotomy... ...	15	15	o		31 10 o and upwards.		
For the operation of Pneumotomy ...	5	5	o		15	15	o
For the operation of Prostatectomy ...	3	3	o		10	10	o
For the operation of Pylorectomy ...	5	5	o		15	15	o
For the operation of Splenotomy... ...	10	10	o		26	5	o

(Medium Fees column, running vertically:) Any sum intermediate between the specified 'Minimum' and 'Maximum' Fees that the practitioner may deem just to his patient, the profession, and himself.

Fig. 5.1 Table taken from the fifth edition of Jukes de Styrap's *The Medico-Chirurgical Tariffs*, a popular reference manual for general practitioners and young surgeons and physicians, published in 1890. Even though ovariotomy was no longer new, it remained more expensive than comparatively riskier operations such as hysterectomy, nephrotomy or splenotomy, and was the only operation to appear on de Styrap's extensive list with a note in the maximum fee column that suggested an almost unlimited price tag upon a private procedure, denoted by the insertion of 'and upwards' (*Credit* Wellcome Collection CC BY)

suggesting prices that doctors of consultant level might charge, where pricing remained at the discretion of the practitioner.[54] Nonetheless de Styrap's pamphlet was warmly welcomed by the profession. As the *Edinburgh Medical Journal* put it, de Styrap's work taught 'the young practitioner promptitude, business habits, and consideration both for his own position and the circumstances of his patient'.[55] Reconceptualising fees was not just about getting the 'right' price but about efficient management of medical practice. This was connected to a broader shift in late nineteenth-century medicine towards managerial efficiency, inspired in part by the increasingly important role of administration and management in hospitals.[56]

De Styrap's work served not only to clarify just how remunerative ovariotomy was but, as it was produced by a branch of the British Medical Association, to morally authenticate it being so. In the 1890 edition, de Styrap suggested as a general guide that ovariotomies were to be charged at between '£15/15 and £31/10 and upwards' and throughout the editions of the pamphlet, ovariotomy and caesarean section were deemed by de Styrap to be the most expensive operations in surgery.[57] But de Styrap also pointedly demarcated between ovariotomy and caesarean section by his use of the phrase 'and upwards' after the suggested price for ovariotomy, seemingly giving practitioners a licence to charge whatever they wanted for the operation. To no other operation or service in his table did de Styrap apply those two telling words. This was despite the appearance by then of operations which were arguably riskier than ovariotomy; splenotomy (incision into the spleen) for example, which had only been introduced into practice in the mid-1880s, was given a suggested price of between £10. 10s and £26. 5s, while nephrotomy (an incision into the kidney), also new and risky, was priced at between £10. 10s and £21, as was hysterectomy. The price of hysterectomy is especially striking, given that by the 1880s, ovariotomy was comparatively safer and more established than hysterectomy, which had replaced the former as the most dreaded of abdominal operations. Like ovariotomy, there had been a chequered history of experimentation with hysterectomy from the mid-century onwards. In the early 1880s, the mortality rate for abdominal hysterectomy remained abysmal, around seventy per cent, far worse than for ovariotomy. Primarily this was due to the complex vascular tissues of the uterus which carried a high risk of haemorrhage.[58] The year 1885 had seen a wisp of hope with Thomas Keith's successes with the operation. He reported that of his total of thirty-eight cases he had had only three deaths—the most successful set of hysterectomies yet to be reported.[59] But the operation remained a fearful prospect, belying the idea that antiseptic and aseptic techniques had acted as some kind of panacea for surgeons who ventured into the abdomen. Even the provocative Robert Lawson Tait, who performed ovariotomy with a certain abandon, quivered at the thought of extirpating the uterus and his mortality rate for the operation reached over thirty-five per cent. This was far beyond any of the other abdominal operations he performed, for which he had achieved some of the lowest mortality rates in the country.[60] The *British Medical Journal* paraphrased Tait translating his horror of the operation into tangible, pecuniary terms: 'he has stated...that the amount of worry which is given him by every case of hysterectomy, even when successful, is such as to be almost beyond the recompense of any fee' the journal reported.[61]

De Styrap's tariff acted only as a guide for practitioners who were not at a consultant level. A well-known ovariotomist like Thomas Spencer Wells, or a successful lithotomist such as Henry Thompson remained at liberty to charge what they wished.[62] Nonetheless the recommendations of *The Medico-Chirurgical Tariffs* had the respect of the profession and its suggestions were taken seriously in light of there being few other similar works for doctors to look to. De Styrap assured readers that the prices were devised using the advice of specialists in each field rather than based solely on his own estimations (suggesting that an ovariotomist had informed de Styrap's judgment of the operation's price).[63] The pricing of ovariotomy by de Styrap poses significant questions about how exactly its pecuniary value was determined and why it continued to be deemed the most expensive operation a practitioner could undertake. Undoubtedly, operative risk was one of the key factors in its pricing, although the risk being compensated for was not so much that to the patient's life but that to the surgeon's professional reputation and even their wellbeing. Despite Keith's assertion about the comparative ease of performing ovariotomy by the 1880s, every performance of it remained mired in risk for the patient. Intertwined with that risk was also a potentially traumatic experience for the surgeon if the operation was difficult or if it failed, and this in itself acted

as a major constraint upon their choice to operate. A high price, therefore, essentially acted as a form of pecuniary compensation for the
anxieties produced by the possible death of a patient and subsequent
damage that might be done to one's reputation. As one American surgeon described his experiences with ovariotomy in 1884, with unusual
candour, 'in 1883, 1881 and 1882....my ovariotomies died right off
as fast as I could operate upon them. It made me so sick, that I could
scarcely bear to hear of a case of ovariotomy'.[64]

The price was also likely inflated by the professional risks specific
to those who performed major surgery upon the female reproductive
organs. All doctors who specialised in diseases of women were susceptible to charges of misconduct, mistreatment or immodesty. As a
consequence, cultivating a professional identity of chivalrous protec-
tor to one's delicate female patients was important.[65] At least three
ovariotomists, Isaac Baker Brown, the scandal surrounding whom
was discussed in the last chapter, Heywood Smith and Francis Imlach,
failed to do so and had their careers brought to virtual ruin by controversies in their practice. Heywood Smith had been revealed in 1886
to have assisted the controversial journalist W. T. Stead in his investigations into child prostitution for the *Pall Mall Gazette*. Stead had
'purchased' a thirteen-year-old girl as part of his exposé into the trade
in young virgins. In an effort to prevent Stead from being accused of
sexually assaulting her, Smith had been drafted in to prove the girl's
virginity through a vaginal examination, in what was seen by the profession as a flagrantly immoral and unprofessional act; Smith only
narrowly avoided expulsion from the Obstetrical Society.[66] Liverpool
surgeon Francis Imlach also received public criticism in 1886 when
he was alleged to have removed both ovaries from a woman without
her consent, an episode which resulted in legal action, and which will
be discussed in more detail in the next section. The financial impact
on all three men was catastrophic. Brown, who at the height of his
powers had received considerable patronage from the wealthy and
elite of London, died virtually penniless, supported in his final years
only by the charity of a few sympathetic members of the profession.
Smith fared a little better, having managed to resurrect a semblance of
a career after the scandal and went on to set up the New Hospital for
Women. But his reputation never quite recovered, and he died with
a comparably paltry £4232 to his name. Imlach also died poor, his
financial worth at death valued at just £125. Imlach's annual earnings

had plummeted from £800 to £37 the year after the controversy surrounding his operations, showing just how drastic the financial impact
of such an episode could be and how rapidly a carefully built-up practice could disintegrate.[67] High prices provided at least some form
of insurance. By the end of the 1880s some ovariotomists, such as
Robert Lawson Tait, had begun to identify themselves as 'abdominal' surgeons. This in part reflected the growing expansion of surgery
into the abdomen as splenotomies and nephrotomies began to be performed more frequently, often by those who had made their names as
ovariotomists. But arguably the term also allowed practitioners to style
themselves as unrestricted by gender, and thus meant their practice
was less loaded with the risky sexual politics which specialists in female
diseases had frequently to negotiate.

The high price accorded to ovariotomy might also be attributed to another aspect not unrelated to risk, that of the time post-
operatively that needed to be spent on a case. De Styrap never specified whether he was factoring in attendance after an operation in his
suggested fees, but the considerable aftercare needed following an
ovariotomy would have contributed significantly to the overall price.
All major operations put demands on a surgeon's time. A lithotomy
case in the 1880s, for example, even if the operation was deemed successful, generally required a month of careful attendance afterwards.[68]
A successful ovariotomy was seen to require slightly less time; most
hospital patients were ready to leave after around eighteen to twenty-four days, although for those who could afford it, this was usually
followed by a stay in a convalescent institution.[69] However, abdominal operations required a depth of care that extended beyond the
remit of most other operations, as surgeons guarded against signs
of any of the array of worrying complications that might occur: septic disease, haemorrhage, fistula, intestinal obstruction and so on. If
an ovariotomy case became complicated, it could mean months of
careful attendance. Much of this care demanded only watchful waiting and dietary regulation on the part of the referring practitioner
and nurses, rather than active treatment. But the burden of responsibility remained heavy on the operating surgeon, whose attendance
was routinely required. Fears of being accused of concealing poor outcomes in ovariotomy remained prevalent and those who performed it
were encouraged to keep abreast of their former patients' condition

for at least a year after the operation, meaning that every case—in theory at least—required serious investment of a surgeon's time.[70] Very little was written about the pricing of aftercare following an ovariotomy, other than the *Lancet's* observation (cited above) that it was the heavy cost of nursing that pushed up the price of the operation. But it seems likely that surgeons often charged separate fees for the operation itself and the aftercare, as the latter's price varied considerably depending on where the patient was convalescing and how frequently their services would be called upon. Charles Clay's preserved case notes, spanning the late 1850s and early 1860s, while detailing an earlier time period, give an important perspective on this particular financial aspect of the operation. Clay charged between £15 and £40 per case, but in his records he often broke these charges down into the constituent parts of the whole process, noting separate fees for 'operation', 'attendance' and on occasion 'lodging' too, all of which required payment.[71] Taking hysterectomy once more as a comparison, it is unclear why there is a difference in their price in de Styrap's table. Technically speaking, ovariotomy was not any more demanding than hysterectomy; in fact, it was probably less so, and the two operations would have likely involved similar regimes of aftercare.[72] Furthermore, those who performed hysterectomy were usually ovariotomists first and foremost, thus liable to the same professional risks and responsibilities that might be endured when performing ovariotomy.

This leads one to speculate that the high fees charged for ovariotomy reflected additional factors, one of which may have been its unique identity as a major innovation. It was ovariotomy that had paved the way for making abdominal surgery safe. Yet early ovariotomists had not been rewarded for their innovations, rather they had been interrogated, scorned and derided for performing the operation. For the newer generation revelling in the acceptance ovariotomy had now gained, and its grand status as the operation that had changed the landscape of surgery, high fees were perhaps compensation for the troubles ovariotomists had been put through before the operation had received acclaim.

There was most likely another factor that was also implicated in the continued expense of ovariotomy: the growing number of conditions that it was claimed could be treated by the operation. By the 1880s, fears were forming in the profession that ovarian surgery was being performed excessively and that women were having their ovaries removed for trivial ailments. As we shall see in the next section, such a possibility not only had professional consequences but financial ones too.

OÖPHORECTOMY, OPERATIVE MANIA AND SURGICAL CONSUMPTION

In the 1880s, ovariotomy continued to be the most common operation performed in women's hospitals. As we have seen, with the emergence of Battey's and Tait's operations, described in Chapter 4, there was also a growing interest among surgeons about how removing both ovaries might alleviate certain conditions other than ovarian tumours.[73] But a backlash against Tait, Battey and their followers was gaining ground, exploding in 1886 in a veritable panic about an apparent 'laparotomy epidemic' which centred almost entirely on the excessive use of ovarian surgery.[74] Fears were growing that surgeons were overenthusiastically removing ovaries for 'trivial' reasons, most often for mild ovarian pain and inflammatory conditions, and usually in conjunction with the removal of the Fallopian tubes. In the closing weeks of 1885, a scandal began to unfold at the Liverpool Hospital for Women. That year, questions had begun to be raised by colleagues regarding the number of major abdominal operations being performed by one of the hospital's surgeons, Francis Imlach. A paper Imlach had given to the Liverpool Medical Institution in December 1885 had cited forty-one cases of salpingo-oöphorectomy (removal of the ovaries and Fallopian tubes) for pyosalpinx (an accumulation of pus in the Fallopian tube) and ovarian abscesses. Despite a comparatively low mortality rate of seven per cent, Imlach's paper sparked questions from his contemporaries, suspicious of the high numbers of patients he was operating upon. An inquiry was duly set up which revealed a substantial increase in the number of abdominal sections undertaken at the hospital between 1884 and 1885.[75] Things went from bad to worse for Imlach when an ex-patient and her husband, a Mr. and Mrs. Casey, began a civil action against the surgeon, claiming that the latter had not properly informed them that they would no longer be able to conceive following the removal of both of Mrs. Casey's ovaries. In a case that brought forth many of the pressing questions of the day surrounding ovarian physiology, Mrs. Casey also cited a loss of sexual desire as a result of the operation.[76] Imlach won the case by the skin of his teeth, after one of the hospital's nurses came forward to claim that she had informed Mrs. Casey of the operation's consequences. But his reputation and his practice were severely compromised.[77] In 1897, even greater controversy would be generated by a similar case involving Charles Cullingworth, a surgeon at St. Thomas' Hospital. Cullingworth was taken to court by a former patient named Alice Jane Beatty. Beatty, who was a nurse, and thus probably more knowledgeable about medical matters than the average patient, alleged Cullingworth had removed both her ovaries without her consent. Beatty had requested an operation to remove one ovary, explicitly expressing her wish that under no circumstance should the other be removed. In a case which highlighted the fragility of patient consent in the surgical encounter, Cullingworth nonetheless had removed the second ovary, claiming he had found it so ravaged with disease upon opening the abdomen, that it was deemed necessary to remove it immediately. The medical profession was split on their judgment of Cullingworth's actions. Remarkably, given the social pressure exerted upon doctors to support and protect their professional peers, several high-profile practitioners publicly acknowledged that Cullingworth had misjudged the case. They included Thomas Spencer Wells, who was called to give expert evidence in court. While Wells cautiously offered support to Cullingworth, whom he believed had 'acted to the best of his ability', he conceded that the removal of both ovaries had been unnecessary and that Cullingworth had not given due consideration to his patient's wishes. Despite the evidence of Wells and others, the plaintiff Alice Beatty eventually lost the case.[78] Nonetheless news of it filtered into the public press.[79] Throughout the last years of the century ovariotomists would remain under intense scrutiny from both the profession and the public about their operating practices.

The fear that hundreds of women's reproductive abilities were being destroyed readily fused with anxieties about degeneration and sterility. That the operation was also, on occasion, being used to treat insanity startled many, even those who were themselves ovariotomists; 'he who cuts mad people must himself be mad' declared Thomas Spencer Wells in his 1886 essay, *On the Castration of Women*, in which he angrily castigated the propensity of some surgeons to preside over questions of mental disease with their knives.[80] This trend was not exclusive to ovarian surgery. In the late nineteenth century, castration and, to a much greater extent, circumcision, were both advocated by doctors to treat male patients for a range of diseases from dyspepsia to rheumatism to insanity.[81] The move towards surgically managing the reproductive organs to treat both physical and mental disease signalled the increasing power of surgeons to monopolise the medical arena. However, ovarian surgery undoubtedly had a much higher profile than male castration and was considered more prevalent. In his essay, Wells questioned whether surgeons would castrate or remove the penis from a man for as trivial reasons as those for which he claimed ovaries were being removed.[82]

Crucial to the argument of Wells and others was that the use of ovarian surgery for an increasingly diverse range of conditions did not seem to be based upon any major developments in physiological under-standings of the ovary. Rather, it rested upon a growing confidence in the safety of removing ovaries, which allowed surgeons to experiment more readily with already-established ideas about the organ's relation to other bodily ills.[83] It was this chasm between a relatively static moment in ovarian physiology and the rapid developments occurring in ovarian surgery that hinted at impropriety, echoing previous cases of surgical abuse like that of Isaac Baker Brown and the clitoridectomy operation. Could it be, as some speculated, that pathologies were being invented by surgeons specifically so that they could be cured for a price?[84] The *Medical Press and Circular* certainly thought so and waged a high-pro-file attack on surgeons leading the trend. An Anglo-Irish publication, it's possible that concerns about removing the female reproductive organs assumed greater importance within the predominantly Catholic Irish medical profession. Even before the Imlach affair, the journal had been the most vocal critic within the medical press of the overuse of ovarian surgery, particularly of oöphorectomy and salpingo-oöphorectomy (or 'the removal of the uterine appendages', as the latter procedure was often termed). As early as 1882 the journal had speculated in regard to the operation that 'greed and the predilection engendered by special and limited study are apt to compel men to unravel all forms of disease'.[85] Thus, the journal reiterated the oft-made accusation that 'specialist' prac-tice was more about money than medicine, and bred an unsavoury cul-ture where diseases were invented simply so that they could be profited from.

The *Medical Press and Circular* revived its attack on oöphorectomy after the revelations about Francis Imlach's practice, but centred its criti-cism upon Robert Lawson Tait, the bombastic Birmingham surgeon who was evidently loathed by the journal. In 1886, it began to make quite clear in a series of articles its opinion of Tait's practice: that his moti-vations were pecuniary rather than medical. Tait, an avid correspondent with many of the medical journals, rarely let sleeping dogs lie when allegations were made about him, and retorted angrily when the jour-nal described his practice as one of the 'large centres in which spaying is practised wholesale'.[86] 'Spaying' was a derogatory term used to describe oöphorectomy by its detractors. Like 'castration', it evoked the idea that women's bodies were being treated as experimental material by doctors in the same vein that animals were. This was a powerful analogy to make at a time when the anti-vivisection movement was flourishing, and narratives of vivisection and ovariotomy were often explicitly brought together by prominent campaigners, who saw both procedures as expressive of cruelty, and the oppression of the weak by medical men.[87] The *Medical Press* refused to retract its inferences about the business aspect to Tait's practice. Instead, they plunged the knife in further: 'if he objects to the word "wholesale" he cannot deny that a very large "retail" business of this kind is done in some very large centres', the journal wrote.[88] Once more Tait responded angrily, claiming that, if anything, his practice in oöphorectomy was costing *him* money, and described how he had been compelled to provide free beds in his private hospital for scores of women who could not afford to fund themselves. Tait claimed that each such case cost him fifteen to twenty guineas and that the patients who came to him—not wealthy, but not so poor as to secure admittance to a general hospital—had already been drained of their resources. Like Isaac Baker Brown before him, Tait claimed that his patients had spent all their money on trying to find a medical rather than surgical solution to their problem, often leaving them in serious financial straits.[89]

Some saw the apparent enthusiasm for gynaecological surgery as little more than a fashion. Thomas More Madden, an Irish surgeon who worried deeply about the spread of excessive surgery of this kind, made the link explicit in his lecture to the Obstetrical Section of the Academy of Medicine in Ireland, Titled 'On the So-Called Laparotomy Epidemic', which he published in 1886 at the height of the controversy.[90] He would go on to expound similar views at the British Medical Association meeting in Brighton the following year.[91] 'No one acquainted with ancient medical literature will question the continually recurring influence of fashion on medical opinion and practice in every age' he wrote, 'nor can it be gainsaid that in successive epochs various forms of disease and methods of treatment come into and go out of vogue with almost as little reason as influences the ever-changing modes of dress'.[92] For Madden, there was a certain alarming inevitability to medicine being swayed by trends, something which had to be kept carefully in check. This was not the first time that ovarian surgery had been described as merely a fashion. As we saw in Chapter 3, similar allegations had been made some forty years before when the justifiability of performing ovariotomy at all was debated.[93]

As a consequence, surgeons like Thomas Spencer Wells were keen to highlight that oöphorectomy was an entirely different operation from ovariotomy. Ovariotomy had proved its worth; oöphorectomy on the other hand, was an innovation upon the original innovation, and an unwelcome one at that. For those outside of the profession, however, and indeed for many within it, the distinction was not clear-cut; oöphorectomy was simply a new unfolding of ovarian surgery's often unnecessary use. When in 1909 playwright and well-known critic of the medical profession, George Bernard Shaw, addressed the Medico-Legal Society on 'the Socialist Criticism of the Medical Profession', Shaw specifically pinpointed the 'fashion' for operations and in particular, ovariotomy, as a symbol of unnecessary profiteering in medicine. Thus, it was not the more recent controversies surrounding oöphorectomy he alluded to but rather the more 'traditional' ovariotomy, indeed he even referred to Spencer Wells.[94] Such depictions led not only to the continued characterisation of ovariotomy as a novelty but also exacerbated already present concerns about ovarian surgery as an immoral money-spinner. The phrases increasingly used to describe it, as a vogue, a fashion, an excess, alluded to the possibility of wastefulness and unthinking consumption.

Regardless of whether these accusations had a solid foundation or not, if the notion of a procedure being fashionable held sway, it at once made it vulnerable, removing any veneer of professional neutrality and imbuing it with worldliness; making it as much the product of whimsical fashion as a style of dress. The use of the word 'fashion' was slippery. It suggested a trend among doctors in their proclivities for performing certain operations. But it also raised once more questions about trends in the demand for operations (explored in Chapter 3). For if there was no demand for an operation, how could there be a fashion? Was it possible, then, that women were, at times, active pursuers, consumers even, of ovarian operations? Reflecting back, George Bernard Shaw took this to be the case, implying that fashionable operations like ovariotomy and tonsillectomy attracted 'ladies and gentleman who had heard and read so much about operations that they felt that they could not live without them. Such people are a tremendous temptation to poor doctors'.[95]

Two polarised perceptions of the ovarian patient were emerging in the eyes of critics. On the one end, the vulnerable victim robbed of her reproductive role by unthinking doctors, on the other, the frivolous woman exercising economic power over the practitioner in pursuit

of an elective operation that put her at unnecessary risk. Both perceptions inhabited dangerous moral ground. This dichotomy has been of
interest to historians. Ornella Moscucci has speculated that oöphorectomies may have been sought by some patients as a method of contracep-
tion. Certainly as Moscucci suggests, in Britain, practitioners discussed
the possibility that oöphorectomy could be extended in its use to produce sterility in women with pelvic deformities as a means of preventing
further obstructed labours.[96] One surgeon also claimed it had become
fashionable in Britain for fertile women to seek out methods of becoming sterile, although he did not link this directly to ovarian surgery.[97]
However, in America, where Britons reckoned oöphorectomy to be far
more widely performed, the connection was made more explicit. The
New York-based journal *The Medical Record* went as far as suggesting
that oöphorectomies were characteristic of a progressive instinct towards
population control and could be economically expedient:

> No woman wants more than two children, many only one, and a large per
> cent, including all the unmarried, not any at all. But in fact the population
> is increasing at a seriously rapid rate, and the modern economist has had to
> revive and readopt the views of Malthus. In this exigency, when society's
> needs are antagonised by infant multiplicity, the laparotomist steps in as a
> kind of modern saviour from the threatened polypedic catastrophe.[98]

This brazen positioning of oöphorectomy as a choice related to life-
style, and as an operation premised upon social concerns, rather than
a medical problem, articulated the deep fears among the profession
regarding the normalisation of serious surgery.[99] Indeed the debate
foreshadowed those which continue today about the ethics of elective surgery; especially in regard to female sterilisation, which remains a contentious issue, particularly when it involves women of reproductive age.[100]
Such comments also require us to examine closely how the female patient
was positioned within this dialogue, as the recipient of the surgical operation on offer. Certainly notions of demand in ovarian surgery should always
be considered in conjunction with risk, which in the 1880s had dropped
significantly but remained at a level where a prospective patient would still
likely be very concerned: somewhere between five to fifteen per cent of
British patients undergoing ovarian surgery died as a result of their operation.[101] We can presume, therefore, that anxieties about operating would
have been as prevalent then as they are today and probably much more
so.[102] Chiefly, critics of the operation were more concerned about lack

of consent or understanding on the part of the patient, than they were about patient demand. But as Regina Morantz-Sanchez and Claire Brock have both argued, even the *possibility* of surgery-by-choice had a significant impact on practitioners; the very notion of it suggested a disempowering of doctors and an increase in the authority of female patients. As Brock argues, it was once more the question of necessity that was central; that an operation might principally be carried out because of a patient's request rather than as a consequence of the surgeon's judgment served only to undermine the idea that the operation was—medically speaking—necessary at all.[103]

These concerns manifested themselves in press reports throughout the 1880s and 1890s. *The Hospital*, a medical magazine with a popular lay readership reported with incredulity a medical society meeting, where 'Two cases were related, in both of which it appeared the patients "insisted on the abdomen being opened"... Where is to be the limit of what a medical man will do at the request of a patient?' inquired the journal.[104] Articles in the *Medical Press and Circular* in particular, emphasised flippancy on the part of patients undergoing oöphorectomy, and included extracts of patients' accounts of their condition. One editorial detailed the case of a woman about to have her ovaries removed by an anonymous operator. Found by an observer to have 'full round rosy cheeks and red lips', under close questioning the patient revealed she suffered pain only three or four days a month. The operation did not go ahead.[105] The *Medical Press* also published a piece by the surgeon Andrea Rabagliati which pondered the justifiability of oöphorectomy. In an article that was to be reprinted in many other journals, Rabagliati reported the case of a consultant friend who:

> ...had been consulted as to the advisability of removing the uterine appendages in a lady who was said to suffer *frightfully*. On coming downstairs, the three doctors met the lady's husband, and the consultant said to him, 'is your wife, do you think, suffering more than usual?" "Well, yes" said the husband, "but she has always suffered a good deal". "Has she been confined to bed?" "Oh no!" "How often has she been out this last week?" "Well, we were three times out for dinner, and twice at the theatre!" The consultant turned and looked at the doctors and said nothing!"[106]

The reference to the couple's glamorous social life was not coincidental. An important class aspect was at work here. The quick fix of an oöphorectomy for painful conditions was believed to have greater worth when

applied to working-class women who had heavier domestic and occupa-
tional duties to contend with—although implicit in this may have been
a judgment on the part of surgeons about the relative worth of reproduction among rich and poor women.[107] Middle-class women, on the
other hand, were seen as having less need to resort to such measures,
as they generally had more time and greater financial resources to
continue with palliative treatments. Thus, the performance of the
operation upon richer women was particularly at risk of appearing lavish:
evocative of the idea of women as consumers, desirous of commodities
and services that would ease their life, regardless of consequences.
In France, in 1909, a caricature appeared of Paris' most fashionable
ovariotomist, Samuel Pozzi, (Fig. 5.2) which reflected these anxieties.
Pozzi, who was gynaecological surgeon at l'hôpital Broca, and who
counted John Singer Sargent and Sarah Bernhardt among his friends,
was a leading light in a field of practice that was considerably smaller
in France than it was in Britain and America.[108] Nonetheless Pozzi was
equally susceptible to allusions regarding the fashionable nature of his
work. The caricature, probably published by the *Académie Nationale
de Médecine*, shows the dapper Pozzi dangling two 'o's, representing
the ovaries, from an épée. Behind him stand three female figures that
appear to be shop mannequins, one of whom, dressed in finery, is labelled
'sterile' or 'sterility'. The cartoon implies the gradual lifelessness of
women following the procedure and the removal of their 'natural' function, but also hints at the consumption of surgical services among fashionable women. It was a perception that increasingly became infused with
turn-of-the-century ideas of women as frivolous, and signalled complex
power relations between the sexes, in which women wielded considerable
economic power but always as part of a social framework built around the
values and preferences of men.[109] It was within this nexus that the high
price of ovarian surgery was constructed; a financial relationship which
saw practitioners at liberty to charge what they wanted, dependent only
upon competition from other practitioners, and where patients, it was
alleged, were pursuing the operation.

How far this was actually the case, that women were indeed allowing themselves to be operated on 'merely' because of minor discomforts
brought to their lives by suspected ovarian disease, or even because they
wished to make reproductive choices, is difficult to know, the dearth of

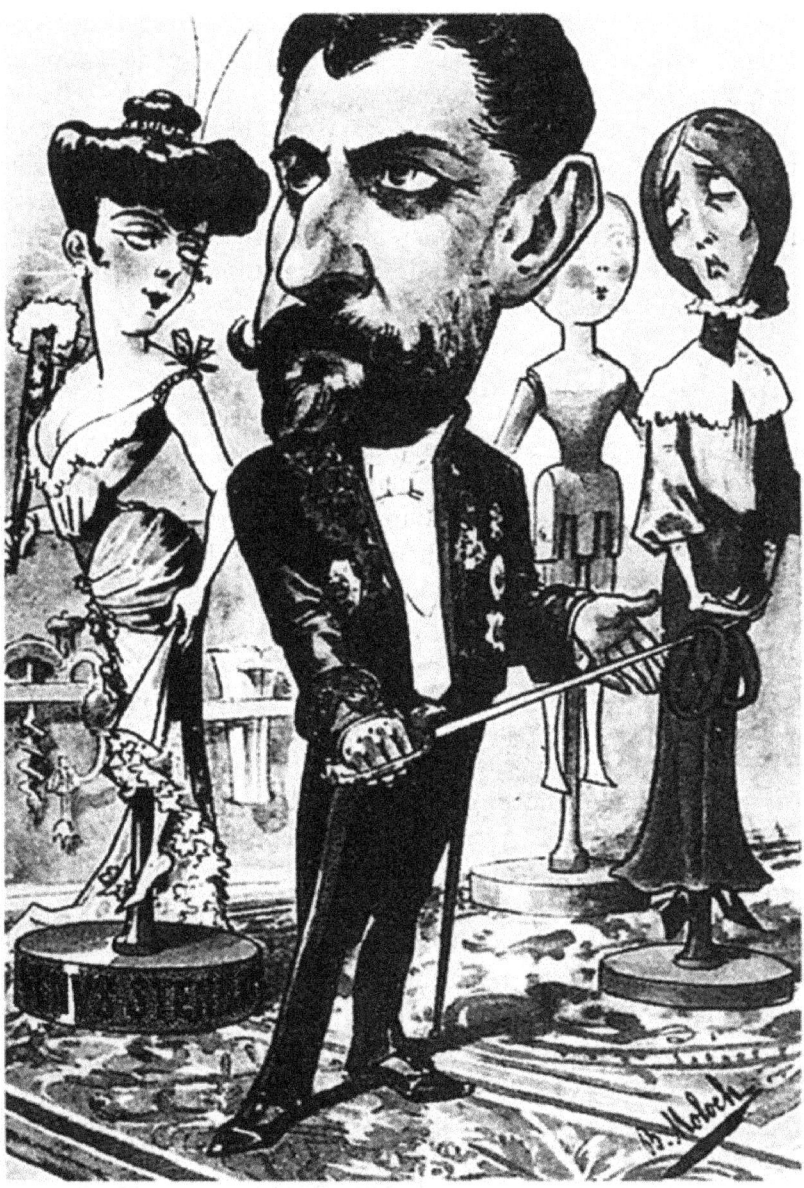

Fig. 5.2 Caricature of the Parisian ovariotomist Samuel Pozzi by the cartoonist Hector Moloch (Alphonse Hector Colomb), 1909 (*Credit* Private collection of Nicolas Bourdet)

female patients' accounts proving here as it does in so many areas of the history of medicine to limit our understanding of the patient experience. But the idea that this was happening was sufficient enough to be played upon by critics of oöphorectomy, who sprinkled their protest pieces with anecdotes to suggest such a trend was occurring. The possibility of female patients as economic actors, their desires acquiesced to by unscrupulous operators, provoked considerable consternation. It served to reaffirm anxieties that both the invention and expansion of ovarian surgery were motivated by profit.

Conclusion

A number of historians have drawn attention to the significant economic implications of ovariotomy. But perhaps none have situated them where they should be: central and absolutely integral to the history of the operation, where the potential financial value of the procedure framed its performance and its representation, and where gender, choice, consumerism and consent were tightly bound together. Ovarian surgery was identified as an innovation of private practice and specialist institutions, both of which suggested financial motivations for the operation. At this time, medical specialists were still on shaky ground in regard to their professional standing, particularly those who specialised in the diseases of women. Yet to become an elite practitioner in ovariotomy also potentially paved the way for a lucrative career because 'ovariotomists' were virtually at liberty to charge what they wanted.

The judgment of Jukes de Styrap in his influential *The Medico-Chirurgical Tariffs* that ovariotomy was the most expensive operation in surgery raises questions about how exactly operative value was determined. While conceptions of risk played a fundamental part, as did the level of commitment that would be required from a surgeon after an operation was performed, so too, perhaps, did a sense of entitlement among ovariotomists. The high price reflected the operation's status as a striking and major innovation. Indeed, even as other equally risky operations began to be practised, such as hysterectomy, it was ovariotomy which was deemed the most expensive operation a surgeon could perform. Its price can also be read in terms of a broader commodification of the operation. During the 1880s, there were widespread concerns about a 'fashion' for ovarian surgery. Ovariotomy and oöphorectomy were permanently informed by a male perspective; male surgeons for the most part organised and executed the operations, and the vulnerability of women against the onslaught of oöphorectomy in particular was a key concern during the so-called 'laparotomy epidemic'. Yet conversely, the use of ovarian surgery for an increasingly diverse range of conditions also raised the spectre of consumer power, of the possibility that women were purchasing risky surgery simply for a more comfortable life, something, according to critics, that unscrupulous practitioners were willing to acquiesce to in their quest to make money. What becomes clear by looking at the financial aspects to ovariotomy is that historians must venture beyond the *explicitly* commercial when looking at business and medicine in the nineteenth century. Ovariotomists did not sell patent medicines or advertise in newspapers but, in the eyes of some in the medical community, their services were as much a commercial enterprise as those who did.

In the late nineteenth century, no surgeon who worked in ovarian surgery outwardly claimed that the lucrative nature of the speciality was what motivated them to operate. Such an assertion would have been unpalatable in that medico-cultural context. Nor is it possible to definitively ascertain what *did* motivate the individual historical actors at play here. The point is that financial issues surrounding ovarian surgery had to be negotiated with great care. That it was lucrative was a double-edged sword; the prices were higher, but so were the stakes. Ovariotomy, still conceived of as a recent innovation, came with its own peculiar risks and responsibilities. Moreover, as new controversies arose with the 'laparotomy epidemic', the possibility that ovarian surgery was an unseemly novelty once more emerged. As we will see in the next chapter, the status of ovarian surgery was not necessarily becoming clearer, in fact it was to become considerably more complex.

NOTES

1. John Gregory, *Observations on the Duties and Offices of a Physician, and on the Method of Prosecuting Enquiries in Philosophy* (London: W. Strahan and T. Cadell, 1770). Gregory observed that medicine could be 'considered either as an art the most beneficial and important to mankind, or as a trade by which a considerable body of men gain their subsistence', 9.
2. G.R. Searle, *Morality and the Market in Victorian Britain* (Oxford: Clarendon Press, 1998), 123–124. As Michael Brown has described

it, 'by the mid-nineteenth century, English medicine and its associated cultural forms had been undoubtedly and irrevocably transformed'. Michael Brown, *Performing Medicine: Medical Culture and Identity in Provincial England, c. 1760–1850* (Manchester and New York: Manchester University Press, 2011), 226.

3. Anne Digby, *Making a Medical Living: Doctors and Patients in the English Market for Medicine, 1720–1911* (Cambridge: Cambridge University Press, 1994), 6.

4. Sally Wilde, *The History of Surgery: Trust, Patient Autonomy, Medical Dominance and Australian Surgery, 1890–1940* (Byron Bay: Finesse Press, 2010), 99–100.

5. Lori Loeb, 'Doctors and Patent Medicines in Modern Britain: Professionalism and Consumerism', *Albion: A Quarterly Journal of British Studies* 33, no. 3 (2001): 404–425; Takahiro Ueyama, *Health in the Marketplace: Professionalism, Therapeutic Desires, and Medical Commodification in Late-Victorian London* (Palo Alto: The Society for the Promotion of Science and Scholarship, 2010). In their explorations of the use of patent medicines in doctors' practices, Loeb and Ueyama have both helped dispel the idea that qualified practitioners and patent medicine vendors were operating in distinct spheres.

6. As Christopher Herbert has eloquently remarked on Victorian attitudes to money, 'writers of the day insistently described their society as a great many-layered system of occluded awareness, one in which *not knowing what one knew* became almost the defining principle of consciousness, at least in the sphere of middle-class life'. Christopher Herbert, 'Filthy Lucre: Victorian Ideas of Money', *Victorian Studies* 44, no. 2 (2002): 186.

7. Anonymous letter quoted in Howard A. Kelly, 'Conservatism in Ovariotomy', *Journal of the American Medical Association* 26, no. 2 (1896): 251.

8. See for example M.W. Weatherall, 'Making Medicine Scientific: Empiricism, Rationality, and Quackery in Mid-Victorian Britain', *Social History of Medicine* 9, no. 2 (1996). Weatherall argues that during this time 'the advancement of medical knowledge was to become concentrated in a few medical schools and hospitals', 180.

9. Guenter B. Risse, *Mending Bodies, Saving Souls: A History of Hospitals* (Oxford: Oxford University Press, 1999), 387.

10. Christopher Lawrence and Richard Dixey, 'Practising on Principle: Joseph Lister and the Germ Theories of Disease', in *Medical Theory, Surgical Practice: Studies in the History of Surgery*, ed. Christopher Lawrence (London and New York: Routledge, 1992), 156.

11. On modifications in Lister's own principles and practice, see Lawrence and Dixey, 'Practising on Principle'.

12. Lawrence and Dixey, 'Practising on Principle', 153–154.

13. William MacCormac, *Transactions of the International Medical Congress, Volume 2* (London: J.W. Kolckmann, 1881), 370–371.

14. Thomas Keith, 'Results of Ovariotomy Before and After Antiseptics', *British Medical Journal* 2, no. 929 (19 October 1878): 591.

15. In 1883 at the London Hospital for example, only six ovariotomies were performed. See 'Surgery Beadle's Return of Operations Performed' (1883) LH/M/3/7 (Royal London Hospital Archives). However at other general hospitals, such as King's College Hospital, surgeons continued to avoid abdominal surgery completely. Joseph Lister's house surgeon St. Clair Thomson recorded in his memoirs that during Joseph Lister's time at King's (between 1877 and 1892) 'I never saw him do an abdominal section. During my term of office, we never heard the word 'appendicitis'; gastric ulcers were diagnosed but never treated surgically; ovarian cysts were tapped and tapped until the patient died; that a calculus could be removed from a ureter or a bile-duct never entered the imagination of the wildest dreamer'. St. Clair Thomson, 'Memories of a House Surgeon', *Lancet* 209, no. 5406 (9 April 1927): 777. Unsubstantiated rumours suggested that ovariotomy was unofficially banned from the hospital at this time; see Berkeley Moynihan, 'Lister as Surgeon', *Lancet* 209, no. 5406 (9 April 1927): 747.

16. Peter D. Mohr, 'Clay, Charles (1801–1893)', in *Oxford Dictionary of National Biography* (Oxford University Press, 2004), Online edn, October 2006, http://www.oxforddnb.com/view/article/5558, accessed 13 April 2018.

17. Keith, 'Results of Ovariotomy', 590; Robert Lawson Tait, 'Removal of the Uterine Appendages', *Medical Press and Circular* 42, no. 2471 (1886): 203; Myrrha Bantock, *Granville Bantock: A Personal Portrait* (London: J.M. Dent, 1972), 27.

18. 'David Lloyd Roberts', *Lancet* 196, no. 5067 (9 October 1920): 767.

19. M. Anne Crowther and Marguerite W. Dupree, *Medical Lives in the Age of the Surgical Revolution* (Cambridge: Cambridge University Press, 2007), 196. At the Samaritan Hospital, virtually every surgeon ever connected to the institution continued their links with it until they retired from hospital practice.

20. For an overview on this see Lindsay Granshaw, '"Fame and Fortune by Means of Bricks and Mortar": The Medical Profession and Specialist Hospitals in Britain 1800–1948', in *The Hospital in History*, ed. Lindsay Granshaw and Roy Porter (London and New York: Routledge, 1989), 199–220. Some also viewed specialist hospitals as detrimental to medical

education, as they stole cases away from general hospitals, thus depriving medical students of experience when walking the wards.

21. James O'Flanagan, *Contradiction! Or English Medical Men and Manners of the Nineteenth Century* (London: Baillière, Tindall and Cox, 1866), 52.

22. Morell Mackenzie, 'Medical Specialism', *Fortnightly Review* 38, no. 224 (1885): 267.

23. Ornella Moscucci, *The Science of Woman: Gynaecology and Gender in England 1800–1929* (Cambridge University Press, 1990), 171.

24. Although the term 'ovariotomist' had first appeared in the medical press in the 1850s. It is not entirely clear who coined the term, although it is possible that like 'ovariotomy' it was Charles Clay, who often used the term to describe himself.

25. Many London ovariotomists were closely associated with the Royal College of Surgeons of England and other London surgical societies. Wells was President of the College in 1882. His assistant both in private practice and at the Samaritan Hospital, Alban Doran, was connected to the College's Hunterian Museum throughout his career.

26. Thomas Schlich, '"The Days of Brilliancy Are Past": Skill, Styles and the Changing Rules of Surgical Performance, ca. 1820–1920', *Medical History* 59, no. 3 (2015): 402–403.

27. King's College Hospital surgeon William Watson Cheyne was described rather politely as 'not a brilliant operator', while Walter Rivington, senior surgeon at the London Hospital was allegedly perceived as a 'poor operator by colleagues'. 'William Watson Cheyne', in *Plarr's Lives of the Fellows*, vol. 3, ed. D'Arcy Power (London: Royal College of Surgeons, 1997), 145; Stephen Trombley, *Sir Frederick Treves* (Routledge, London and New York, 1989), 12.

28. 'Obituary—Alban Henry Griffiths Doran', *British Journal of Obstetrics and Gynaecology* 34, no. 3 (1927): 547.

29. 'Royal Medical and Chirurgical Society, Tuesday November 11th 1862', *Lancet* 80, no. 2047 (22 November 1862): 569.

30. *The American Practitioner and News* reported that Robert Lawson Tait, who along with Thomas Spencer Wells was probably the British ovariotomist of greatest renown in America, charged from 'five guineas to one hundred for an ovariotomy'. 'Notes and Queries', *The American Practitioner and News* 3 (1887): 224. Guineas were no longer a form of currency by this time, having been replaced in 1816 by the pound. However 'guinea' was still used to refer to a payment of twenty-one shillings (around £70 in today's money). The term was thought to give transactions an air of refinement and was popularly used by doctors when charging fees.

31. 'Within the Hospital Walls: A Matter of Fact Narrative', *Lancet* 127, no. 3277 (19 June 1886): 1202.

32. 'Notes and Queries', *The American Practitioner and News* 16 (1877): 59.

33. Moscucci, *The Science of Woman*, 170.

34. R.V. Jackson, 'The Structure of Pay in Nineteenth-Century Britain', *Economic History Review* 40, no. 4 (1987): 563.

35. 'Within the Hospital Walls: A Matter of Fact Narrative', 1202. In her popular volume, *Lectures on General Nursing* (1884), London Hospital matron Eva Lückes warned nurses of the careful and exacting care that would be expected from those looking after ovariotomy cases, which was 'one of the most important operations of which you can ever have charge'. Eva Lückes, *Lectures on General Nursing* (London: Kegan Paul, 1884), 133.

36. 'Within the Hospital Walls: A Matter of Fact Narrative', 1202. Acting as a nurse in ovariotomy cases was considered difficult work and both those employed in public and private institutions were expected to spend many hours watching over their patients. Ideally one or two specialist nurses were appointed to a case. 'Nursing Echoes', *Nursing Record* 1, no. 25 (1888): 337.

37. Keith, 'Results of Ovariotomy', 593.

38. Regina Morantz-Sanchez also addresses the impact of ovariotomy's daring and bold nature as a means of explaining resistance to the operation by many American surgeons; Regina Morantz-Sanchez, *Conduct Unbecoming of a Woman: Medicine on Trial in Turn-of-the-Century Brooklyn* (Oxford: Oxford University Press, 1999), 92.

39. *Proceedings at the Seventh Annual Meeting of the London Surgical Home* (London: Savill & Edwards, 1865), 34. Lawson Tait used a similar argument when his motives for performing oöphorectomy were questioned. Tait, 'Removal of the Uterine Appendages', 202–203.

40. Charles K. Harley, 'Trade, 1870–1939: From Globalisation to Fragmentation', in *Cambridge Economic History of Modern Britain, Vol. 2: Economic Maturity, 1860–1939*, ed. Roderick Floud and Paul Johnson (Cambridge: Cambridge University Press, 2004), 168.

41. Overcrowding in the medical profession was a perpetual source of anxiety among doctors throughout the nineteenth century. Historians have tended to focus on the middle decades when, as Irvine Loudon has argued, the expansion of the middle classes and an increase in graduates from the Scottish medical schools were believed to have increased the number of practitioners vying for positions. This led to deepening stigmatisation of irregular practitioners and growing anxieties about competition, that were in part expressed through the establishment of the 1858 Medical

Act; Irvine Loudon, *Medical Care and the General Practitioner* (Oxford: Clarendon Press, 1986), 208–227.

42. 'The Prospects of the Profession', *Medical Press and Circular* 40, no. 2420 (1885): 257.

43. Keir Waddington, *Medical Education at St. Bartholomew's Hospital, 1123–1995* (Woodbridge: The Boydell Press, 2003), 299.

44. Despite the concern many doctors had that the profession was over-crowded, statistics compiled by Walter Rivington in 1888 in his exhaustive account of the state of the medical profession during the late nineteenth century suggested that proportionally there was a decline in the num-ber of doctors within the general population between 1851 and 1881. Walter Rivington, *The Medical Profession of the United Kingdom* (Dublin: Fannin & Co, 1888), 2. This was also picked up on by the *British Medical Journal*, 'Review: The Medical Profession of the United Kingdom', *British Medical Journal* 1, no. 1474 (30 March 1889): 717–718.

45. The lithotomist Henry Thompson, a surgeon renowned for his pol-ymathic bent and cultivation of fine tastes in art and literature, com-mented in one of his pseudonymous novels that 'it is not a curious fact, for it is an indispensable one, that almost every medical man of ordinary intelligence, who achieves a fair share of success in his profession—and unluckily the taste sometimes exists without success enough to war-rant its cultivation—becomes a fine art collector of some sort, and has a hobby, which when you know him, and not until then, you are per-haps astonished to discover'. Pen Oliver (Henry Thompson), *Charley Kingston's Aunt* (London: Macmillan, 1885), 14.

46. Digby, *Making a Medical Living*, 193.

47. In a publication in 1879, the Manchester Medico-Ethical Association wrote that it was 'convinced that the subject of medical charges must ever remain a somewhat open one, so long as the profession, unlike all other trades and professions, continues to claim its remuneration not according to the abstract worth of its services alone, but also accord-ing to the ability of its clients'. Manchester Medico-Ethical Association, *Tariff of Medical Fees Issued by the Manchester Medico-Ethical Association* (Manchester: J. E. Cornish, 1879), 3.

48. 'Consultation-Fees', *British Medical Journal* 2, no. 923 (7 September 1878): 376. See also 'Physicians, Practitioners, Patients and Fees', *British Medical Journal* 1, no. 889 (12 January 1878): 56–57.

49. 'Consultation-Fees', *British Medical Journal* 2, no. 927 (5 October 1878): 539.

50. Manchester Medico-Ethical Association, *Tariff of Medical Fees*, 10. The tariff's only concession to this was to include the Poor Law's scale of surgical fees as a guide to minimum charges.

51. 'Professional Fees', *British Medical Journal* 1, no. 737 (13 February 1875): 223. Some physicians expressed admiration for surgeons for charging such disparate fees, as it directly opposed the uniform guinea-fee payment they were subjected to.

52. Jukes de Styrap, *A Code of Medical Ethics* (London: J. & A. Churchill, 1878).

53. Jukes de Styrap, *The Medico-Chirurgical Tariffs* (*Prepared for the Late Shropshire Ethical Branch of the British Medical Association*) (London: H. K. Lewis, 1890).

54. The *Edinburgh Medical Journal* noted that de Styrap's pamphlet 'did not profess to be a guide as to how the wealthy should be charged by their ordinary attendant, or how consultants should estimate the value of their own services'. 'Review: The Medical-Chirurgical Tariffs', *Edinburgh Medical Journal* 34, no. 1 (1888): 62.

55. 'Review: The Medical-Chirurgical Tariffs', 62.

56. Steve Sturdy and Roger Cooter, 'Science, Scientific Management, and the Transformation of Medicine in Britain c. 1870–1950', *History of Science* 36 (1998): 422.

57. De Styrap, *The Medico-Chirurgical Tariffs*, 20–27. For the highest socio-economic class listed, de Styrap suggested between 315 and 610 shillings could be charged for a caesarean section.

58. For a detailed discussion of uterine surgery in the nineteenth century, see Ilana Löwy, '"Because of Their Praiseworthy Modesty, They Consult Too Late": Regime of Hope and Cancer of the Womb, 1800–1910', *Bulletin of the History of Medicine* 85, no. 3 (2011): 356–383. Statistical studies of hysterectomy mortality rates were sparse around this time as so few were being performed. But a table of 365 hysterectomies performed by surgeons across the world, compiled by American surgeon Theodore Gaillard in 1880, put the mortality rate of hysterectomy at seventy per cent; Theodore Gaillard, *A Practical Treatise on the Diseases of Women* (London: Henry Kimpton, 1880), 547. By the end of the 1880s, vaginal as well as abdominal hysterectomy was being practised, although this too had a high mortality rate. De Styrap does not specify which method of hysterectomy he is referring to.

59. Thomas Keith, 'Thirteen Cases of Hysterectomy, With Remarks on Carbolic Acid Spray in Abdominal Surgery', *British Medical Journal* 1, no. 1257 (31 January 1885): 214; 'Editorial: Ovariotomy, Hysterectomy and Oöphorectomy', *British Medical Journal* 1, no. 1257 (31 January 1885): 240.

60. Lawson Tait, 'Abstract of an Address on One Thousand Abdominal Sections', *British Medical Journal* 1, no. 1257 (31 January 1885): 218.

61. 'Editorial: Ovariotomy, Hysterectomy and Oöphorectomy', 240.

62. Thompson was well-known for commanding huge fees for his services, spurred on by the prestige he had garnered from treating King Leopold of Belgium for bladder stones in 1863. Zachary Cope notes that in 1865, Thompson earned £2000 for treating a high-ranking British Admiral in Paris. Zachary Cope, *The Versatile Victorian: Being the Life of Sir Henry Thompson, 1820–1904* (London: Harvey & Blythe, 1951), 45.

63. De Styrap, *The Medico-Chirurgical Tariffs*, 4.

64. 'Essay on Desperate Surgery in Its Relation to Women: The Proper Place for It; Who Should and Who Should Not Attempt It', *Journal of the American Medical Association* 3, no. 12 (20 September 1884): 322.

65. Ornella Moscucci, 'Clitoridectomy, Circumcision and the Politics of Sexual Pleasure in Mid-Victorian Britain', in *Sexualities in Victorian Britain*, ed. Andrew H. Miller and James Eli Adams (Bloomington: Indiana University Press, 1996), 75–76.

66. 'Obstetrical Society of London', *Lancet* 127, no. 3258 (6 February 1886): 255–256. Stead was well-known for his crusade against child prostitution. This case, however, in which Stead had attempted to 'buy' a child prostitute, was considered scandalous and led to his conviction for child abduction.

67. J.J. Rivlin, 'Francis Imlach (1851–1920) and the Liverpool Medical Establishment', *Medical Historian* (1999): 48. All probate information cited is taken from the UK index of probate records at www.ancestry.com.

68. William Cadge, 'Lithotomy', in *Dictionary of Practical Surgery*, vol. 1, ed. Christopher Heath (London: Smith, Elder & Co., 1889), 937.

69. John Knowsley Thornton, 'Ovariotomy', in *Dictionary of Practical Surgery*, vol. 2, ed. Christopher Heath (London: Smith, Elder & Co., 1886), 158.

70. Alban Doran, *Handbook of Gynaecological Operations* (Philadelphia: P. Blakiston & Son, 1887), 271. The American ovariotomist Edmund Peaslee claimed to have rejected over 100 ovariotomy cases on the basis that he wouldn't be able to adequately oversee their aftercare, writing in 1867 that the after-treatment of an operation constituted 'three fourths the responsibility, and nine-tenths the anxiety'. Edmund Peaslee, 'Ovariotomy, When and How to Operate; After-Treatment', *Southern Journal of the Medical Sciences* 2 (1867): 551.

71. Charles Clay's case book, M/C Medical Collection—cat.9.11.54 MNB (Manchester Medical Collection, University of Manchester).

72. Keith, 'Results of Ovariotomy', 593.

73. As seen in the operative statistics of the Samaritan Free Hospital, where between 1878 and 1897, of the 1643 abdominal sections undertaken at the hospital, exactly 1000 were ovarian operations. Hysterectomies

comprised just 163 of the procedures. Alban Doran, 'Classification of Abdominal Sections in Index Form, 187–1897' (c. 1924) MSO155/2/2 (Royal College of Surgeons of England).

74. The terms oöphorectomy and laparotomy tended to be used interchangeably in this context. Technically laparotomy was any incision into the abdomen, but the 'laparotomy epidemic' almost always referred to procedures where the ovaries, often in conjunction with the Fallopian tubes, were being removed. The rapidly changing terminology in operative surgery will be explored in more detail in the next chapter.

75. J.J. Rivlin, 'Francis Imlach', 44; 'Editorial', *Lancet* 128, no. 3285 (14 August 1886): 304–307. Imlach's colleague Thomas Grimsdale stated that the number of abdominal sections at the hospital in 1884 was 44, compared to 111 in 1885.

76. Whether women lost their sexual desire after having both ovaries removed was one of the biggest issues of the oöphorectomy debate. Lawson Tait was always adamant that this was not the case and publicly supported Imlach throughout the episode. Robert Lawson Tait, 'Casey vs Imlach', *Lancet* 128, no. 3286 (21 August 1886): 375.

77. Rivlin, 'Francis Imlach', 48–49.

78. Claire Brock, 'Risk, Responsibility and Surgery in the 1890s and Early 1900s', *Medical History* 57, no. 3 (2013): 330–333.

79. 'Remarkable Action Against a London Surgeon', *Sheffield and Rotherham Independent*, no. 13150 (17 November 1896): 8; 'Action Against a Doctor', *Dundee Courier and Argus*, no. 13537 (17 November 1896): 4; 'Nurse v. Doctor: A Claim for Damages', *Hampshire Telegraph and Sussex Chronicle*, no. 6010 (21 November 1896), 2.

80. Thomas Spencer Wells, *Modern Abdominal Surgery: The Bradshaw Lecture Delivered at the Royal College of Surgeons of England December 18th, 1890 with an Appendix on the Castration of Women* (London: J. & A. Churchill, 1891), 49. *On the Castration of Women* was originally published in America in 1886 but Wells insisted on republishing it in 1891.

81. Robert Darby, *A Surgical Temptation: The Demonization of the Foreskin and the Rise of Circumcision in Britain* (Chicago and London: University of Chicago Press, 2005), 10–11.

82. Wells, *Modern Abdominal Surgery*, 47.

83. For example, the connection between the ovaries and hysteria was intimated earlier in the century in the physiological writings of Thomas Laycock; Thomas Laycock, *A Treatise on the Nervous Diseases of Women* (London: Longman, Orme, Brown, Green and Longmans, 1840), 144.

84. Henry Coe of the Women's Hospital in New York was reported by the *Medical Press and Circular* to have remarked that a peculiarity in the growth of abdominal surgery was that 'it owes its impetus to the surgeons rather than to the pathologists'. 'The Frequency of Diseases of the Uterine Appendages', *Medical Press and Circular* 42, no. 2463 (1886): 30.

85. 'Editorial: Questionable Surgery', *Medical Press and Circular* 33 (1882): 385.

86. 'The Frequency of Disease of the Uterine Appendages', 31.

87. Mary Ann Elston, 'Women and Anti-Vivisection in Victorian England, 1870–1900', in *Vivisection in Historical Perspective*, ed. Nicolaas A. Rupke (London and New York: Routledge, 1990), 278–279. Although interestingly, Tait himself vehemently opposed vivisection.

88. 'The Frequency of Disease of the Uterine Appendages', *Medical Press and Circular* 42, no. 2464 (1886): 58.

89. 'Removal of the Uterine Appendages', 203. In Tait's case the accusation may have been unfair. As Regina Morantz-Sanchez has shown, Tait was known for using money he earned from treating rich patients to fund his work with the poor. Morantz-Sanchez, *Conduct Unbecoming of a Woman*, 152.

90. Thomas More Madden, 'On the So-Called Laparotomy Epidemic', *Dublin Journal of Medical Science* 82, no. 1 (1886): 2.

91. Thomas More Madden, 'Observations on Removal of the Uterine Appendages', *British Medical Journal* 1, no. 1358 (8 January 1887): 52–54.

92. Madden, 'On the So-Called Laparotomy Epidemic', 2.

93. 'Extirpation of Ovarian Tumors', *Medico-Chirurgical Review* 40 (1 April 1844): 557.

94. 'I cannot believe that all the ovariotomies that were performed after Spencer Wells found out how to do it were necessary', George Bernard Shaw, 'The Socialist Criticism of the Medical Profession', *Transactions of the Medico-Legal Society* 6 (1909): 216.

95. Shaw, 'The Socialist Criticism of the Medical Profession', *Transactions*, 216–217. Tonsillectomy was performed with increasing frequency in the early twentieth century. See Sally Wilde, *The History of Surgery: Trust, Patient Autonomy, Medical Dominance and Australian Surgery, 1890–1940* (Byron Bay: Finesse Press, 2010), 79.

96. Moscucci, *The Science of Woman*, 149.

97. Thomas M. Dolan, 'Gynaecological Specialism and General Practice', *British Gynaecological Journal* 5, no. 19 (1889): 296.

98. 'The Usefulness of Spaying', *Medical Record* 29, no. 15 (1886): 419. As quoted in the *Medical Press and Circular*. 'Editorial: The Virtues of

Laparotomy', *Medical Press and Circular* 41, no. 2457 (1886): 502–503. 'Polypedic' referred to multiple children.

99. 'Editorial: The Virtues of Laparotomy', 502–503. See also Mary J. Hall-Williams, *Ovariotomy Averted* (Plymouth, 1899).

100. Holly Brockwell, 'Why Can't I Get Sterilised in My 20s?' *The Guardian* (28 January 2015), http://www.theguardian.com/commentisfree/2015/jan/28/why-wont-nhs-let-me-be-sterilised#comment-46773414, accessed 11 December 2017.

101. By 1883, the mortality rate at the Samaritan Hospital in London was about one in eighteen. Not all surgeons were able to claim such results, though. In 1887, the surgeon Charles Cullingworth, who would shortly after move from Manchester to take up a position at St. Thomas' Hospital in London, reported that he had lost 13.5% of his thirty-seven ovariotomy patients during the first half of the 1880s. Thomas Spencer Wells, 'An Inaugural Address on the Revival of Ovariotomy, and Its Influence on Modern Surgery', *Lancet* 124, no. 3194 (15 November 1884): 857; Charles Cullingworth, 'A Tabular Statement of Sixty-Four Abdominal Sections; Including Forty-Five Completed Ovariotomies with Remarks', *Lancet* 130, no. 3335 (30 July 1887): 205.

102. Patients' anxiety about undergoing an operation remains virtually universal. E. Carr et al., 'Patterns and Frequency of Anxiety in Women Undergoing Gynaecological Surgery', *Journal of Clinical Nursing* 15, no. 3 (2006), 341–352.

103. Brock, 'Risk, Responsibility and Surgery', 330.

104. 'The Patient Insisted Upon Abdominal Section!', *The Hospital* 23 (12 March 1898): 412.

105. Morantz-Sanchez, *Conduct Unbecoming of a Woman*, 106–107; Editorial response to correspondence from Robert Lawson Tait, *Medical Press and Circular* 42, no. 2471 (1886): 203.

106. Andrea Rabagliati, 'Notes on Abdominal Section for Ovariotomy, Oophorectomy, and Hysterectomy', *Medical Press and Circular* 41, no. 2455 (1886): 445.

107. Morantz-Sanchez, *Conduct Unbecoming of a Woman*, 50. Morantz-Sanchez cites the American experience specifically, but contemporary reports suggest a similar attitude prevailed in Britain. In 1879 Heywood Smith wrote 'Where a patient is able to afford to lie up and have every appliance for the relief of pain, when, at the same time, her general health is not suffering much, she might be advised to wait and tide over the time till the menopause. But when a patient is poor and dependent upon others who are equally poor, when her sufferings extend over at least three weeks out of every four, when she is quite unable to earn her living, and when she prefers running a certain amount of risk to

continuing in her wretched and useless state, then we are bound to listen to her pleading, and do what improved science places in our power to do to relieve pain'. Heywood Smith, 'Successful Case of Battey's Operation or Oöphorectomy', British Medical Journal 2, no. 967 (1879): 42.

108. On Samuel Pozzi, see Caroline de Costa and Francesca Miller, *The Diva and Doctor God: Letters from Sarah Bernhardt to Doctor Samuel Pozzi* (Bloomington: Xlibris, 2010).

109. Judith Walkowitz, *City of Dreadful Delight: Narratives of Sexual Danger in Late Victorian London* (Chicago: University of Chicago Press, 1992), 48; see also Mary Louise Roberts, 'Review Essay: Gender, Consumption and Commodity Culture', *American Historical Review* 103, no. 3 (1998): 817–844.

6

The Afterlife of an Operation

'The perfecting of ovariotomy has resulted in the saving and prolonging the lives of multitudes', surgeon John Halliday Croom declared in 1896, adopting a salvational tone that was common among surgeons as they reflected upon the triumphs of their craft over the previous decades.[1] Surgeons of the late nineteenth century had seen remarkable changes in their field and to Croom's mind, as to many others', it was ovariotomy that most evocatively conveyed the remarkable ability of surgeons to cure. The lengthy battle for the operation's acceptance reinforced a narrative of victory among the profession, augmented by the fact that it was women—the wives, mothers and daughters of Britain, the Empire and beyond—who were being drawn away from the clutches of disease. This fitted with broader understandings Victorian surgeons had of themselves as a civilising force, their life-saving work a melding of sagacity and selflessness. Already by 1877 Thomas Spencer Wells had proclaimed that his ovariotomy operations alone had added eighteen thousand years to the lives of European women, a claim that was duly repeated by the medical and general press over the following years.[2] By the end of the century, the fruits of ovariotomists' labour appeared manifest in the many hundreds of successful cases that continued to be reported in the medical literature. Gatherings of medical societies in the final decades of the century frequently give rise to speeches similar to Wells' and Croom's, which weaved together the success of ovariotomy with a broader narrative of sur-gery which stressed the craft's unprecedented progress from a dark age of butchery to its present incarnation of modern wonderment. Connecting contemporary practices with their historical lineage brought doctors into contact with the cultural value which came with longevity and tradition. Historicising the craft was a way to restore equilibrium between science and art, which some felt was threatened by the growing centrality of the laboratory to medicine. In the last years of the century, there was a resur-gent interest in the role of history within medical education as a means of ensuring students became well-rounded doctors, able to look beyond the laboratory and recognise the value of history, as well as literature and philosophy, in shaping the modern medical man; in essence, many doctors sought to reclaim the gentleman-physician ideal for the profession.[3]

Underneath the celebratory stories of surgeons there lurked, how-ever, a rather more complex status to ovariotomy and what it repre-sented. Through it, the past, present and future of surgery intermingled uneasily, as the operation—while still in use—was also utilised by sur-geons to try and understand both the controversial past of surgery and its recent progress. Surgery before this time was increasingly viewed with a sense of disbelief: how, some wondered, could surgeons have worked under circumstances where there was no anaesthesia, no antisepsis and no abdominal surgery? How could practitioners of the early nineteenth century have been so blind to the possibilities of ovariotomy? Such senti-ments were entangled with an apprehension as to where the future of sur-gery lay and a desire on the part of many to look back at the past decades for guidance. By the turn of the century, the history of ovariotomy gave rise to both disbelief as to the way surgery had been only a few decades earlier, as well as nostalgia for an era that had passed. Moreover, while thought by many to have revolutionised surgery, ovariotomy was also beginning to lose some of its pre-eminence as a versatile surgical tool that could be used to rectify an array of medical problems. Increasingly, the value of the operation—as well as the theories which underpinned it— were challenged by new ideas in physiology. All the while, ovarian sur-gery continued to be a central part of surgical practice, sometimes even flourishing in new ways. In fact, despite the controversies of the 1880s explored in Chapter 5, procedures involving the removal of one or both ovaries were being performed more than ever. Up until the late 1930s, the term 'ovariotomy' remained common in medical parlance, although the meaning of the word, long a source of confusion and contention, was becoming ever more complicated. For these reasons, the transition of ovariotomy from a 'contemporary' practice to an 'historical' one was without any definitive lines of demarcation. Yet, fast forward to today and 'ovariotomy' is a word seldom used by surgeons and rather more by historians. What then happened to ovariotomy after the controversies surrounding it peaked in the late nineteenth century? And how did it shift from being a contemporary phenomenon to an historical one?

Evaluating this transition is useful in that it goes beyond a simplistic account of the 'decline' of ovariotomy. What I offer instead is something more akin to exploring the 'afterlife' of the operation. By doing so I intend to show how circularity operated—and continues to operate—between contemporary and historical accounts of the procedure, while also seeking to problematise our understanding of innovation in terms of acceptance or rejection. The broader point I make is that histories constructed by turn-of-the century surgeons should be recognised for their historiographical significance rather than only as whiggish constructs. The 'traditional' doctor-authored account of medical history often remains grist for the mill to social historians of medicine, 'a simplistic straw figure, cited only that it may be trounced', as Frank Huisman and John Harley Warner have put it.[4] This chapter instead conceives of surgeons' turn to history as a significant *part* of ovariotomy's innovation, rather than merely reflections upon an already-established innovation. For it was through the production of historical accounts that the operation's identity as a striking and significant moment in medicine was moulded. Furthermore, surgeons' reflections on the operation revealed a difficult relationship with the concept of innovation that was not merely read in terms of triumph. As Victorian surgeons grappled with connecting past, present and future, so too this chapter interlaces their sense of history with contemporary historians', emphasising connectivity between understandings then and now of ovariotomy which are often underplayed. This chapter is about both ends and beginnings.

ALL IN A NAME? DECLINE, DIFFUSION AND SURGICAL LINGUISTICS

Medical innovations are often historicised as either diffused and accepted or definitively rejected. Surgery is no exception. Writing on the history of gynaecological operations, Ann Dally argued that 'new operations were invented and either flourished and developed or declined into oblivion'.[5]

In the case of ovariotomy however, neither option is sufficiently explanatory as to what happened to it towards the end of the nineteenth century. There has been a tendency for histories of the operation to conclude with the outcries that came from many in the profession in the 1880s and 1890s that ovarian surgery was being performed excessively, an episode which acts as a convenient and dramatic endpoint to its historical narrative. Ornella Moscucci, for instance, describes the continued echoes of the ovariotomy controversy in ensuing debates as to whether obstetricians or general surgeons had the 'right' to perform pelvic surgery.[6] But it was, she argues, the Imlach affair in 1886 which 'brought into relief not only beliefs about the biological basis of femininity, but also profound tensions within the obstetrical profession over the propriety of radical operations'.[7] Lawrence Longo and Regina Morantz-Sanchez, albeit looking at the American experience, conclude similarly that there was a decline in radical ovarian surgery in the 1890s, followed by a shift to more conservative procedures.[8] As will be shown here, in Britain at least, the transition in surgical style was not necessarily so smooth.

In part, the difficulty of unpacking this moment in the history of the operation is because further consideration is needed of how exactly we measure decline and dissemination in surgery, and the extent to which such a framework is even useful. Sally Wilde has applied the 'career' innovation path—a characteristic approach in innovation studies—to surgical operations. As she sees it, 'operations have careers, and the processes through which they are developed have many parallels to the processes through which other technological innovations are developed'.[9] Wilde separates operations into those which might be classed as 'production line operations' and those which are 'unstable objects'. In the former category she locates procedures such as tonsillectomy, performed with increasing frequency from the early twentieth century onwards and, despite going through various fashions and periods of decline, has been continually practised from the time of its inception. If not completely standardised, the operation has at least become a stable part of surgical culture. In the other category are operations that enjoyed a brief vogue before disappearing entirely. Wilde suggests as examples Battey's operation and nephropexy, the latter a moderately controversial operation which became popular in the late nineteenth century and involved surgically treating the condition commonly known as 'floating kidney'.[10] Thus, Wilde establishes a dichotomy between those surgical novelties that 'succeed' and those that 'fail'.

Wilde is right that some operations have identities more durable than others. But surgical operations are inherently unstable entities and the staged 'career' approach to technological innovation can oversimplify understandings of 'new' surgery. Meanings of operations shift continually, no matter how long and established their history. A tonsillectomy is performed, experienced and interpreted quite differently today than from how it was in the 1920s. Nephropexy as well, once ridiculed by much of the surgical profession, is in fact in use again today, but framed by an entirely difference medico-cultural context.[11] Even if the technical objective remains the same, there is a continual negotiation between surgical nomenclature and the meaning of an operation, which complicates notions of success and failure.

Ovariotomy similarly belies the staged career model. In the last decades of the nineteenth century, the question was less whether ovariotomy was accepted or rejected but what it had come to mean. Such concerns, as we have seen, were not new; the definition of ovariotomy was often in flux and, in particular, defining the difference between ovariotomy and oöphorectomy had significant ethical ramifications. But during the late nineteenth century, the relationship between nomenclature and procedure grew steadily more unwieldy and was subject to increasing linguistic complexity. By the end of the 1880s, the terms used to describe ovarian operations had expanded so greatly that it left many surgeons unsure about what the original and most popular term, 'ovariotomy' actually meant. 'Ovariotomy' *usually* indicated the treatment of tumours and cysts. Oöphorectomy tended to signal treatment for inflammatory conditions, diseases of the Fallopian tubes and the removal of the ovaries as a means of bringing on the menopause. But these definitions were by no means hard and fast and could be used interchangeably. For example, 'oöphorectomy' could also be taken to indicate the removal of both ovaries, while 'ovariotomy' could refer to the removal of just one of them, regardless of the pathological reason behind the operation. Intermingled with this were other terms, including 'double ovariotomy', 'removal of the uterine appendages', 'Battey's Operation', and 'salpingo-oöphorectomy', and which together, served to further complicate the language of ovarian surgery.

Surgical textbooks, which might be expected to offer a degree of nuance, did little to clarify the definition of ovariotomy. In their 1897 monograph *Diseases of Women: A Handbook for Students and Practitioners,* Arthur Giles and John Bland-Sutton, surgeons at the Chelsea Hospital for Women, who were by the 1890s two of the most prolific performers of the operation in London, described ovariotomy as 'the removal through an incision in the abdominal wall of tumours and cysts of the ovary and parovarium'.[12] Fourteen years later, Victor Bonney and George Comyns Berkeley, colleagues of Giles and Bland-Sutton, gave an even vaguer definition, referring to ovariotomy simply as 'the removal of an ovarian tumour, either cystic or solid', omitting to mention whether the term could be applied to operations where both ovaries were affected, or only to those where just one ovary was removed.[13] Lay conceptions of the operation were undoubtedly even cloudier. This was significant. Intertwined with the issues of patient consent and surgical abuse of power that cases such as Beatty versus Cullingworth had raised, was the question of the right a surgeon had to change and adapt a procedure mid-operation, as had occurred in the case of Alice Jane Beatty when her second ovary was removed, she claimed, without her consent. Sally Wilde has suggested that surgeons' freedom to adapt in this way highlights hierarchical structures within medicine, demonstrating the power surgeons have historically wielded in moulding new procedures as they saw fit.[14] Implicit in this hierarchical structure was also a power over patients: what might seem to be a simply a question of nomenclature was, through the experience of those who actually underwent the operation, equally an ethical one.

This did not mean the issue didn't trouble some in the profession too; 'the nomenclature is so various, and some of its terms so ambiguous, that all will concur in the advisability for the adoption of certain words which will indicate clearly particular operations', wrote one surgeon on the matter in a letter to the *British Medical Journal* in 1886. 'What is "ovariotomy?"' he appealed.[15] A response a few weeks later from an anonymous Fellow of the Royal College of Surgeons indicated concern was prevalent: 'with every succeeding advance, fresh difficulties in division and in nomenclature have arisen' the author argued, 'the question, "what is ovariotomy?" is one which, at the present moment, it is perfectly impossible to give a definite and scientific answer to'.[16] The author's implication that 'ovariotomy' failed to provide an adequately scientific definition suggested that the proliferation of different types of procedure was not the only issue at hand. By the end of the 1880s, the term was beginning to appear outdated, unscientific and unhelpful; in part because it did little to indicate the pathology of the tumour being treated by the operation. Younger surgeons were increasingly cognisant of the importance histology held in their clinical calculations.

Ovarian pathology was fertile ground in this respect. Histological investigations had only reinforced the long-held notion among medical
practitioners that the ovaries were an extremely common site of disease,
and this was reflected in surgical pathology, a field that was led by John
Bland-Sutton at the turn of the century. It is no coincidence that Bland-
Sutton combined his specialism in ovarian surgery with a strong interest in the histology of tumours, asserting in 1906 that it was because of
the structural complexity of the organ with its multiplicity of tissues that
the ovaries were with 'extraordinary frequency the source of tumours'.[17]
Although 'ovarian tumour' and 'ovarian cyst' continued to be used,
more precise terms were increasingly employed to describe the variety of
growths that could occur, including adenomas, paraovarian cysts, fibro-
mas and sarcomas. Regardless of speciality, many surgical terms in use
were perceived to fail in reflecting precise pathology; 'ovariotomy', with
its misnomered suffix, highlighted how scientifically imprecise popular
surgical terms could be.[18]

On a purely lexical level, a decline in the use of the term ensued from
the 1880s. Though a slightly crude approach—looking as it does at the
quantity rather than content of conversation—the volume of discussion
regarding ovariotomy in the medical weeklies provides a useful overview in this regard (Fig. 6.1). Looking at the number of times the word
'ovariotomy' was cited in an article of any type in the *Lancet* and *British
Medical Journal* during the six decades between 1880 and 1939, we see
a continuous decline in the use of the word. There is a sharp drop in
particular from the first to the second decade of the 1900s, during which
'oöphorectomy' was increasingly favoured to describe ovarian operations
of all types. By the 1940s, 'ovariotomy' had almost entirely disappeared
from medical publications in Britain, excepting where older cases were
cited as supporting evidence to new developments in physiology and surgery, or where doctors prefaced their work with a brief historical introduction. While the term was in clear decline, that decline was arguably
slow, considering its acknowledged imperfections. In 1933, the eminent
obstetrician Herbert Spencer used the term to give a 'Review of 658
Ovariotomies' that he had performed in his career. He described ovariotomy as 'the removal of an ovarian or paraovarian tumour, including
the excision of a tumour from the ovary, with the retention of the rest of
the organ' (although not including the removal of 'normal or small cystic
ovaries').[19] Spencer's definition alluded to the greater use of conservative

	Lancet	British Medical Journal
1880–1889	440	541
1890–1899	391	441
1900–1909	229	266
1910–1919	78	100
1920–1929	58	70
1930–1939	31	41

Fig. 6.1 Number of articles in which 'ovariotomy' is cited in the *Lancet* and *British Medical Journal* (1880–1939) (*Source* Elsevier Science Direct Database (http://www.sciencedirect.com) and *The BMJ* online archives (http://www.bmj.com/archive) (accessed 29 August 2013))

techniques that was by then occurring in ovarian surgery and his 658 cases included a range of technically distinct procedures. Yet given the nature of the publication—a review of his surgical work that spanned over forty years—it was only 'ovariotomy', it seems, that could adequately convey his practice during that time, in what was both a contemporary medical report and an historical account of his career.

The continued sensitivity surrounding 'oöphorectomy'—a word deeply associated with over-operating—that continued into the 1890s may explain why 'ovariotomy' did not shift easily from medical language, even as its meaning became uncertain, and where 'oöphorectomy' was technically a more accurate term for any operation that involved the removal of the whole ovary, as the majority of 'ovariotomies' did. The structure of the word offered a degree of ambiguity which potentially protected surgeons from being associated with radical interventions, the suffix 'otomy' denoting surgical interference but not surgical removal. Medical nomenclature is not easily changed once it has become common parlance, nor are clarity or technical accuracy the only factors which occasion its use. As one medical commentator reflected in 1940, medical terminology is a 'mixture in which historical and sentimental factors play a large part'.[20] Ovariotomy, which had come to represent a poignant and triumphant episode in surgery and which was deeply steeped in history and emotional resonance, retained a powerful symbolism that was not easily lost.

Indeed, 'ovariotomy' never quite disappeared from scientific use. Looking internationally, it is noticeable that medical researchers still occasionally use the term today, showing that, as Stuart Hall has described it, 'we never cleanse language completely', as well demonstrating the subtle linguistic shifts that can occur translationally in medicine.[21] 'Ovariotomy' remained deeply embedded in medical language even after concerns began to be raised as to its clarity in the 1880s. Well into the twentieth century meaning was shifting to accommodate the term, rather than terminology being promptly altered to reflect changing understandings of the operation. The historic achievements that had occurred in ovarian surgery were indelibly associated with that one word: 'ovariotomy'. Nonetheless by the end of the century, the reputation of ovariotomists for remarkable success was coming under threat, as the long-term effects of ovarian surgery began to be scrutinised more closely. Past triumphs were now being challenged by fears for the future.

AFTERLIVES: PATIENT EXPERIENCES AFTER OVARIAN SURGERY

In the 1890s and early 1900s, serious concerns began to arise about the fates of those who had undergone ovariotomy. In part this was a continuation of anxieties already present by the 1880s, about the probable sterility of those who had had both ovaries removed and the consequences this might have upon the general health and wealth of the populace, closely bound up as it was with the politics of reproduction. In the 1890s concerns widened out to the general long-term health of the patient; 'what is the condition, mental and physical, which obtains in a castrated woman? I care not if it be said that mortality is small. But what are the symptoms in after life?' asked Charles Routh, physician to the Samaritan Free Hospital, in 1894.[22] As has been discussed already, the importance of tracking the post-operative outcomes of those who underwent abdominal surgery was already acknowledged by surgeons, who recognised that the risk of complications and subsequent death in the weeks after an operation often remained high. But by the end of the century surgical mortality rates were sufficiently low so as to make serious discussion about the longer-term effects of such operations worthwhile. Medical texts such as John Lockhart-Mummery's *The After-Treatment of Operations* (1903) were novel in that they focused wholly on the recovery period and called for surgeons to give greater attention to the health and individual needs of their patients after an operation was complete.[23]

The interest in the long-term consequences of operations intersected with the growing attention of life insurance companies to the risks of further ill-health in surgical patients.[24] Insurance companies were well-established by the mid-nineteenth century, as was doctors' involvement in the life assurance business.[25] But the interest of such companies in surgery in the early twentieth century was a new departure. In the 1900s, the Life Assurance Medical Officers' Association published pamphlets which brought surgery into the fold of insurance claims, acknowledging that the field had until recently been led by physicians. The inclusion of surgery was based partly on an understanding that there was an increase in serious but survivable operations taking place, making surgery a potentially lucrative market for insurance policies. The encroachment of the insurance industry upon surgery generated vigorous discussion about the influence of both pre-operative health and the postoperative period upon surgical risk. At a meeting of the Life Assurance Medical Officers' Association, surgeon Alfred Pearce Gould identified three possible risks that needed to be considered: first, the loss of function that came with the removal of certain parts of the body—Gould echoing the debates eighteenth-century practitioners had entered into regarding the effect of organ removal upon the body's physiology—second, the risks of additional injuries and diseases that the operation entailed, and third, the effects of surgery upon the nervous system.[26]

Having been performed so prolifically over the last three decades, and with an ever-present degree of controversy, the long-term effects of ovariotomy were exemplary of the type beginning to be studied in more detail by the 1890s, and some of the conclusions being reached about the operation were worrying. Most concerning of all was that the operation appeared to be implicated in the development of cancer.[27] Understandings of cancer were considerably transformed in the nineteenth century, during which time malignancies came to be understood as local in origin rather than constitutional. As Ornella Moscucci has shown, this had a significant impact upon cultural perceptions of the disease. By the early twentieth century, Moscucci argues, cancer had become a potent public health issue, as doctors and other concerned parties strove to high-light that if the disease was caught early, it was possible to cure it, challenging the sense of fatalism that lingered around the 'dread disease'.[28] The long-held assumption that women were more susceptible to cancer than men only intensified during this time; cancer was thought to attack women's breasts and reproductive organs with peculiar aggression.[29] In general, cancer deaths were thought to be increasing. The phenomenon was linked with modern lifestyles; cancer was the physical price of the industrialised, fast-paced, nervous life of Western society.[30] Doctors discussed the possibility that a nervous disposition in a woman could cause cell disruption, which in turn increased the risk of cancer, particularly breast cancer. A potent metaphorical reciprocity between degeneration and cancer began to play out unhappily and the language used to describe cancerous change was often that of inescapable decline.[31]

A source of great suffering for those afflicted with them, malignancies of the womb were the focus of a turn towards surgery for treating cancer in the 1890s.[32] Gynaecologists soon demonstrated the potential for surgery to provide a solution to cancer as the curative rates for cancer of the cervix, including advanced cases, begin to increase substantially following the introduction of new procedures for the disease.[33] In stark contrast, ovarian malignancies remained virtually untouched by such developments. The difficulties in detecting ovarian tumours in their early stages continued to be a problem for surgeons, to whom cancer of the ovary remained as it always had been: a fearful and insidious disease. Surgeons in part rested the justifiability of radical surgery for ovarian tumours on the possibility that a growth might be an early malignancy or might become malignant.[34] But in cases of undoubted and advanced cancer, operations carried very little hope and were rarely performed. As surgery for cancer of the cervix became a symbol of hope in the battle against the disease, surgery for ovarian malignancies remained 'an operation…of a desperate character…only carried through because the removal of the growth offers at least a small chance of life, while the alternative to removal is certain death'.[35] The continued difficulties in both diagnosing and treating ovarian cancer would cement the disease's reputation as a 'silent killer'.[36]

Indeed, it seemed plausible to some that ovarian surgery was in fact a cause of rather than a cure for cancer. Surgeons began to cast a critical eye upon the records of past ovariotomists, arguing that the procedure increased the chances of a woman developing cancer. The most avid proponent of this theory was William Roger Williams, who had previously been surgeon at the Middlesex Hospital, one of the few hospitals to have specialist cancer wards.[37] Like others, Williams connected cancer to ageing. Breast cancer, for example, seemed more likely to occur after the menopause when the ovaries were no longer active. By this logic, Williams argued, removing the ovaries caused a premature ageing of the reproductive system and thus increased the risk of malignancy. Controversially, he used Thomas Spencer Wells' records to show what appeared to be a dramatically high incidence of cancer among women who had had ovaries removed by Wells, particularly—but not exclusively—those who had had both removed. Of the eighty-eight patients of Wells' that had died since the operation and where the cause of death was known, Williams reported that thirty-two had perished from cancer, a mortality rate of over one in three. This he compared to cancer mortality in the general population of women, which he placed at one in fifteen.[38] Williams' analysis brought an unwelcome angle not only to the much-revered legacy of Thomas Spencer Wells but to ovariotomy as a whole. By Williams' estimation, there were two possibilities: the first was that Wells had operated on more malignancy cases than he had admitted to, whether knowingly or unknowingly. The second was that surgical treatment for local disease had potentially devastating effects on the rest of the body, especially if performed upon the reproductive organs.[39]

Williams's views did not gain widespread acceptance. But they mingled uneasily with other concerns that were being raised about the long-term consequences of ovarian surgery, one of the most widely discussed of which was whether the operation might be responsible in causing insanity when performed upon women who already exhibited tendencies towards mental fragility. If this was the case, it not only undermined the panacean optimism of the 1880s, which had led some practitioners to remove the ovaries in an attempt to cure madness, but it completely reversed the relationship between surgery and insanity, positing the former as a cause rather than a cure. Surgeons and alienists alike were producing cases where operations of all types appeared to have triggered a severe mental reaction. Various arguments were put forward as to the cause of post-operative insanity, from septic shock to the effect of anaesthesia to the anxiety of the patient undergoing the operation.[40] Many feared operations of the reproductive organs came with the greatest risk to the nerves; in regard to women, this idea hinged upon the connection between the ovaries, the menopause, and the mental precariousness which the latter was thought to induce.[41] In 1906, the Life Assurance Medical Officers' Association issued a pamphlet warning of the risk of acute melancholia following ovariotomy and castration.[42] It was yet another permutation of the perpetual dialogue between the reproductive organs and the wider bodily economy that was expressed through the operation.

The passing of time and accumulation of cases meant that a plethora of information on the post-operative lives of ovariotomy patients was available by the early 1900s. The most exhaustive study was that authored by the Chelsea Hospital surgeon Arthur Giles. Published in 1910, *A Study of the After-Results of Abdominal Operations on the Pelvic Organs* recorded one thousand operative cases, mainly operations upon the ovaries, Fallopian tubes and uterus, performed by Giles since 1894, and which included follow-up information on 728 of the cases where he'd been able to trace the patient. Giles built upon the already present networks of informal correspondence that existed between patients, their usual medical attendants and operating surgeons, and which often saw the latter attempt to follow up on former cases at a later date; his work anticipated a general trend among surgeons towards more consistent reporting of the 'remote' results of operations.[43] Giles' former patients were asked a series of questions ranging from the operation's physical effects ('have you had any pain since the operation?') to its impact on sexual relations ('have marital relations been the same as before the operation?') to the vexed question of its impact upon mental health ('are you usually cheerful, irritable, or depressed?').[44] Where possible, patients were asked to submit to a medical examination too. (see Fig. 6.2).[45] Giles was able to follow up on eighty per cent of his cases, a remarkable endeavour given that locating and corresponding with former patients was not always easy and there was not necessarily a motivation on the part of patients to participate in the exercise.[46] If the results were to be believed—some were hesitant about Giles' self-reporting of his own cases[47]—they appeared to show just how significant the impact of an operation could be on a patient's life; twelve months after their operation, ninety per cent of Giles' patients reported that their health was better than it had been before the procedure. Giles also allayed some of the more extreme fears about what happened to women who had both ovaries removed. Reflecting on two hundred such cases, he reported that '70 per cent of the patients regained perfect health and rigour and retained their sex-instincts; that the legends of women developing bass voices and growing beards were pure romance; and that there was no more tendency to insanity after double ovariotomy than there was after any other abdominal operation', thus challenging the concerns voiced about the physiological and psychological effects of removing the ovaries.[48]

188   AFTER-RESULTS OF ABDOMINAL OPERATIONS   TABLE M   189

TABLE M. Total Extirpation for Ovarian Tumours.

Initials Age C.S.	Date.	Place.	Doctor.	Operation Notes.	Wound.	General Health.	Local Conditions.	Remarks.	Date.
1 J.O. 49 S	1905 Dec. 11	C.H.W.	—	Left ovarian (?parovarian) cyst; uterus and right ovary previously removed for fibroid	—	Not very good; has headaches; "much better than before"	Uterus absent; vagina normal	Spinster. Depressed sometimes	Oct. 10, 1907
2 R.H. 26 M	1907 June 27	P.W.H.	Dr. D. McArdie	Large right parovarian cyst, densely adherent to floor of pelvis; left salpingo-oophoritis	S.A.	Very good; "much better"	Normal stump of cervix; vagina normal	Has normal feelings and desire. Cheerful	Mar. 10, 1909
3 A.C. 32 M	1908 Feb. 20	Do.	Dr. W. H. Howlett	Left ovarian cyst in broad ligament and hydrosalpinx; right tubo-ovarian cyst; hysterectomy for dense adhesions	—	Indifferent; has indigestion; "worse in myself at times"	Normal stump of cervix; vagina normal	No difference in marital relations. Gets depressed	Feb. 20, 1909
4 A.C. 53 W	Oct. 14	P.	Dr. Mcare Dr. W. R. Orr	Right ovarian cyst with papilloma; left ovarian cyst	S.A.	Very good	Not examined	Cheerful	Oct. 13, 1909
5 L.B. 34 S.	Nov. 2	C.H.W.	Dr. A. T. Scott Dr. W. Paul Jones	Large left ovarian cyst (15 lbs.); cystic right ovary; uterine fibroids	11½" long	"Very good indeed"	Normal small stump of cervix; vagina normal	Cheerful. Spinster	Oct. 21, 1909
6 M.A.L. 55 M	Nov. 5	P.W.H.	Dr. W. Love	Large left ovarian cyst; smaller right; small fibroids in uterus	—	"Very...good; much better"	Vagina atrophic; normal small stump of cervix	Menopause 8 years before operation. Marital relations unaltered. Cheerful	Dec. 14, 1909
7 A.L. 51	Nov. 19	Do.	—	Double ovarian carcinoma; hydroperitoneum	—	Patient died of recurrence, May 12th, 1909.			
8 H.S. 48 S.	Dec. 12	Do.	Dr. C. R. Salisbury	Large left intraligamentary ovarian cyst with grumous contents; right cystic ovary; uterine fibroids	H.	"Very good indeed; I feel perfectly well"	Normal small stump of cervix; vagina normal	Cheerful. Spinster	Dec. 16, 1909
9 J.M. 40 M	1909 Feb. 15	C.H.W.	Dr. R. H. Marjoribanks	Large right ovarian cyst with intra-cystic haemorrhage; left cystic ovary; multiple small fibroids	—	"Very well; as well as before operation; was not ill before"	Normal small stump of cervix; vagina normal	Desire and feeling never much developed, but both diminished since operation. Cheerful	Jan. 23, 1910
10 C.S. 57 W	May 13	P.W.H.	—	Large left ovarian multilocular cyst; extensive adhesions, multiple fibroids, flattened over cyst	9" long	Good, but still rather weak; much better altogether than before	Small atrophic stump of cervix; some atrophy of vagina	Menopause in 1903. Cheerful. widow	Jan. 21, 1910

◀ **Fig. 6.2** Arthur Giles, *A Study of the After-Results of Abdominal Operations on the Pelvic Organs: Based on a Series of 1000 Consecutive Cases* (1910). Part of Giles' table showing the results of operations that involved the 'Total Extirpation for Ovarian Tumours'. Giles provided one of the most detailed accounts yet of the long-term effects of ovariotomy and other forms of ovarian surgery (*Credit* Wellcome Collection CC BY)

Giles' study broadly corroborated similar reports about abdominal and gynaecological surgery published during this period, but it provided perhaps the most exhaustive analysis.[49] By dint of the sheer detail of his work, the shimmers of heroism associated with ovariotomy could only be eroded by what was an in-depth examination of patients' lives after the operation. While most women confirmed they had experienced a general improvement in health, Giles' study also showed the variation in post-operative experience. Those such as A.C., who complained of being 'worse in myself at times' or C.S., who, although better than before the operation was 'still rather weak', were statistically successes, but for whom the long-term outcome had been rather less good. Giles' results also showed just how long and drawn out the process of recovery from an abdominal operation was; one year on from their procedure, only sixty-eight per cent of his patients had fully recovered, while a further eight to ten per cent were 'incapacitated during all this time'.[50] Giles' work also addressed the question of how risky it was to leave behind the second, healthy ovary, in case it later became diseased, something which had been a source of contention in the Beatty versus Cullingworth case. Disease recurrence had only occurred in ten per cent of Giles' cases, which some practitioners viewed as a relatively small risk, but it would have been a risk, nonetheless, that not all surgeons would have been willing to take.[51]

Assessments of the long-term effects of ovarian surgery allayed some of the fears about its consequences. But it also compelled surgeons to consider more carefully the implications of removing the organ. By the early 1900s new trends in medicine internationally were once more challenging and changing the techniques of British ovariotomists.

COULD OVARIOTOMY EVER HAVE BEEN CONSERVATIVE?

It has been suggested by Annmarie Adams and Thomas Schlich that during the late nineteenth century a significant shift occurred—a new paradigm even—in which surgery came to be principally based upon physiology.

They argue that surgical innovation was increasingly centred upon restoring or correcting physiological function through surgical measures, exemplified by the growing interest among surgeons in experimental organ transplantation.[52] Applying this to ovarian surgery, Regina Morantz-Sanchez has contended that while 'moral qualms may have produced the most dramatic of the critiques of over-operating' it was in fact these 'ongoing attempts to explore the chemical, physiological, and pathological processes of the female reproductive system' that was the *coup de grâce* for the regular use of radical ovarian surgery at the end of the nineteenth century.[53] Historians have highlighted a deeply symbiotic relationship between physiology and clinical practice that was at the centre of this; both Schlich and Chandak Sengoopta argue that it was increasing concerns about the long-term effects of ovarian surgery that in fact spurred on experimental ovarian transplants by European gynaecologists in the early 1900s. At the heart of this was the work of Viennese gynaecologist Emil Knauer, whose experimentation with re-grafting transplanted ovarian tissue in rabbits was prompted by his concerns about the acute menopausal-like symptoms some women experienced after having both ovaries removed.[54] Although ultimately abandoned by the 1930s, Knauer's experiments inspired numerous performances of ovarian transplants in Europe and America over the next three decades, not only to restore ovarian function in women who had had ovaries removed, but also to treat a vast range of other conditions, including mental illnesses. As Schlich notes, during this early phase of transplantation surgery it was ovarian transplantations that were the most common form of the procedure.[55] Thus, the early decades of the century saw a striking turnaround in physiological understandings of the ovary, which—in theory at least—saw the introduction of ovarian tissue replace its removal as a cure-all for the maladies of women; if the rationale and technique of surgery had changed, one thing was consistent: the identity of the ovary as an organ highly amenable to surgical interference and which saw it, once more, prominent in the formulation of new surgical techniques.

From these physiological experiments—both animal and human—an idea was gaining traction that the ovary produced 'internal secretions', somewhat mysterious products of the organ which appeared to influence the development and maintenance of the reproductive system. It was this, Regina Morantz-Sanchez has contended, that precipitated a shift towards conservative ovarian surgery in the 1890s, characterised by 'the trend among younger students to resect (cut away parts) of organs wherever possible', and by increasing divisions between 'conservative' and 'radical' ovariotomists.[56] Here, however, the British and American experiences seem to have differed. In Britain, not only was there considerable scepticism as to the usefulness of taking a more conservative approach, but what exactly constituted conservative surgery of the ovary was not clear. 'Conservative surgery' is a rather problematic term which has received surprisingly little attention from historians since Gert Brieger addressed the shift between 'radical' and 'conservative' types of operative surgery in late nineteenth-century America. Principles of conservative surgery were of course not novel to the late nineteenth century: John Hunter's aphorism that operations were 'the defect of surgery' had long been embedded in surgical philosophy.[57] But, as Brieger contends, by the end of the nineteenth century the meanings attached to both 'radical' and 'conservative' surgery were complicated, the latter, in particular, having a number of meanings. Generally, it alluded to the preservation of as much bodily tissue from the surgeon's knife as possible; but, Brieger argues, 'in the last decades of the nineteenth century radical could also mean conservative in the sense of complete or finally curative; conservative of life'.[58] To add a further complication, it was also possible for tissue-preserving techniques to be potentially curative. Thus, 'radical' and 'curative' were no longer necessarily equated with one another as they had been earlier in the century; the conservative could also be the curative.[59]

Brieger's fine-grained analysis concludes with his assertion that during the middle and late decades of the nineteenth century, technically conservative surgery prevailed in America, with resection deemed considerably more effective and desirable than radical surgery. But the most important aspect of his analysis is that it shows that competing surgical philosophies of radicalism and conservatism did not necessarily form the basis of a hard and fast professional schism; the definitions of both were simply too elastic, especially when it came to ovariotomy. In part this was because conservative surgery had thus far been defined through operations on the external parts of the body, such as amputations, making any kind of relationship between operations of the internal organs and conservative surgery a novel concept.[60] From the early decades of its innovation, ovariotomy had been conceived of and understood as radical; radical ethically in that it represented a major shift away from surgical norms, and radical in that, up until this time, surgical removal of the whole ovary had been seen as the only sure way to cure an ovarian tumour, and where therapeutics likes tapping and medicines were viewed as the more conservative alternative. But being conceived of as 'conservative' had its appeal to ovariotomists, keen to distance themselves from the unfortunate associations between 'radical' surgery and unnecessary operating. Aided by its rather flexible definition, some began to depict ovariotomy as a conservative procedure. Samaritan Free Hospital surgeon George Granville Bantock argued that there could be a multitude of meanings to conservative ovarian surgery; that it could apply equally to the removal of the second ovary in cases of suspected double disease, removal of just one ovary if the second was not thought sufficiently pathological to necessitate removal, or could also mean resection of the diseased part of the organ to ensure the preservation of healthy tissue.[61] 'Conservative surgery of the ovary' also at times referred to hysterectomies where ovarian tissue was preserved, as it had become relatively common practice for surgeons to remove the ovaries along with the womb during hysterectomy, the logic being that without the womb the ovaries would become useless and possibly dangerous appendages.

Chief among the early champions in Britain of resectioning was Christopher Martin, a Birmingham-based gynaecological surgeon and protégé of Robert Lawson Tait at the Birmingham and Midland Hospital for Women. Tait had retired from hospital practice in the mid-1890s, following controversies in his private and professional life, and had died aged fifty-four in 1899.[62] His death, which had been preceded by those of Thomas Keith in 1895 and Thomas Spencer Wells in 1897, marked the end of an era in abdominal surgery. This gave greater intellectual space to young surgeons like Martin to innovate. Martin began to experiment with conservative techniques for diseased ovaries and Fallopian tubes, spurred on by the claims about the various physiological after-effects of oöphorectomy. Publishing his results in 1898, Martin was cautiously optimistic about his findings.[63] Among his operations were five resections of the ovary for cystic, dermoid and fibrous disease, histological tissues that, it appeared, were relatively easy for the surgeon to 'shell out' from the rest of the ovary (see Fig. 6.3). All five cases had been successful and that the patients were aged between twenty and thirty-three, and thus of childbearing age, gave extra weight to Martin's argument for more conservative measures.

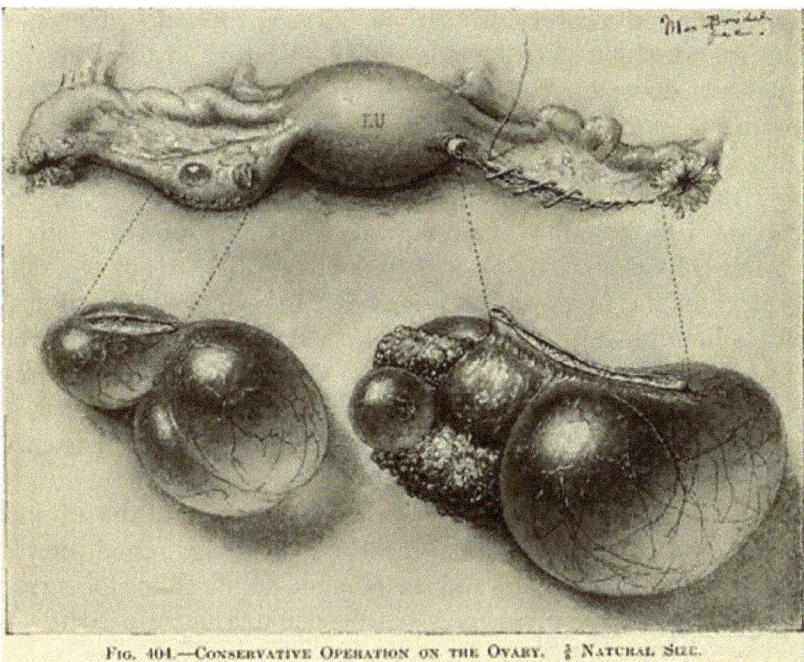

FIG. 404.—CONSERVATIVE OPERATION ON THE OVARY. ⅔ NATURAL SIZE.

Fig. 6.3 Illustration showing the difference between conservative section-ing with preservation (left) and radical extirpation (right) of the ovary, from American surgeon Howard A. Kelly's *Operative Gynecology, vol. 2* published in 1906. This image, taken from a fairly straightforward case of enlarged cysts, belied the frequent complexities that arose in conservative surgery, particularly concerns that diseased tissue was often being inadvertently preserved (*Credit* Wellcome Collection CC BY)

Urging 'gynaecologists to give a fair and unbiased trial to the con-servative surgery of the ovary', he referenced similar operations that were already being performed by surgeons in Paris and Berlin.[64] In fact, there was a striking difference between the uptake of tissue-preserving surgery in Britain compared to France, Germany and America, where by the 1890s, it had become relatively well-established.[65] This may have been in part to do with a reluctance within the British medical commu-nity to embrace fully the new understandings of ovarian physiology that were emerging, or at least, to applying them to clinical practice. Schlich has noted that despite the great interest in ovarian transplantation in the early twentieth century, British practitioners took little interest in it, making the idea of a paradigmatic shift in practice, in the British context at least, debatable.[66] Until the 1910s, the 'internal secretions' of the ovaries were oblique enough that prominent ovariotomists remained dubious about their existence; 'there is not a particle of evidence to support this view of an internal secretion', asserted George Granville Bantock in 1903.[67] John Bland-Sutton, speaking four years later, was less dismissive, acknowledging that 'modern research tends to exalt the importance of the ovary and indicates that its ovigenous function is by no means the only duty it performs'; like Martin he believed that retaining a small piece of ovarian tissue where possible was in the interest of patients.[68] However, Bland-Sutton admitted that precisely what these secondary functions were remained mysterious and the existence of internal secretions was only 'hypothetical'.[69]

It seems unlikely that surgeons were actively resisting the advance of physiology into their professional territory; plenty expressed interest in the role of internal secretions and the possible ramifications for surgery.[70] Developments in ovarian physiology, for example, were used to justify the experimental use of oöphorectomy to treat breast cancer. A procedure that stood in direct contrast to that which would be advocated by William Roger Williams a few years later (who, as discussed above, had believed removing the ovaries could cause the disease), the logic behind this procedure was distinctly physiological: if the ovaries were responsible for influential actions and secretions around the body, as well as the primary seat of reproductive action, then it seemed quite possible that they played a part in controlling physiological changes in the breast, and thus by removing the former, cancerous degeneration in the latter could be halted. There was a flurry of interest around the potentiality of the procedure before it was ultimately deemed ineffective in treating the disease.[71] Nonetheless, that it occurred at all suggests that British surgeons' comparative reluctance to embrace conservative surgery was not necessarily to do with a disbelief in its physiological logic but an unwillingness to give up radical surgery regardless. The advantages of retaining ovarian tissue needed to be balanced against the risks of doing so. Extirpation of the entire ovary, if nothing else, virtually ensured that a diseased organ was obliterated; resectioning ovaries potentially meant that the pathological tissue might not be fully eradicated. The vigilant aftercare that such cases would need weighed heavily on surgeons' minds, as did the potential technical complexities of conservative surgery. Where once it had been the removal of the ovary that had required the utmost surgi-cal courage, it was now the choice to conserve—to run the risk of not curing or of missing diseased tissues—that called for prowess, skill and nerve; 'as experience grows no doubt conservatism will be more prac-tised' concluded the surgeon Stanley Boyd in 1900, 'but there are some cases in which it needs a certain amount of courage to leave within the abdomen diseased structures which may prove by no means harmless'.[72]

Despite the conversations taking place as to the varying worth of different ovarian procedures, for many patients at the turn of the cen-tury, the experience of being diagnosed and treated for ovarian disease was not hugely changed from that of patients twenty years previously. The records of the London Hospital for the first decades of the twen-tieth century show patterns in patient experience and presentation that had remained stubbornly unchanged; women who had suffered the slow onset of symptoms for years, before presenting with grossly diseased ova-ries that had grown to huge sizes. When sixty-five-year-old Eliza Hold was brought into the London Hospital in 1900, she was found to have an ovarian cyst the 'size of a pumpkin'; not so different from the cases of patients with huge tumours which had warranted practitioners' atten-tion back in the eighteenth century.[73] Patients also continued to report lengthy histories of suffering before seeking surgical treatment. The same year that Hold was treated at the London Hospital, twenty-seven-year-old Annie Wright was also admitted to the institution, having first noticed an abdominal swelling seven years previously. She sought help only after the tumour began to increase in size and cause more pain.[74] It would be the 1930s before cases involving very large tumours became a comparative rarity, as women began to report symptoms earlier.

Patients with large tumours still mostly continued to receive 'radi-cal' surgery in the early decades of the twentieth century; Annie Wright, as well as having her large tumour removed, also had her second ovary taken out by the surgeon after it was found to be cystic; her notes, as is so often the case, provide few clues to whether she had fully consented to the additional procedure. Records at two hospitals which retain full surgi-cal registers support the notion that 'radical' surgery remained dominant. At the Chelsea Hospital for Women, for example, of the one hundred and eighty or so ovarian operations performed in 1912, the vast majority of these were salpingo-oöphorectomies, where the ovaries and Fallopian tubes were removed. Many more—at least a third—involved the removal of both ovaries, sometimes as part of treatment for uterine disease, in which both the uterus and ovaries were removed. Resection, on the other hand, remained comparatively uncommon at the hospital.[75] The records for the London Hospital reveal a similar picture; general hospitals, as we have seen, tended to undertake few ovariotomies in the earlier decades of the nineteenth century, the majority being performed in private practice or in specialist hospitals. At the London Hospital, at least, it was only in the 1890s, *after* the panic about 'operative mania', that the operation flourished within its walls, suggesting that the Imlach affair and other controversies in fact did very little to quell the supply of or demand for ovariotomies. In 1883, just five were undertaken; in 1895, over forty ovarian operations were performed, the majority of which were described as 'ovariotomy' or 'double ovariotomy'. This was compared to approximately twenty-eight appendectomies and eleven major operations of the uterus, showing it to be by far the most common abdominal operation performed at the hospital at that time.[76] It would be the 1920s before radical ovarian surgery grew less common at the hospital—only thirteen bilateral oöphorectomies occurred in 1925, compared to 111 total hysterectomies.[77] Nonetheless operations upon the ovary were increasing as a whole, in line with other operations; altogether 114 procedures were performed upon the ovary that year.[78] Such records suggest that while the rhetoric of 'conservative' surgery was appealing to ovariotomists, in practice, radical surgery remained the favoured form of treatment for ovarian disease well into the twentieth century.

Ann Dally has characterised the 'decline' of ovariotomy at the end of the nineteenth century as intimately connected with the 'rise' of hysterectomy in the early twentieth. She has argued that hysterectomy became the new focal point for the medical profession's preoccupation with operating upon women's pelvic organs.[79] The number of hysterectomies did increase greatly during this period, eclipsing the number of ovariotomies, as the indications for removing the womb expanded and the operation became safer. But the trajectory of ovariotomy suggests a more complicated diffusion of surgical ideas and ethics than one where it was simply replaced by hysterectomy. The legacy of ovariotomy, the enduring idea that the ovaries are organs which are especially amenable to surgery, continues. Ovaries remain uncertain and dangerous entities, the treatment of which errs on the side of radical, surgical caution. Nowhere is this more apparent than in the growing management of 'precancer', a field where by far the most common and well-known procedures are prophylactic mastectomy and oöphorectomy for women with the faulty BRCA gene, a trend Ilana Löwy has linked to 'the tradition of surgical management of gynaecological problems'.[80] It is problematic to assume that radical ovarian surgery disappeared as surgeons' interests moved from the anatomical to the physiological, or from the ovaries to the uterus. In Britain especially, there was no neat shift from the radical to the conservative in surgery; indeed, the move towards conserving ovaries was markedly slow, despite genuine concerns about the long-term effects of removing them.

Disbelief and Nostalgia: How Surgeons Used History to Make Sense of Ovariotomy

Towards the end of the nineteenth century, another type of ovariotomy was appearing regularly in the medical periodicals, alongside radical and conservative ovariotomies; an ovariotomy that was principally an historical artefact. Looking back at the past decades to assess the rapid changes that had occurred in the field, the operation began to feature heavily in the reflective narratives of doctors. The 'history' of ovariotomy was not, of course, a particularly new topic; as we have seen, priority disputes regarding the operation often took the form of historical accounts, as surgeons attempted to ascertain the order in which various developments in ovarian surgery had occurred. Establishing an historical element to the operation gave it a sense of authority and weakened its associations with the tainted notion of 'novelty'. Nor was it new that surgeons were using history in the forging of their group identity. Historical narratives were already in use as a way of making sense of the perceived 'barber to brain surgery' rise of the profession, and surgeons often used history as a tool for shaping their perceptions of themselves.[81]

But at the turn of the century, doctors' historicising of their recent past intensified dramatically. Surgeons were notable in their production of these narratives, using the opportunities for reflection afforded by the close of the nineteenth century. Much of their content attempted to sum up what appeared to be the considerable—perhaps incomparable—legacy that their era had bequeathed to surgery. In 1902, just before he moved to London from Leeds, where he had been learning, teaching and practising surgery for over thirty years, the abdominal surgeon Arthur Mayo Robson delivered an opening speech to new students of his alma mater, the Leeds School of Medicine, that exemplified this historicising impulse.

Addressing a mixed sex crowd—a new characteristic of many early twentieth-century medical schools—Robson chose as his topic 'the Advance in Surgery during 30 Years':

> In comparing the present with the past of medicine and surgery and in attempting to forecast the future I have the advantage of being able from my own experience to contrast the work of 1870 with that of 1902. During that interval of 32 years so great have been the changes and so marked have been the advances that one cannot but feel a profound sense of gratitude that it has fallen to our lot to have lived and worked through this important period in the world's history and to have contributed in however so small a degree to the reformation which has occurred in our noble profession.[82]

Robson imagined himself as living history, connecting his own long career with the profound changes that had occurred. He intimated that the impact of medical and surgical advance over the past thirty years went far beyond the professional world but was part of the monumental societal and technological changes that had occurred during the late nineteenth century on a global scale. In a manner which echoed the sentiments of many of his fellow surgeons, Mayo Robson declared the nineteenth century to have been 'the surgical century'.[83] Ovariotomy was hugely important to these accounts. Like antisepsis it was symbolic of the progress that had been made in surgical practice. But perhaps even more than the former, ovariotomy signalled an image of Britain as the producer of robustly utilitarian innovations, its success clearly measurable through the publication of thousands of successful cases where patients had been cured from debilitating disease. It demonstrated Britain's prowess in the development of new, practical inventions, contributing to a group identity among the nation's doctors that they were, if not leaders in scientific research, the mantle of which lay with continental Europe, nonetheless at the vanguard of practical medicine, and who at the ground level of the doctor–patient encounter, were fixing bodies and saving people's lives.[84]

Progress was so great that it made the anxieties surrounding the operation earlier in the century seem almost inconceivable; 'the younger generation of to-day could not realise the wonder which a successful case of ovariotomy then excited or the dread of opening the peritoneal sac', reflected one gynaecologist in 1906, looking back on his student days forty years previously.[85] This powerful sense of disbelief at the past—disbelief at what had come before changes like ovariotomy and antiseptics, as well as disbelief at those who had stood in the way of what was now conceived of as progress—coloured much of this rhetoric. 'Can we to-day believe', commented the physician Lionel Weatherly in an address to the Bristol branch of the BMA in 1898, in a reference to the old pejorative used to describe ovariotomists, 'that it was only a comparatively short time ago that the benches of the Royal Medical and Chirurgical Society rang with excited cries of "Down with the belly-rippers!"'[86] Weatherly's words evoked an almost unimaginable era—yet one only fifty years before—in which ovariotomy was castigated rather than celebrated. Surgery of the past came to function as a convenient straw man for narratives of progress, serving to build a subtle distinction between two generations of surgeons.[87]

Reinforcing this was a frequent recourse to envisioning how doctors from other eras would experience the surgical present.[88] Imagining both how those from the past and the future would experience the Victorian era was a common literary device during this time and played an important role in defining what, exactly, 'Victorian' constituted.[89] These accounts are at once insightful and curious in their shifting of surgeons across time. In a talk given by the abdominal surgeon James Greig Smith in 1894, the mid-century surgeon and ardent opponent of ovariotomy Robert Liston was relocated to the 1890s. Smith imagined Liston would have 'revelled in all our "otomies," "ectomies" and "ostomies" of today!'—this despite Liston's fierce opposition to the most well-known 'otomy' of them all.[90] Liston was cast as a victim of the circumstances of his time, rather than a contributor towards those circumstances. Another interesting account which employed a temporal shift came in the form of a speech delivered by the physician James Lindsay on the penultimate day of the nineteenth century. Lindsay played upon the turning year to imagine the sparse medical world of his counterpart of 1799:

> He knew of the virtues of opium and quinine, of iron and mercury, but he had never heard of digitalis, or of salicin or of cocaine. He knew almost nothing of the physiology of the nervous system and had never heard of reflex action or of cortical centres. He had never counted the corpuscles in his own blood or seen a radiogram of his own vertebral column. He probably regarded ovariotomy as criminal.[91]

Lindsay's words are interesting in regard to ovariotomy. While he mainly describes therapeutics and practices that were yet to be discovered or invented, with ovariotomy, he imagined instead an innovation already in existence but with criminal connotations. Extirpation of the ovary had of course been suggested by 1799, but the operation was not well-known, and certainly not by the name 'ovariotomy', suggesting that Lindsay's reference to ovariotomy in this context was in part for the dramatic effect of imagining a distant past where removing ovaries would have been considered murderous. Unlike the other innovations mentioned, it was not a question of that which was 'waiting' to be understood or discovered, but one which remained morally dubious until it was perfected by the Victorians. This aspect was hugely important to the historicisation of ovariotomy; perhaps even more important than the intellectual victory of technically perfecting the procedure.

Looking back, these narratives can seem triumphant, whiggish and perhaps a little bit silly; they are often taken as evidence of the limited powers of Victorian surgeons for a robust and honest assessment of their practices—at least in public. Certainly, these narratives clearly had a role to play in boosting the self-confidence of surgeons and providing a spirited rallying call to a younger generation—it is no coincidence that many of the speeches were given in front of crowds of medical students—as well as to provide a metaphorical pat on the back to those surgeons who had dared to innovate; similar rhetoric has been important to many group identities, regardless of profession, cause or time period. But as various historians have delineated, these narratives were by no means unmitigated celebrations; for surgeons they were an important way, perhaps the most important way, through which to understand the immense changes that had occurred in their field.[92] Looking back enabled them to look forward and inward too; what they found was not always a cause for optimism. Surgeons' intense retrospection around the turn of the century was characterised by fear, pessimism and nostalgia as much as it was progress and advance. The culture of triumphant histories of the era and celebratory accounts of individual surgeons who had been part of it often caused unease as the two melded together to an uncomfortably close degree. As one American surgeon privately complained to his British counterpart D'Arcy Power in 1926, upon a public celebration in his honour, 'these are trying occasions; more especially when one has to speak after hearing his obituary and is actually buried,—even though it be under a bank of flowers'.[93] As a collective, the production of historical narratives read as an obituary to an age gone by.

The sense of fractured endings and doubtful beginnings which characterised the Victorian fin de siècle percolated into surgery. The feeling of many was that surgical innovation was beginning to dwindle, or at least, was not occurring at the startling pace that it had been in the previous few decades; '[the] wave of progress has largely spent itself, or reached its full height', opined the *Lancet* in 1891.[94] This idea had been gaining momentum since the late 1880s, most famously encapsulated in a speech given by John Erichsen, surgeon at University College London, in 1886. 'That the final limits of surgery have been reached in the direction of all that is manipulative and mechanical there can be little doubt' Erichsen argued, noting as John Halliday Croom did ten years later, that ovariotomy had reached 'perfection'.[95] Erichsen did not go as far as to suggest that surgery had reached its most advanced state but that surgical *technique* at least could not be improved upon, having reached a state of accomplishment through the vast array of operations now performed and which collectively made the human body in its entirety surgical territory.[96] Erichsen's comments hinted at the dying embers of an unprecedented era of surgery—which ovariotomy was symbolic of—where new operations for each internal organ had represented the inching grasp of surgical hands. It was difficult for surgeons to look beyond the survival rates for each of these operations to ascertain where surgery could possibly go from there. Writing in 1888, Bristol surgeon James Greig Smith cited Thomas Keith's achievement of a two per cent mortality in ovariotomy as the pinnacle of surgical achievement; 'surely this is the *ne plus ultra*, not only of abdominal surgery but of all surgery' Smith wrote.[97] The idea that surgical innovation had peaked, or that it would have to be completely reconceptualised to continue, undermined more optimistic rhetoric which imagined the progress of surgery as one of steady and continual advance. As Erichsen saw it, future generations of surgeons would have to be content with being mere imitators of his generation.[98]

Not everyone agreed with Erichsen's position.[99] Well into his sixties when he made his speech, Erichsen's perspective was that of one coming to the end of his professional life, which, chronologically speaking, was closely aligned with the period of highly visible surgical success that was passing; younger surgeons were unlikely to have viewed the future in such stark terms. Nonetheless the idea rippled through the profession; if surgeons had perfected the manual techniques of their craft, what was left to do that was original? Advances in physiology and bacteriology, the latter signalled most remarkably by Robert Koch's discovery of the tubercle bacillus in 1882, might initiate a new phase of surgery, but any innovations in the field would be increasingly reliant on medical knowledge and rather less on surgical skill. This set apart any forthcoming advances from the high era of 1880s surgery, during which many surgeons had seemed almost entirely independent from their physician counterparts, their work based on a 'surgical' rationale of local pathology. By this logic, Arthur Mayo Robson predicted, while the nineteenth century was the 'surgical century', the twentieth would be the medical one.[100]

The changes afoot influenced surgeons' identity. As much as ovariotomy called upon particular conceptions of femininity, it was built upon notions of masculinity too. Victorian surgeons aspired to being gentlemen and scientists while retaining a strong masculine identity, which relied on 'physical endurance, courage, solidity and honesty'.[101] Ovariotomy had fulfilled the multiple demands upon surgeons' complex selfhood: while the operation was not always technically complicated, it was physically and emotionally demanding, its performance requiring strength of body and mind, as both medical and moral challenges presented themselves with each case. What had previously been considered the reckless bravado of ovariotomists in the mid-century had, by the 1880s, been re-imagined as heroic behaviour in the face of female suffering. Thomas Spencer Wells recalled in 1884 his thoughts about continuing with ovariotomy after his first attempt in 1858 had ended in the death of the patient, revealing that the fatality had led him to 'fear that I might be entering upon a path which would lead rather to an unenviable notoriety than to a sound professional reputation'. Wells went on, 'if I had not seen increasing numbers of poor women hopelessly suffering, almost longing for death, anxious for relief at any risk, I should probably have acquiesced in the general conviction…rather than have hazarded anything more in the way of ovariotomy'.[102] An increase in surgery based on physiology and technical conservatism suggested an identity more in line with surgeons' understandings of themselves as scientists; but it was, perhaps, at the cost of the courageous qualities demonstrated by surgeons like Wells. Now that manual skill, stamina and physical strength appeared to be of diminishing importance, some expressed serious concerns as to how this would impact on the type of person who would be attracted to the profession. In 1892, the *St. Thomas's Hospital Gazette*, the hospital's in-house magazine for staff and students, used the death of the hospital's high-ranking surgeon Frederick Le Gros Clark to lament that 'in these days of Chloroform and bloodless surgery, when time, though more precious in every other department, can yet be more lavishly expended at the operating table, almost any "pudding headed, leaden hearted man" (to use a Carlyian epithet) can if he acquired sufficient technical knowledge, operate successfully, nay more guarded and defended by Antiseptics'.[103] The entry of women into medicine in the late 1860s likely played implicitly into narratives centred upon a decline in physical prowess. The question of whether women had the strength of body and mind to perform medicine, and especially surgery, with its demand on manual skill and emotional resilience, was often at the crux of debates about the justifiability of their place within the medical world. As Claire Brock has discussed, while by the 1890s female medical practitioners had begun to assimilate into varying sectors of the profession, surgery was still considered an inappropriate practice for women, and the Royal College of Surgeons of England continued to bar women from its ranks. A small pool of women, including the first female practitioner to qualify in Britain, Elizabeth Garrett Anderson, did perform ovariotomy during the nineteenth century in Britain, but, as Brock notes, the operation similarly raised questions around self-identity for female surgeons as it did their male counterparts. Those such as Garrett Anderson who performed the operation received criticism from female colleagues for seemingly aping the self-glorification of male surgeons, by participating in a culture of excessive gynaecological surgery.[104]

The *Gazette's* opinion on the impact of antiseptics upon the quality of surgeons also highlighted the continued, complicated relationship between ovariotomy and antisepsis. Surgeons turned to history to elucidate the connections between what were perhaps the two greatest surgical successes of the second half of the nineteenth century. But accounts differed as to how exactly they interrelated. Some surgeons gave pride of place to advancements in scientific knowledge when historicising surgical innovation, primarily by lauding the achievements of Joseph Lister.[105] In these, ovariotomy—or at least the success of ovariotomy—was carefully reconfigured as the product of broader changes in surgery, rather than an innovation itself. Arthur Mayo Robson's speech in 1903 to the British Medical Association, which reflected upon surgery since 1870, centred upon the notion that antiseptics had liberated surgery from many of its ills, saving 'more lives each year than Napoleon destroyed in all his wars'.[106] Robson disregarded almost entirely any developments in abdominal surgery before this date, claiming that 'surgery had then no business inside the abdomen'.[107] The appeal of such a narrative was that it prioritised the all-encompassing and scientifically theorised innovation of antisepsis over the practical, manual work of operative surgery. Together with the reification of Joseph Lister the individual—by the end of the century a peer of the realm and the embodiment of the gentleman-surgeon—the 'rise' of antiseptics was a hugely appealing grand narrative. At the turn of the century, Lister's successes and popular public image were a vital constituent of the profession's projection of itself.[108]

Yet for those more personally invested in ovariotomy, a historical stocktake of the operation also allowed for quite the opposite—to conceptualise the operation as an innovation which ran independently of other developments. Thomas Spencer Wells' historical account of ovariotomy, written in 1884, had the operation at the centre of its narrative:

> One hundred years ago, it was but a germ that might be described in a lecture by John Hunter. Ten years later, it was seed that fell from the hand of Bell. In little more than another decade it germinated as a living vitalising reality in Kentucky. Sixty years ago, it was transplanted to the land of its philosophical conception. In twenty years more we find it a sapling on English soil, growing slowly at first, and up to 1858 looking as if it might prove no more than a withering gourd. But by 1865, its root had struck firm, its stem stood erect, its branches were wide and strong, known and sought as a refuge by the sick and dying. That it was no withering gourd has been proved by all that the world has since seen.[109]

Indeed, throughout Wells' entire piece on the history of ovariotomy, he made little reference to the effects of anaesthesia and antiseptics on the operation. In line with many ovariotomists, Wells tended to view these developments as reinforcements to the advance of ovariotomy rather than its cause—something which perhaps tied in with the scepticism of many late-century ovariotomists about the benefits of the Listerian system of surgery. Robson's and Wells' contrasting viewpoints attest to the flexibility already apparent in the historicisation of ovariotomy by the turn of the century. For some, the success of the operation was simply the product of 'greater' innovations like antiseptics. But for others, the decisive and practical success of the operation made it alone an ideal symbol of recent surgical progress.

Conclusion

In surgery, where the physical performance of the operation takes centre stage, the role of language remains under-explored and underestimated. But during the late nineteenth century, surgical taxonomy came to the fore amid changing conceptions of ovariotomy. 'Ovariotomy' had an increasingly vague definition; the variety of meanings attached to the term by the early twentieth century attest to the conceptual elasticity underlying it. This elasticity precludes any kind of simplistic picture of the operation's conclusive acceptance or rejection. Ovariotomy, insofar as it was understood to constitute radical ovarian surgery, began to experience a degree of decline in the 1920s, as did use of the term; but in Britain a shift towards more conservative measures was both slow and incomplete, despite changing ideas in physiology which seemed to confirm that removing the ovaries could have implications for the patient's health. These risks had to be carefully weighed against the opposing risk of retaining diseased ovarian tissue within the body.

At the turn of the century, the ways in which ovariotomy related to the past, present and future of surgery were widely discussed among doctors. At this time, ovariotomy still continued to be practised. But contemporaneously, it was also becoming an historical phenomenon. This played out in dual ways. The passage of time and the operation's vastly diminished mortality rate gave scope for surgeons to perform wide-scale follow-ups to their cases and ask questions concerning its impact previously considered of secondary importance to the business of ensuring the patient's survival. The foundational work of Arthur Giles, assessing the impact of abdominal operations on hundreds of his patients, marked out a transitional moment. His work allayed certain fears about the detrimental effects of ovariotomy upon mental and physical health. But Giles' account also gave a platform to patients' narratives of postoperative experience, some of which were characterised by disappointing results, highlighting a lack of congruity between the operation's reputation as a quick fix for chronic disease and the reality of some women's experiences.

The historicisation of the procedure played out on a more explicitly cultural level too, as it was transformed into an artefact of the passing Victorian era. Should these histories be considered merely triumphant and 'whiggish'? Certainly, they could be both those things. Speeches like John Erichsen's on the 'finality' of operative surgery and the 'perfection'

of ovariotomy seem to betray the worst excesses of laudatory nineteenth-century history, buttressing a story of surgery in which continual
advance peaked in the hands of Victorian surgeons. But to say the function of these narratives was merely to be self-congratulatory is rather lim-
iting. The historical narrative crafted around the operation was as much a
part of the innovation process as technical developments; it allowed surgeons to shape the lineage of the operation, define its meaning and make
sense of the mixture of jubilation, anxiety, disbelief and nostalgia that its
success precipitated. Deriding as simplistic the use of history in this way
does little justice to what was playing out; as historian William Cronon
has advised when dealing with 'progressivist' histories of the past, 'we still
cannot evade the storytelling task of distilling history's meaning'.[110] The
historicisation of ovariotomy encapsulated the struggles to define a surgical age that was passing, of which the operation had become emblematic.

NOTES

1. John Halliday Croom, 'Obstetrics', *Lancet* 148, no. 3805 (1 August
   1896): 343.
2. Thomas Spencer Wells, 'The Address in Surgery', *Lancet* 110, no. 2815
   (1877): 193.
3. John V. Pickstone, 'Medical History as a Way of Life', *Social History
   of Medicine* 18, no. 2 (2005): 310; Frank Huisman and John Harley
   Warner, 'Medical Histories', in *Locating Medical History: The Stories
   and Their Meanings*, ed. Frank Huisman and John Harley Warner
   (Baltimore and London: The Johns Hopkins University Press, 2004),
   11.
4. Huisman and Warner, 'Medical Histories', 2.
5. Ann Dally, *Women Under the Knife: A History of Surgery* (London:
   Hutchinson Radius, 1991), 210.
6. Ornella Moscucci, *The Science of Woman: Gynaecology and Gender in
   England 1800–1929* (Cambridge University Press, 1990), 181–184.
7. Moscucci, *The Science of Woman*, 164.
8. Lawrence D. Longo, 'The Rise and Fall of Battey's Operation: A
   Fashion in Surgery', *Bulletin of the History of Medicine* 53, no. 2 (1979):
   265; Regina Morantz-Sanchez, *Conduct Unbecoming of a Woman:
   Medicine on Trial in Turn-of-the-Century Brooklyn* (Oxford: Oxford
   University Press, 1999), 110.
9. Sally Wilde, *The History of Surgery: Trust, Patient Autonomy, Medical
   Dominance and Australian Surgery, 1890–1940* (Byron Bay: Finesse
   Press, 2010), 61.

10. This was the common name for nephroptosis, a condition which sees the kidney detach from surrounding connective tissues and sink down into the pelvis.

11. S.J. Srirangam, et al., 'Nephroptosis: Seriously Misunderstood?' *BJU International* 103, no. 3 (2009): 296–230.

12. John Bland-Sutton and Arthur Giles, *Diseases of Women: A Handbook for Students and Practitioners* (Philadelphia: W. B. Saunders, 1897), 387. 'Parovarium' refers to a group of small ducts located next to the ovary.

13. George Comyns Berkeley and Victor Bonney, *A Textbook of Gynaecological Surgery* (London: Cassell & Company, 1911), 452.

14. Sally Wilde and Geoffrey Hirst, 'Learning from Mistakes: Early Twentieth-Century Surgical Practice', *Journal of the History of Medicine and Allied Sciences* 64, no. 1 (2009): 67.

15. Charles Jennings, 'Nomenclature for Operations Upon the Ovaries', *British Medical Journal* 2, no. 1331 (3 July 1886): 49.

16. 'F.R.C.S.', 'Nomenclature for Operations Upon the Ovary', *British Medical Journal* 2, no. 1334 (24 July 1886): 187.

17. John Bland-Sutton, *Tumours, Innocent and Malignant* (London: Cassell & Company, 1906), 478.

18. 'F.R.C.S.', 187.

19. Herbert R. Spencer, 'A Review of 658 Ovariotomies', *Proceedings of the Royal Society of Medicine* 26, no. 11 (1933): 1435.

20. 'H.E.M.', 'Medical Nomenclature', *Canadian Medical Association Journal* 43, no. 6 (1940): 597–598.

21. Stuart Hall, 'The Work of Representation', in *Representation: Cultural Representations and Signifying Practices*, ed. Stuart Hall (Milton Keynes: Open University, 1997): 33. The term 'ovariotomy' is occasionally used by medical researchers in China and India. Recent examples include: Xin Zhao et al, 'Ovariotomy and persistent pain affect long-term Fos expression in spinal cord', *Neuroscience Letters* 375, no. 3 (2005): 165–169, and B. Chakrabarti and N. Mondal, 'Adolescent Ovarian Malignancy', *International Journal of Gynecology and Obstetrics* 107, Supplement 2 (2009): S138.

22. Charles H.F. Routh, 'The Conservative Treatment of Disease of the Uterine Appendages', *British Gynaecological Journal* 10 (1894): 59.

23. Lockhart-Mummery commented that 'the after-treatment of operation cases is a subject of such importance that it is not a little surprising to find how little has hitherto been written about it. What has been written is to be found, for the most part, in a somewhat fragmentary form in the larger text books'. J.P. Lockhart-Mummery, *The After-Treatment of Operations: A Manual for Practitioners and House Surgeons* (London: Baillière, Tindall & Cox, 1903), v.

24. Thomas Schlich, *Surgery, Science and Industry: A Revolution in Fracture Care, 1950s–1980s* (Basingstoke: Palgrave Macmillan, 2002), 12.

25. Marguerite W. Dupree, 'Other Than Healing: Medical Practitioners and the Business of Life Assurance During the Nineteenth and the Early Twentieth Centuries', *Social History of Medicine* 10, no. 1 (1997): 86–88.

26. Alfred Pearce Gould, *The Influence of Surgical Operations upon the Expectation of Life* (Lecture for the Life Assurance Medical Officers' Association, C.E. Gray: London, 1906), 102–103.

27. Gould was himself a cancer specialist.

28. Ornella Moscucci, 'Gender and Cancer in Britain, 1860–1910: The Emergence of Cancer as a Public Health Concern', *American Journal of Public Health* 95, no. 8 (2005): 1319.

29. Ornella Moscucci, *Gender and Cancer in England, 1860–1948* (Basingstoke: Palgrave Macmillan, 2017), 2.

30. Moscucci, *Gender and Cancer*, 34.

31. Patricia Jasen 'Breast Cancer and the Language of Risk, 1750–1950', *Social History of Medicine* 15, no. 1 (2002): 3; James T. Patterson, *The Dread Disease: Cancer and Modern American Culture* (Cambridge and London: Harvard University Press, 1987), 13–26. In 1895, abdominal surgeon Arthur Mayo Robson described one of the causes of cancer as 'senility and decadence of tissues which have passed the period of their usefulness and are about to undergo physiological rest'. Arthur Mayo Robson, 'The Bradshaw Lecture on the Treatment of Cancer', *British Medical Journal* 2, no. 2292 (3 December 1904): 1501.

32. Ilana Löwy, '"Because of Their Praiseworthy Modesty, They Consult Too Late": Regime of Hope and Cancer of the Womb, 1800–1910', *Bulletin of the History of Medicine* 85, no. 3 (2010): 368–371.

33. This was principally to do with the introduction of 'Wertheim's Hysterectomy' into practice to treat cancer of the cervix. Pioneered by Austrian gynaecologist Ernst Wertheim, the operation involved the removal of the entire womb as well as surrounding cellular tissue and lymph nodes. By 1905, Wertheim could claim that thirty per cent of his cases were free from recurrence five years later. Ornella Moscucci, '"The 'Ineffable Freemasonry of Sex"': Feminist Surgeons and the Establishment of Radiotherapy in Early Twentieth-Century Britain', *Bulletin of the History of Medicine* 81, no. 1 (2007): 142–145.

34. Berkeley and Bonney, *A Textbook of Gynaecological Surgery*, 452.

35. Arthur E. Giles, 'Meditation on 1000 Consecutive Abdominal Operations at the Prince of Wales's General Hospital, Tottenham', *Lancet* 184, no. 4740 (4 July 1914): 9.

36. Patricia Jasen, 'From the "Silent Killer" to the "Whispering Disease"': Ovarian Cancer and the Uses of Metaphor', *Medical History* 53, no. 4 (2009): 495–496.

37. In the late eighteenth century, the Middlesex Hospital opened the first dedicated ward for cancer patients, going on to become a leading institution in cancer research; for a detailed account of this see R.S. Handley, 'Gordon-Taylor, Breast Cancer and the Middlesex Hospital', *Annals of the Royal College of Surgeons of England* 49, no. 3 (1971): 153–159.

38. Roger W. Williams, 'Some Reasons for Believing That Oophorectomy Tends to Favour Rather Than to Prevent the Development of Cancer', *British Medical Journal* 2, no. 2081 (17 November 1900): 1472.

39. By 1902, Williams had begun to suspect that radical operations on the uterus could have a similar effect. Roger W. Williams, 'Correspondence', *British Medical Journal* 1, no. 2141 (11 January 1902): 111.

40. John Halliday Croom, 'Edinburgh Obstetrical Society: Psychoses Following Pelvi-Abdominal Operations', *Lancet* 157, no. 4044 (2 March 1901): 517; A.C. Butler-Smythe, 'Acute Mania Following Rupture of the Rectum by Enema Thirteen Days After Ovariotomy. Recovery', *Journal of Mental Science* 39, no. 166 (1893) 395–396; C.T. Dent, 'Insanity Following Surgical Operations', *British Journal of Psychiatry* 35, no. 149 (1889): 12.

41. Edward Tilt, *The Change of Life in Health and Disease* (Philadelphia: P. Blakiston, Son & Co, 1882): 103–132. The Edinburgh gynaecologist John Halliday Croom argued in 1901 that by removing the ovaries 'for disease or other cause, one placed the woman in all the possible risks of climacteric trouble', John Halliday Croom, 'Edinburgh Obstetrical Society: Psychoses Following Pelvi-Abdominal Operations', *Lancet* 157, no. 4044 (2 March 1901): 517.

42. Gould, 'Surgical Operations and Life Assurance', 106. Gould does not specify as to whether he means 'castration' of men, but it seems probable.

43. This was particularly the case in abdominal surgery, seen in the work of Britain's leading surgeon in the field in the 1920s, Berkeley Moynihan. Moynihan espoused a view of surgery as 'the pathology of the living', a way to collect data on internal disease. Writing on his practice of gastro-enterostomy (the surgical creation of a connection between the stomach and jejunum) he advocated the long-term follow-up of cases. In 1910, Moynihan wrote that 'we are all accustomed to be asked by the relatives of patients who are interviewed when an operation is immediately over, whether the operation has been "successful". That is

a question which may be answered satisfactorily only after the lapse of many months. In an operation of the severity of gastro-enterostomy— an operation, moreover, by which certain physiological principles seem to be set at naught—the lapse of two years is certainly not too much to allow us to speak with confidence as to its success'. Berkeley Moynihan, *The Pathology of the Living and Other Essays* (Philadelphia and London: W.B. Saunders Company, 1910), 82.

44. Arthur E. Giles, *A Study of the After-Results of Abdominal Operations on the Pelvic Organs: Based on a Series of 1000 Consecutive Cases* (London: Baillière, Tindall and Cox, 1910), 5.

45. Berkeley and Bonney, *A Textbook of Gynaecological Surgery*, 701.

46. Berkeley and Bonney claimed that patients, once they became outpatients, retained little interest in staying in contact with a hospital, or with their surgeon, unless the operation had not fully restored their health. Participating in follow-ups could also be timely and expensive for the patient, and thus an unappealing prospect for all but a self-selecting few; Berkeley and Bonney, *A Textbook of Gynaecological Surgery*, 700.

47. 'Reviews and Notices of Books: A Study of the After-Results of Abdominal Operations', *Lancet* 177, no. 4562 (4 February 1911): 310.

48. Arthur E. Giles, 'Address in Surgery', *Canadian Medical Association Journal* 2, no. 9 (1912): 760.

49. See for example the report published by the anaesthetist to the New Hospital for Women, May Thorne. May Thorne, 'After-Effects of Abdominal Section', *British Medical Journal* 1, 1988 (4 February 1899), 264–265. As also discussed in Claire Brock, 'Risk, Responsibility and Surgery in the 1890s and Early 1900s', *Medical History* 57, no. 3 (2013): 330–333.

50. Giles, *A Study of the After-Results of Abdominal Operations*, 96.

51. Berkeley and Bonney, *A Textbook of Gynaecological Surgery*, 702.

52. Annmarie Adams and Thomas Schlich, 'Design for Control: Surgery, Science, and Space at the Royal Victoria Hospital, Montreal, 1893–1956', *Medical History* 50, no. 3 (2006): 313.

53. Regina Morantz-Sanchez, *Conduct Unbecoming of a Woman: Medicine on Trial in Turn-of-the-Century Brooklyn* (Oxford: Oxford University Press, 1999): 108–109.

54. Chandak Sengoopta, 'The Modern Ovary: Constructions, Meanings, Uses', *History of Science*, 38, no. 122, part 4 (2000): 442; Thomas Schlich, *The Origins of Organ Transplantation: Surgery and Laboratory Science, 1880–1930* (Rochester and Woodbridge: University of Rochester Press, 2010): 85–98.

55. Schlich, *The Origins of Organ Transplantation*, 95.

56. Morantz-Sanchez, *Conduct Unbecoming of a Woman*, 110.

57. John Hunter's Lectures (c. 1775–1786): Western Manuscripts MS5598 (Wellcome Collection), 2; see also Stephen Jacyna, 'Physiological Principles in the Surgical Writings of John Hunter', in *Medical Theory, Surgical Practice: Studies in the History of Surgery*, ed. Christopher Lawrence (London: Routledge, 1992): 135–152.

58. Gert H. Brieger, 'From Conservative to Radical Surgery in Late Nineteenth-Century America', in *Medical Theory, Surgical Practice: Studies in the History of Surgery*, ed. Christopher Lawrence (London and New York: Routledge, 1992): 216.

59. A further intricacy was that conservative and radical techniques often converged in a surgeon's practice. Brieger cites the work of the American surgeon William S. Halsted, for example, who was prominent in the surgical community for his work at the Johns Hopkins Hospital in Baltimore during the late nineteenth and early twentieth centuries. As a general surgeon, Halsted was known for his emphasis on tissue preservation and controlling blood loss. However, he was equally well-known for pioneering radical mastectomy, which involved removing the whole breast as well adjoining muscular tissue. Brieger, 'From Conservative to Radical Surgery', 226–229. See also Jasen, 'Breast Cancer and the Language of Risk', *Social History of Medicine* 15, no. 1 (2002): 30; Terrie M. Romano, 'Halsted, William Stewart', http://www.anb.org/articles/12/12-00365.html, American National Biography Online February 2000, accessed 25 May 2013.

60. In Britain it was often associated with the practice and publications of King's College Hospital surgeon William Fergusson, active during the middle of the century. William Fergusson, *Lectures on the Progress of Anatomy and Surgery During the Present Century* (London: John Churchill and Sons, 1867), 37.

61. George Granville Bantock, 'The Conservative Treatment of Lesions of the Uterine Appendages', *Lancet* 162, no. 4169 (25 July 1903): 221.

62. Tait was involved in several libel cases and, towards the end of his life, was embroiled in a scandal when one of the nurses in his employment claimed that he had made her pregnant. He became seriously ill with renal disease and died aged fifty-four in 1899.

63. Christopher Martin, 'On the Conservative Surgery of the Ovary', *British Medical Journal* 2, no. 1968 (17 September 1898): 791–792.

64. Specifically, August Martin in Berlin and Samuel Pozzi in Paris.

65. For an overview of conservative surgery in America see A. Palmer Dudley, 'The Trend of Gynecologic Work To-Day', *Journal of the American Medical Association* 41, no. 25 (19 December 1903): 1527–1532; esp. 1530. Dudley gave statistics collated from the work of a

number of surgeons. Of a total of 1276 operations that were performed upon diseased ovaries, he found that 754 had been conservative (resection or puncture) and 522 were radical (removal). Like many other surgeons, Dudley saw the ovaries as more amenable than the Fallopian tubes to resection. The latter organ was thought to be liable to becoming the seat of returning disease, especially inflammatory conditions such as pyosalpinx. See also the surgeon Florence Nightingale Boyd's 1903 overview of conservative surgery which records numerous cases from France, Germany and America that had occurred in the 1890s. Boyd notes that 'when we come to enquire into the work done in this direction in Great Britain it is difficult to acquire accurate information, as so few results have been published'; Florence Nightingale Boyd, 'Conservative Surgery of the Tubes and Ovaries', *British Gynaecological Journal* 3, no. 3 (1903): 254.

66. Schlich, *The Origins of Organ Transplantation*, 95. For more on physiological surgery in Austria see Tatjana Buklijas, 'Surgery and National Identity in Late Nineteenth-Century Vienna', *Studies in History and Philosophy of Biological and Biomedical Sciences* 38, no. 4 (2008). Buklijas contends that a physiologically based approach to surgical practice was present in the teachings and followers of Theodor Billroth during the mid-nineteenth century, suggesting that physiological surgery was already much more well-established in central Europe than it was in Britain.

67. Bantock, 'The Conservative Treatment of Lesions', 221.

68. John Bland-Sutton, 'A Clinical Lecture on the Value and Fate of Belated Ovaries', *Medical Press and Circular* 135 (31 July 1907): 111.

69. Bland-Sutton, 'A Clinical Lecture', 108.

70. For example, the Leicester surgeon C.J. Bond conducted numerous experiments into ovarian and uterine physiology in the early 1900s. This included research studying possible compensatory hypertrophy in cases where one ovary remained after surgery. C.J. Bond, 'Some Points in Uterine and Ovarian Physiology and Pathology in Rabbits', *British Medical Journal* 2, no. 2377 (21 July 1906): 121–127.

71. Sengoopta, 'The Modern Ovary', 437–440. Initial experimentation with oöphorectomy in breast cancer patients in the late 1890s appeared to garner some success. In 1897, the surgeon Stanley Boyd presented five cases which he used to tentatively argue that the lives of those suffering from breast cancer might be considerably extended by treatment with oöphorectomy. However, optimism surrounding the procedure was short-lived. By the following year, experiments with the same operation by Joseph Lister's former right-hand man, William Watson Cheyne, had ended in disappointment and Cheyne reported only a brief regression

in the size of breast cancer tumours in his patients before the condition worsened once more after a short period. See Stanley Boyd, 'On Oöphorectomy in the Treatment of Breast Cancer', *British Medical Journal* 2, no. 1918 (2 October 1897): 890–896. W.W. Cheyne, 'Two Cases of Oöphorectomy for Inoperable Breast Cancer', *British Medical Journal* 1, no. 1194 (7 May 1898): 1194–1195.

72. Stanley Boyd, 'Conservative Surgery of Tubes and Ovaries', *British Medical Journal* 2, no. 2072 (15 September 1900): 734.

73. Surgical In-patients (1900), case 228 LH/M/15/4 (Royal London Hospital Archives).

74. Surgical In-patients (1900), case 1096 LH/M/15/4 (Royal London Hospital Archives).

75. Chelsea Hospital for Women—Register of Major Operations (1912) H27/CW/B/10/03/014 (London Metropolitan Archives). In cases where disease was clearly confined to one side, there seemed to be little logic in attempting to preserve part of that ovary, it being established by then that a woman's physiology or fertility should not be affected if she had one ovary remaining. See Martin, 'On the Conservative Surgery of the Ovary', 791.

76. Surgical Beadles Register of Operations performed (1895) LH/M/3/112 and the Surgical Index of the same year (1895) LH/M/2/1 (Royal London Hospital Archives). The nature of the records means that only approximate statistics can be given.

77. Obstetric and Gynaecology case indexes (1925) LH/M/2/142 (Royal London Hospital Archives).

78. Obstetric and Gynaecology case indexes (1925) LH/M/2/142 (Royal London Hospital Archives).

79. Dally, *Women Under the Knife*, 220.

80. Löwy, 'Because of Their Praiseworthy Modesty', 237.

81. Christopher Lawrence, for example, notes the re-configuration of anaesthesia into 'a significant historical moment' in the 1860s; Christopher Lawrence, 'Democratic, Divine and Heroic: The History and Historiography of Surgery', in *Medical Theory, Surgical Practice: Studies in the History of Surgery*, ed. Christopher Lawrence (London: Routledge, 1992): 8.

82. Arthur Mayo Robson, 'An Introductory Address on the Advance in Surgery During 30 Years', *Lancet* 160, no. 4127 (October 4 1902): 914.

83. Mayo Robson, 'An Introductory Address', 913.

84. Michael Worboys, 'British Medicine and Its Past at Queen Victoria's Jubilees and the 1900 Centennial', *Medical History* 45, no. 4 (2001): 472.

85. W. Stephenson, 'The British Association Meeting at Swansea: Obstetrics and Gynaecology', *Lancet* 162, no. 4170 (1 August 1903): 350.

86. Lionel Weatherly, 'Remarks on Medical Progress', *Lancet* 152, no. 3918 (1 October 1898): 853.

87. Lawson Tait, 'The Evolution of the Surgical Treatment of the Broad Ligament Pedicle', *Lancet* 147, no. 3794 (16 May 1896): Tait remarked on the 'slow and tardy' evolution of abdominal surgery, 1338.

88. Mayo Robson, 'An Introductory Address', 914.

89. Although principally looking at the ways Victorian era writers imagined how future generations would look back at them, Kelly J. Mays' analysis of this form of literary device—as a way to 'apprehend the present as a coherent "age"', can be equally applied to the use of invoking figures from the past. Kelly J. Mays, 'Looking Backward, Looking Forward: The Victorians in the Rearview Mirror of Future History', *Victorian Studies* 53, no. 3 (2011): 453.

90. James Greig Smith, 'The Art of the Surgeon, and How We Train Men to Practise It', *Lancet* 144, no. 3701 (4 August 1894): 248.

91. James A. Lindsay, 'An Inaugural Address on Our Position and Outlook', *Lancet* 154, no. 3983 (30 December 1899): 1798.

92. Worboys, 'British Medicine', 473–474; Christopher Lawrence and Michael Brown, 'Quintessentially Modern Heroes: Surgeons, Explorers and Empire, c. 1840–1914', *Journal of Social History* 50, no. 1 (2016): 156–157.

93. Letter from Rudolph Matus to D'Arcy Power, Dec 31st 1926; (MS0289/6; Royal College of Surgeons of England).

94. 'The Annus Medicus 1891', *Lancet* 138, no. 3565 (26 December 1891): 1447.

95. John Eric Erichsen, 'An Address Delivered at the Opening of the Section of Surgery', *British Medical Journal* 2, no. 1337 (14 August 1886): 314.

96. Operations of the appendix, liver and gallbladder were relatively common by the end of the century. The brain too had become surgical territory. The surgeon Rickman Godlee, Joseph Lister's nephew, first performed an operation to remove a brain tumour in 1884. Although the procedure was ultimately unsuccessful, Godlee's attempt paved the way for the work of other surgeons, such as Victor Horsley of University College Hospital, who in the 1880s began to successfully perform brain surgery in London.

97. James Greig Smith, *Abdominal Surgery* (London and Bristol: J. & A. Churchill & J. W. Arrowsmith, 1880), 120.

98. Erichsen, 'An Address', 314.

99. Sir William Stokes, President of the Royal College of Surgeons of Ireland, described Erichsen's views, in an address to the Academy of Medicine in Ireland, as 'a dismal view of the present as well as the future'. Stokes pointed out the continued 'infancy' of brain and abdominal surgery (inferring its probable growth) as well as the developments awaiting that might enable the treatment of organs still untouched by surgeons, such as the lungs. W. Stokes, 'An Address on Finality in Surgery', *Lancet* 128, no. 3299 (20 November 1886): 961.

100. Robson, 'An Introductory Address', 916.

101. Christopher Lawrence, 'Medical Minds, Surgical Bodies', in *Science Incarnate: Historical Embodiments of Natural Knowledge*, ed. Christopher Lawrence and Steven Shapin (Chicago and London: University of Chicago Press, 1998), 194. See also Christopher Lawrence and Michael Brown's exploration of the analogies between explorers and surgeons and their 'shared culture of heroism and muscular masculinity'; Lawrence and Brown, 'Quintessentially Modern', 153.

102. Thomas Spencer Wells, 'An Inaugural Address on the Revival of Ovariotomy, and Its Influences on Modern Surgery', *Lancet* 124, no. 3193 (8 November 1884): 812.

103. 'Obituary of Frederick Le Gros Clark'. *St. Thomas' Hospital Gazette* 7, no. 2 (October 1892): 110; TH/PUB2/1 (Kings College London). See also Sally Frampton 'Applause and Amazement': Social Identity and the London Surgical Elite, 1880–1905 (MA thesis University College London, accessible from the Wellcome Library London, http://www.wellcomelibrary.org): 21–23.

104. Claire Brock, *British Women Surgeons and Their Patients, 1860–1918* (Cambridge: Cambridge University Press, 2017), 7–8, 50–51. As Brock discusses, Garrett Anderson was publicly criticised by Elizabeth Blackwell, the British-born physician who was the first woman to receive a medical degree in the United States and who had returned to Britain in 1869. Blackwell spoke openly of her belief that female practitioners were equally susceptible to 'operative madness'.

105. Frederick Treves, 'Address in Surgery: The Surgeon in the Nineteenth Century', *Lancet* 156, no. 4014 (4 August 1900): 316.

106. Arthur Mayo Robson, 'Address in Surgery: Observations on the Evolution of Abdominal Surgery from Personal Reminiscences Extending Over a Third of a Century and the Performance of 2000 Operations', *Lancet* 162, no. 4170 (1 August 1903): 292.

107. Mayo Robson, 'Address in Surgery', 293.

108. Marguerite Wright Dupree, 'From Mourning to Scientific Legacy: Commemorating Lister in London and Scotland', *Notes and Records of the Royal Society* 67, no. 3 (2013): 262.

109. Thomas Spencer Wells, 'An Inaugural Address on the Revival of Ovariotomy, and Its Influences on Modern Surgery', *Lancet* 124, no. 3194 (15 November 1884): 857.

110. William Cronon, 'Two Cheers for the Whig Interpretation of History', *Perspectives on History* 50, no. 6 (2012), http://www.historians. org/perspectives/issues/2012/1209/Two-Cheers-for-the-Whig-Interpretation-of-History.cfm, accessed 6 June 2013.

7

Conclusion

In his monograph, *The Shock of the Old*, David Edgerton laments the tendency within the history of technology towards 'innovation-centric history'. Hugely successful innovations, he argues, are mined for historical value while those that fail, which in fact make up a greater proportion of science and technology's past, are sidelined. Addressing technology in general, rather than medicine specifically, Edgerton nonetheless, like John Pickstone before him, calls attention to the easy slippage between histories of innovation and histories which simply document advance. For Edgerton, this calls into question the whole value of using innovation as an historical framework.[1]

But this argument sets up a straw man. Such criticisms of innovation-focused history rely on a simplistic notion of what innovation is and how it is experienced. In fact, the history of innovation is only this narrow if we let it become so: if we make it our business as historians to shoehorn innovations into immutable categories of successful diffusion or ultimate failure, depict those associated with innovations as either winners or losers, and if we assume that the process of innovation is an ordered one. In the preceding chapters, I have sought to show that in the case of ovariotomy no such order or simplicity can be found, nor is this a desirable way to frame the negotiation of the operation into medical practice. Rather, what it shows is that no aspect of the innovation process in surgery can be treated as self-evident; that which we might initially take for granted as being unambiguous about an innovation: its beginning, its ending, its definition, are not necessarily so. Moreover, innovation in operative surgery comes with its own unique set of problems and peculiarities, which neither broader histories of medicine nor of technology adequately convey. Caught between overlapping but distinct worlds of theory and performance, the physical invasiveness of surgery has, historically, amplified tensions around the introduction of new procedures. When a new operation succeeded, the potentiality of innovation to restore the body to health was made dramatically visible. But so too, were the devastating physical consequences of surgery when an operation failed.

As a means of showing this, I have set out with the objective of examining one surgical procedure, the removal of the ovary, making the operation itself central to the narrative. It may seem odd to claim an operation-centred approach to surgery as novel within the historiography, but, a few notable exceptions aside, it is.[2] And yet an operation-centred approach can do valuable work in helping us understand innovation. It serves to magnify the deficiencies that remain in the history of surgery: patients' journeys through referral networks, understandings of surgical responsibility, the pre- and post-operative periods, the negotiation of an operation's financial cost: all these are issues that are nuanced through a close reading of ovariotomy.

By addressing the complex genealogy of a single operation over a lengthy time period, this study also obliges reconsideration of the temporality of surgical innovation. John Pickstone long ago drew attention to distinctions between invention and innovation, insisting that innovation involves not just a new product or phenomenon but its negotiation into medicine.[3] But it is the 'new' that studies of innovation remain indelibly linked to. I do not deny this association, nor that ovarian surgery represented genuine and significant novelty among the historical actors under scrutiny here; for better or worse, the entry into the peritoneum was viewed as a striking innovation by many contemporary surgeons. But by reviewing the lengthy process of negotiation that ovarian surgery underwent, we see that the 'new' is as much a representation as it is an essential quality of a product or process, fixed to a specific period. Surgical innovation did not necessarily begin with the first performance of a procedure. In the case of ovariotomy, the shift from theoretical possibility to surgical practice was a slow process—about as distant from modern-day conceptions of innovation as lightning-quick that one can get. As described in Chapter 2, Ephraim McDowell's canonical operation in 1809 was preceded by decades of discussion as to the feasibility and ethicality of removing diseased ovaries, coupled with reports of numerous procedures where the ovary or part of the ovary had been removed, both intentionally and unexpectedly. Notions of ovarian surgery's novelty and longevity were constantly shifting and did not pertain to any self-evident, linear temporality. When the possibility of the operation was discussed in the late eighteenth century, for example, precedents of ovarian extirpation from the ancient world were emphasised in a bid to improve its credibility and show that the procedure was not simply a dangerous novelty. But when at the tail end of the nineteenth century ovariotomy was historicised by some as the pinnacle of Victorian surgery's achievement, as described in Chapter 6, it was its identity as a novelty of *that* era which became increasingly valued. Furthermore, in Chapter 6, I teased apart the idea of an innovation's 'ending'. Generally, medical innovations are considered to have two possible destinies: integration or rejection. But the history of ovariotomy shows operations can have a different fate. By the beginning of the twentieth century, elements of both integration *and* rejection were part of ovariotomy's status. Changing and inconsistent nomenclature further complicated matters, as the definition of 'ovariotomy' became increasingly uncertain. In this chapter, I also probed the idea of endings by considering how the medical profession sought to historicise recent innovations in ovariotomy, even as the operation remained in contemporary use. The historicisation of past achievements tangled uneasily with anxieties about the future of surgery. The significance of taking a chronologically expansive view of ovariotomy has other implications too. Recent literature on the history of surgical innovation has generally focused on the late nineteenth century onwards. But if the chronological focus remains this way then 'innovation' and attendant concerns of risk, responsibility, credit and so forth, remain invariably wedded to recent times when, as the history of ovariotomy shows, such concerns were already considered highly important by surgeons.

Throughout this study I have attempted to elucidate the operation's constantly shifting, malleable identity, which runs throughout its history; over the nineteenth century, ovariotomy could be depicted both as a murderous procedure performed by immoral 'belly-rippers' and the dazzling beginning of a new era of surgery. Diverse methodologies, from patient narratives to ambitious statistical accounts, were employed by doctors to try and ascertain just how risky the operation was. With the emergence of a new term for the operation, 'ovariotomy', in the 1840s, as detailed in Chapter 3, a transitional moment occurred in which the operation was reconceptualised from a range of diverse acts—often private endeavours—to a single identity, in which all occurrences of the procedure were expected to be relayed through print and thus available for public comparison and consumption. The term 'ovariotomy' helped to make sense of the developments taking place, but underneath the label there struggled multiple identities and meanings. When situating surgical procedures historically, it seems useful to think of an operation as a network in itself, and one that perhaps more closely resembles a cobweb, formed of gossamer thin threads that constitute an unstable whole. This factored into almost every key debate around ovariotomy, from the differing definitions of the operation used to calculate its risks, to disputes over the intellectual property of the procedure, to the discussions around the justifiability of performing it for a growing range of pathologies. All were impacted by the varying definitions ascribed to ovariotomy by different actors.

To an extent, my conclusions speak to those of other historians. Thomas P. Hughes, in his extensive explorations of innovation in technology, most notably through the work of Thomas Edison, understood inventions as being incorporated into large-scale technological systems, which involve various stages of development, growth, competition and consolidation, although not necessarily in that order. Hughes cautions against a reliance on models of innovation which suggest a one-size-fits-all staged career, alluding instead to the messiness and complexity of the process of innovation.[4] Focusing on surgery specifically, Thomas Schlich has elaborated further, pointing to the unhelpfulness of a 'sharp distinction between innovation, invention and diffusion, which is so typical of economic models of innovation', when both the context and the technology of a surgical innovation are, in fact, liable to change.[5] A further deconstructive step, however, can be taken in understanding the fragile identity of surgical operations. Twenty-five years ago, Charles E. Rosenberg and Janet Golden's seminal work, *Framing Disease*, powerfully put forward the case for unravelling the intricacies of disease categories. In it Rosenberg argued that biological events were continually being re-framed in response to cultural change.[6] Their work has been influential on medical history (and beyond) ever since. Given the constructivist bent of the discipline, it is then remarkable that little has been done to understand surgical operations in the same way. But as the history of ovariotomy shows, new surgical operations are equally subject to continual reframing and even reconceptualisation.

As Thomas Schlich has noted, historians of medicine have focused predominantly on 'concepts and practices that are obviously influenced by culture and society'.[7] The connections between operative surgery and broader cultural concerns may seem less immediately obvious. But as I have sought to show, ovariotomy channelled a spectrum of wider issues pertinent particularly to Victorian society, from preoccupations with financial success, honour and reward, to gender normativity and the pernicious effects of fashion upon society. These issues often converged through the operation. Chapters 4 and 5 reveal a rather complicated picture of the economics of nineteenth-century surgery. Professional and surgical risks, expectations of aftercare, ovariotomists' self-identity, as well as patient demand, all factored into the pricing of the operation. Meanwhile, those practitioners able to claim a role in the operation's innovation, following its growing success in the middle decades of the century, were able to capitalise financially on their connection with it. Implicit within the financial benefits of performing ovariotomy were multiple professional and ethical questions, as the prolific performance of the operation led to fears that unnecessary surgery was taking place and that patients were demanding what was by the late 1880s perceived by some as a 'fashionable' operation. This factored into understandings of the operation's performance as economically motivated. For some doctors, it also signalled excessive amounts of power on the part of female patients—facilitated by professional acquiescence—to shape their treatment, potentially to the detriment of their health.

Indeed, questions of sex and gender course through the history and historiography of ovariotomy. A long-held supposition within the historical literature has been that surgical innovation around the ovaries, in comparison with the relative *lack* of surgical innovation around less obviously gendered abdominal organs, reflected upon the susceptibility of women's bodies to becoming experimental material for doctors, particularly in the Victorian era. Undeniably, this is part of the story. Enmeshed within contemporary concepts of womanhood, which were also framed by ideas of class and race, an exclusively female set of patients suited and shaped the narrative many surgeons wished to project of the operation as a life-saving necessity for vulnerable and suffering women, restoring them to health so that they could perform their familial and societal duties. Moreover, in some cases, the existence of the patient's full consent to undergo the procedure is doubtful. But the gendering of ovariotomy was also more complex than previous works have suggested, and the controversies surrounding ovarian surgery by the end of the nineteenth century can be read within a broader and longer history of disease and therapeutics. The burgeoning fields of reproductive physiology and morbid anatomy in the eighteenth century found common ground in the ovary and its pathological complexities, which revealed itself in practitioners' interest in the large tumours many female patients were afflicted with. But it was also the relative expendability of the ovaries that made them a potential site of surgical intervention, as the male testicles were already; and a growing understanding that it was possible for women to go on to live a healthy life without their reproductive organs—although this idea would come under scrutiny once more at the end of the nineteenth century. Moreover, a close reading of the operation paints a more nuanced picture of power relations between practitioners and patients, ever-fluctuating in the face of the operation's own evolution. Ovarian disease could be a painful, humiliating and life-threatening condition; the possibility of a complete cure that ovariotomy offered meant that while patients felt fear and trepidation about its risks, some also pursued the operation regardless in their quest for relief. Indeed, there is ample space for further work in this area. Traditionally, it is the 'pioneering' surgeon we see as pushing the boundaries of surgical innovation, but what about the role some patients played, not just in enduring operations but in initiating and shaping them? New research is bringing the surgical patient into the history of innovation.[8] Although most work has so far been focused on the twentieth century, if relevant primary sources could be unearthed, such work could be done in a nineteenth-century context as well, helping to refine our conceptualisations of the symbiosis involved in the patient–practitioner relationship.

No one operation could ever seamlessly reflect the unfolding of all surgical innovations during the period in question, and there is no doubt that ovariotomy in many respects occupied a singular place in surgery during this time. Its acceptance into established practice was based upon a profound shift in the ethics of surgery; the operation portended a significant reframing of major surgery from last resort to elective treatment. But the controversies surrounding the operation leveraged it to a status that meant through it, conceptions and concerns about surgical innovation were visibly channelled. These conceptions and concerns can be read more widely into the negotiation of surgical novelty during this time, where innovation did not simply equate to progress and where a single surgical procedure, the removal of the ovary, gave rise to deep-seated questions about the objectives—and even the very meaning—of surgery.

Notes

1. David Edgerton, *The Shock of the Old: Technology and Global History Since 1900* (London: Profile, 2006), xiv.
2. Thomas Schlich, *Surgery, Science and Industry: A Revolution in Fracture Care, 1950s–1980s.* (Basingstoke: Palgrave Macmillan, 2002); Thomas Schlich and Christopher Crenner, 'Technological Change in Surgery: An Introductory Essay', in *Technological Change in Modern Surgery*, ed. Thomas Schlich and Christopher Crenner (Rochester: University of Rochester Press, 2017). Both Schlich, and Schlich and Crenner in their edited volume, make individual procedures central to their historical investigation.
3. John V. Pickstone, 'Introduction', in *Medical Innovations in Historical Perspective*, ed. John V. Pickstone (Basingstoke: Macmillan, 1992), 1.
4. Thomas P. Hughes, 'The Evolution of Large Technological Systems', in *The Social Construction of Technological Systems: New Directions in the Sociology and History of Technology*, ed. Wiebe E. Bijker and Thomas P. Hughes and Trevor Pinch (Cambridge, MA: MIT Press, 2012), 50–51.
5. Schlich, *Surgery, Science and Industry*, 241.
6. Charles E. Rosenberg, 'Framing Disease, Illness, Society and History', in *Framing Disease: Studies in Cultural History*, ed. Charles E. Rosenberg and Janet Golden (New Brunswick: Rutgers University Press, 1992), xiii–xv.
7. Thomas Schlich, *The Origins of Organ Transplantation: Surgery and Laboratory Science* (Rochester and Woodbridge: University of Rochester Press, 2010), 8.
8. Cynthia L. Tang and Thomas Schlich, 'Surgical Innovation and the Multiple Meanings of Randomized Controlled Trials: The First RCT on Minimally Invasive Cholecystectomy (1980–2000)', *Journal of the History of Medicine and Allied Sciences*, 72, no. 2: 117–141; Beth Linker, 'Prosthetic Imaginaries: Spinal Surgery and Innovation from the Patient's Perspective', in *Technological Change in Modern Surgery*, ed. Thomas Schlich and Christopher Crenner (Rochester: University of Rochester Press, 2017), 100–128.

Primary Literature

Abernethy, John. (1827). 'Mr. Abernethy's Physiological, Pathological and Surgical Investigations.' *Lancet* 7 (187): 817–827.

Adams, Thomas. (1616). *Diseases of the Soule: A Discourse Diuine, Morall, and Physicall.* London: George Purslowe for John Budge.

'Aesculapius Scalpel' (Edward Berdoe). (1887). *St. Bernards: The Romance of a Medical Student.* London: Swan Sonnenschein, Lowrey & Co.

Aitken, John. (1784). *Principles of Midwifery, or Puerperal Medicine.* Edinburgh: Edinburgh Lying-In Hospital.

Allen, Elizabeth, J.L. Turk, and Sir Reginald Murley. (1993). *The Case Books of John Hunter FRS.* London: Royal Society of Medicine Services Limited.

Anonymous. (1670). *An Account of the Causes of Some Particular Rebellious Distempers.* London: s.n.

———. (1739). 'A Cure for Dropsy.' *Gentleman's Magazine* 9: 299.

———. (1760). 'A Receipt for Dropsy.' *Gentleman's Magazine* 30: 416.

———. (1764). 'General Bills of Mortality for the Year 1764.' *Scots Magazine* 26: 72.

———. (1790). 'Médicine-Pratique.' *Histoire de la Société Royale de Médecine* 8: 7.

———. (1799). 'Account of Diseases in London.' *Monthly Magazine* 7 (41): 68–69.

———. (1825). 'Review: Observations on Extraction of Diseased Ovaria.' *Lancet* 4 (103): 327.

———. (1826a). 'Extirpation of the Ovaria.' *The Medico-Chirurgical Review* 6: 215–217.

———. (1826b). 'Ovarian Dropsy.' *Medico-Chirurgical Transactions* 3: 588.

———. (1826c). 'Review: On the Extirpation of Diseased Ovaries.' *The London Medical Repository and Review* 3: 135–145.

———. (1828). 'Extirpation of Ovarian Tumors.' *London Medical and Physical Journal* 59: 175–176.

———. (1830). 'Review: Illustrations of Some of the Principal Diseases of the Ovaria.' *Edinburgh Medical and Surgical Journal* 34: 123–140.

———. (1833). 'German Medicine: Extirpation of a Diseased Ovary.' *London Medical and Surgical Journal* 4: 32.

———. (1837). 'Editorial.' *Lancet* 28 (726): 669–670.

———. (1838). 'Physical Society, Guy's Hospital.' *London Medical Gazette* 23: 313–314.

———. (1842). 'Review of Mr. Eagle's Proposition to Excise the Spleen.' *Lancet* 39 (999): 130–131.

———. (1843). 'Review: Cases of Peritoneal Section.' *British and Foreign Medical Review* 16: 387–402.

———. (1844a). 'Review: A Practical Treatise on Midwifery by M. Chailly.' *The Medico-Chirurgical Review* 41: 403–410.

———. (1844b). 'Ovarian Dropsy.' *Medical Times* 10: 11.

———. (1844c). 'Extirpation of Ovaria.' *Lancet* 43 (1074): 45–47.

———. (1844d). 'Extirpation of Ovarian Tumors.' *The Medico-Chirurgical Review* 40: 557–562.

———. (1846). 'Medico-Chirurgical Society of Edinburgh.' *The Monthly Journal of Medical Science* 6 (4): 53–67.

———. (1847a). 'To Correspondents.' *Medical Times* 15 (381): 307.

———. (1847b). 'Westminster Medical Society.' *Lancet* 50 (1261): 451–478.

———. (1847c). 'The Blessings of Chloroform.' *Punch* 13: 232.

———. (1849). 'Results of the Operation for the Extirpation of Diseased Ovaria: Review.' *London Medical Gazette* 44: 899–900.

———. (1850a). 'Royal Medical and Chirurgical Society.' *Lancet* 56 (1421): 583–587.

———. (1850b, December 6). 'Editorial.' *The Times* no.20665: 4.

———. (1851a). 'Royal Medical and Chirurgical Society.' *Lancet* 57 (1432): 147–172.

———. (1851b). 'Biographical Sketch of Robert Lee, M.D., F.R.S.' *Lancet* 57 (1438): 332–337.

———. (1860). 'The Late Professor John Lizars.' *Edinburgh Medical Journal* 6: 101–103.

———. (1861). 'Le Prix Barbier ses Métamorphoses.' *Revue de Thérapeutique Medico-Chirurgicale* 2 (21): 561–563.

———. (1862a). 'The Week.' *British Medical Journal* 1 (55): 69.

———. (1862b). 'Royal Medical and Chirurgical Society, November 11th 1862.' *Lancet* 80 (2047): 565–569.

———. (1862c, March 12). 'Bankrupts.' *The Standard* no.11726: 5.

———. (1862d). 'Medical Annotations: A Laurel for English Surgeons.' *Lancet* 79 (2001): 12.

———. (1863a). 'Obstetrical Society of London.' *Lancet* 81 (2067): 417.

———. (1863b). 'Obstetrical Society of London.' *Medical Times and Gazette* 1: 407–408.

———. (1863c). 'Dublin.' *Lancet* 82 (2098): 578–579.

———. (1864a). 'Progress from the French Point of View.' *The New Monthly Magazine* 131: 253–269.

———. (1864b). 'The Week.' *British Medical Journal* 2 (201): 528.

———. (1865a). 'Reviews and Notices of Books.' *British Medical Journal* 2 (239): 121.

———. (1865b). 'Review: Diseases of the Ovaries, Their Diagnosis and Treatment.' *British Medical Journal* 1 (214): 117.

———. (1865c). *Proceedings at the Seventh Annual Meeting of the London Surgical Home*. London: Savill & Edwards.

———. (1865d). 'Freedom V License.' *British Medical Journal* 2 (259): 637–638.

———. (1866). 'Ovariotomy in New Zealand.' *Medical Times and Gazette* 1: 640.

———. (1867a). 'Obstetrical Society of London.' *Lancet* 89 (2275): 429–441.

———. (1867b). 'Review: Diseases of the Ovaries—Their Diagnosis and Treatment.' *Edinburgh Medical Journal* 13 (1): 565–568.

———. (1868). 'The Theory of Professional Remuneration.' *British Medical Journal* 1 (371): 122–123.

———. (1870). 'Medical Fees in Prussia.' *British Medical Journal* 1 (484): 370–371.

———. (1872). 'Review Essay.' *Edinburgh Review, or Critical Journal* 136 (278): 488–515.

———. (1874). 'Obituary: Frederic Bird.' *Medical Times and Gazette* 1: 520.

———. (1875). 'Professional Fees.' *British Medical Journal* 1 (737): 223.

———. (1877a). 'Professional Ethics and Etiquette.' *Edinburgh Medical Journal* 23 (4): 333–338.

———. (1877b). 'Notes and Queries.' *The American Practitioner and News* 16: 59.

———. (1878a). 'Consultation-Fees.' *British Medical Journal* 2 (923): 375–376.

———. (1878b). 'Consultation-Fees.' *British Medical Journal* 2 (927): 539.

———. (1878c). 'Physicians, Practitioners, Patients and Fees.' *British Medical Journal* 1 (889): 56–57.

———. (1880). 'Ovariotomy.' *British Medical Journal* 1 (1016): 931–932.

———. (1881). 'Letter from London.' *The Boston Medical and Surgical Journal* 104 (6): 142–143.

———. (1882a). 'Canadian Medical Fees.' *Lancet* 119 (3065): 897.

———. (1882b). 'Editorial: Questionable Surgery.' *Medical Press and Circular* 33: 385–386.

———. (1884a). 'Essay on Desperate Surgery in Its Relation to Women: The Proper Place for It; Who Should and Who Should Not Attempt It.' *Journal of the American Medical Association* 3 (12): 318–325.

———. (1884b). 'An Inaugural Address on the Revival of Ovariotomy, and Its Influence on Modern Surgery.' *Lancet* 124 (3194): 857–860.

———. (1885a). 'Editorial: Ovariotomy, Hysterectomy and Oöphorectomy.' *British Medical Journal* 1 (1257): 239–240.

———. (1885b). 'The Prospects of the Profession.' *Medical Press and Circular* 40: 256–257.

———. (1885c). 'Ovariotomy, Hysterectomy and Oöphorectomy.' *British Medical Journal* 1 (1257): 239–240.

———. (1885d). 'Reviews and Notices of Books: The Story of My Life by J. Marion Sims.' *Lancet* 126 (3232): 247.

———. (1886a). 'Editorial.' *Lancet* 128 (3285): 304–307.

———. (1886b). 'Editorial: The Virtues of Laparotomy.' *Medical Press and Circular* 41: 502–503.

———. (1886c). 'The Usefulness of Spaying.' *Medical Record* 29 (15): 419.

———. (1886d). 'Within the Hospital Walls: A Matter of Fact Narrative.' *Lancet* 127 (3277): 1194–1205.

———. (1886e). 'Obstetrical Society of London.' *Lancet* 127 (3258): 255–256.

———. (1886f, August 23). 'The Shaw Street Hospital.' *Liverpool Mercury* no.12050: 7.

———. (1886g). 'The British Gynaecological Society, November 11th 1885.' *British Gynaecological Journal* 1 (4): 371–387.

———. (1886h). 'The Frequency of Diseases of the Uterine Appendages.' *Medical Press and Circular* 42: 30–31.

———. (1887). 'Notes and Queries.' *The American Practitioner and News* 3: 224.

———. (1888a). 'Nursing Echoes.' *Nursing Record* 1 (25): 336–338.

———. (1888b). 'The Militant Spirit in Gynaecology Societies.' *Medical Press and Circular* 45: 495.

———. (1888c). 'Review: The Medical-Chirurgical Tariffs.' *Edinburgh Medical Journal* 34 (1): 62.

———. (1889). 'Review: The Medical Profession of the United Kingdom.' *British Medical Journal* 1 (1474): 717–718.

———. (1891). 'The Annus Medicus 1891.' *Lancet* 138 (3565): 1443–1462.

———. (1893). 'Obituary: Charles Clay.' *Lancet* 142 (3657): 846.

———. (1895). 'Obituary: Thomas Keith.' *British Gynaecological Journal* 11 (43): 394–397.

———. (1896a, November 17). 'Action Against a Doctor.' *Dundee Courier and Argus* no. 13537: 4.

———. (1896b, November 17). 'Remarkable Action Against a London Surgeon,' *Sheffield and Rotherham Independent* no. 13150: 8.

———. (1896c, November 21). 'Nurse v. Doctor: A Claim for Damages.' *Hampshire Telegraph and Sussex Chronicle* no. 6010: 2.

———. (1897). 'The Address in the Section of Obstetrics and Gynaecology.' *British Medical Journal* 2 (1916): 726–727.

———. (1898). 'The Patient Insisted Upon Abdominal Section!' *The Hospital* 23: 412.

———. (1911). 'Reviews and Notices of Books: A Study of the After-Results of Abdominal Operations.' *Lancet* 177 (4562): 308–311.

———. (1916). 'Obituary—W.A. Meredith.' *Lancet* 188 (4860): 727.

———. (1920). 'Obituary: David Lloyd Roberts.' *Lancet* 196 (5067): 766–767.

———. (1927). 'Obituary—Alban Henry Griffiths Doran.' *British Journal of Obstetrics and Gynaecology* 34 (3): 546–547.

———. (1933). 'Obituary: Christopher Martin.' *British Journal of Obstetrics and Gynaecology* 40 (2): 305–309.

Ashwell, Samuel. (1845). 'Extirpation in Ovarian Dropsy.' *The Boston and Medical and Surgical Journal* 45: 357–359.

Astruc, John. (1767). *A Treatise on the Diseases of Women*, Vol. 3. London: J. Nourse.

Baillie, Matthew. (1789). *An Account of a Particular Change of Structure in the Human Ovarium from the Philosophical Transactions*. London: s.n.

———. (1793). *The Morbid Anatomy of Some of the Most Important Parts of the Human Body*. London: J. Johnson.

Ball, John. (1762). *The Modern Practice of Physic*, Vol. 1. London: A. Millar.

———. (1770). *The Female Physician, or Every Woman Her Own Doctress*. London: L. Davis.

Bantock, George Granville. (1887). 'One Hundred Consecutive Cases of Abdominal Section.' *Lancet* 129 (3315): 518–521.

———. (1903). 'The Conservative Treatment of Lesions of the Uterine Appendages.' *Lancet* 162 (4169): 220–221.

Bantock, Myrrha. (1972). *Granville Bantock: A Personal Portrait*. London: J.M Dent.

Battey, Robert. (1873). *Normal Ovariotomy*. Atlanta: Herald Publishing.

Bell, Benjamin. (1783). *A System of Surgery*, Vol. 1. Edinburgh: Charles Elliot and G. Robinson.

Bell, Charles. (1798). *A System of Dissection, Explaining the Anatomy of the Human Body, the Manner of Displaying the Parts, and Their Varieties in Disease*. Edinburgh: Mundell and Son.

Bell, John. (1795). *Discourses on the Nature and Cure of Wounds*. Edinburgh: Bell and Bradfute.

Bell, John, and Charles Bell. (1816). *The Anatomy and Physiology of the Human Body*, Vol. 3. London: Longman.

Bell, Joseph. (1866). *Manual of the Operations of Surgery*. Edinburgh: MacLachlan and Stewart.

Berkeley, Comyns, and Victor Bonney. (1911). *A Textbook of Gynaecological Surgery*. London: Cassell.

Bird, Frederic. (1851). 'Diagnosis, Pathology and Treatment of Ovarian Tumours.' *Medical Times* 24 (57): 120–123.

Black, C. (1857). 'On a Case of Ovarian Disease: Ovariotomy; Death on the Third Day from Destruction of the Bronchial Mucous Surface.' *Lancet* 69 (1745): 138–140.

Blackmore, Richard. (1725a). *A Critical Dissertation Upon the Spleen*. London: J. Pemberton.

———. (1725b). *A Treatise of the Spleen and Vapours*. London: J. Pemberton.

Bland-Sutton, John. (1891). *Surgical Diseases of the Ovaries and Fallopian Tubes.* Philadelphia: Lea Bros.

———. (1906). *Tumours, Innocent and Malignant.* London: Cassell.

———. (1907). 'A Clinical Lecture on the Value and Fate of Belated Ovaries.' *Medical Press and Circular* 135: 108–111.

———. (1930). *On Faith and Science in Surgery.* London: William Heinemann.

Bland-Sutton, John, and Arthur Giles. (1897). *Diseases of Women: A Handbook for Students and Practitioners.* Philadelphia: W.B. Saunders.

Blundell, James. (1829a). 'On the Surgery of the Abdomen.' *Lancet* 12 (303): 353–356.

———. (1829b). 'Lectures on the Diseases of Women and Children.' *Lancet* 11 (290): 769–772.

———. (1837). *Observations on Some of the More Important Diseases of Women.* Edited by Thomas Castle. London: E. Cox.

Bond, C.J. (1906). 'An Inquiry into Some Points in Uterine and Ovarian Physiology and Pathology in Rabbits.' *British Medical Journal* 2 (2377): 121–127.

Boyd, Florence Nightingale. (1903). 'Conservative Surgery of the Tubes and Ovaries.' *British Gynaecological Journal* 3 (3): 241–261.

Boyd, Stanley. (1900). 'Conservative Surgery of Tubes and Ovaries.' *British Medical Journal* 2 (2072): 727–734.

Brickett, George E. (1877). 'History of Ovariotomy in Maine.' *Transactions of the Maine Medical Association* 6: 73–96.

Brown, Isaac Baker. (1844). 'Practical Remarks on the Cure of Ovarian Dropsy Without Abdominal Section.' *Lancet* 43 (1083): 306–307.

———. (1854). *On Some Diseases of Women Admitting of Surgical Treatment.* London: John Churchill.

———. (1862). *On Ovarian Dropsy: Its Nature, Diagnosis & Treatment; the Result of Thirty Years Treatment.* London: John W. Davies.

———. (1866). 'Management of the Pedicle in Ovariotomy.' *British Medical Journal* 2 (302): 421.

Bryant, Thomas. (1867). *On Ovariotomy.* London: John Churchill.

Burton, John. (1751). *An Essay Towards a Complete New System of Midwifery, Theoretical and Practical.* London: James Hodges.

Butcher, Richard G. (1865). 'On Ovariotomy, and the After-Treatment of the Patient.' *Dublin Quarterly Journal of Medical Science* 40 (80): 257–284.

Butler-Smythe, A.C. (1893). 'Acute Mania Following Rupture of the Rectum by Enema Thirteen Days After Ovariotomy. Recovery.' *Journal of Mental Science* 39 (166): 389–397.

Cadge, William. (1889). 'Lithotomy.' In *Dictionary of Practical Surgery*, Vol. 1, ed. Christopher Heath, 934–943. London: Smith, Elder & Co.

Cheston, Richard Browne. (1766). *Pathological Inquiries and Observations in Surgery, from the Dissections of Morbid Bodies. With an Appendix Containing Twelve Cases on Different Subjects.* Gloucester: R. Rakes.

Cheyne, William W. (1898). 'Two Cases of Oöphorectomy for Inoperable Breast Cancer.' *British Medical Journal* 1 (1194): 1194–1195.

Chiene, John. (1908). *Looking Back, 1907–1860*. Edinburgh: Darien Press.

Churchill, Fleetwood. (1841). *Researches on Operative Midwifery*. Dublin: Martin Kenne and Son.

———. (1844). 'Ovariotomy.' *The Medico-Chirurgical Review* 42: 528–532.

Clarke, J.F. (1874). *Autobiographical Recollections of the Medical Profession*. London: J. & A. Churchill.

Clay, Charles. (1842a). *Cases of Peritoneal Section for the Extirpation of Diseased Ovaria by the Large Incision from Sternum to Pubes*. London: Munro & Congreve.

———. (1842b). 'Cases of Peritoneal Section.' *Medical Times* 7 (160): 43–45.

———. (1842c). 'Cases of Peritoneal Section.' *Medical Times* 7: 139–142.

———. (1843a). 'Dr. Clay's Reply to Dr. Granville on Ovarian Extirpation.' *Medical Times* 8 (204): 326–327.

———. (1843b). 'Ovariotomy.' *Medical Times* 9 (211): 4–5.

———. (1848). *The Results of All Operations for the Extirpation of Diseased Ovaria*. Manchester: W.M. Irwin.

———. (1865a). 'On Ovariotomy and Ovariotomists.' *Lancet* 85 (2165): 200–202.

———. (1865b). 'On Ovariotomy and Ovariotomists.' *Lancet* 85 (2166): 226–228.

———. (1865c). 'The Ovariotomy Controversy.' *Lancet* 85 (2171): 380.

———. (1880). 'History of Ovariotomy.' *British Medical Journal* 2 (1020): 109–110.

Clay, John. (1860). *Chapters on Diseases of the Ovaries translated, by Permission, from Kiwisch's Clinical Lectures*. London: Churchill.

———. (1862). 'Adhesion Clam: A New Instrument for Aiding the Removal of Ovarian Tumours Etc.' *Medical Times and Gazette* 1: 640–641.

———. (1865). 'Ovariotomy: Clay's Adhesion Clam.' *British Medical Journal* 1 (225): 418–419.

———. (1866). 'On Management of the Pedicle in Ovariotomy.' *British Medical Journal* 2 (303): 449–450.

Cleghorn, James. (1787). 'The History of an Ovarium, Wherein Were Found Teeth, Hair and Bones. By James Cleghorn M.B. Communicated by Robert Perceval M.D.' *Transactions of the Royal Irish Academy* 1: 73–89.

Cole, F.J. (1930). *Early Theories of Sexual Generation*. Oxford: Clarendon Press.

Collins, Wilkie. (1994). *Heart and Science: A Story of the Present Time*. Peterborough: Broadview Press.

Cope, Zachary. (1951). *The Versatile Victorian: Being the Life of Sir Henry Thompson, 1820–1904*. London: Harvey & Blythe.

Croom, John Halliday. (1896). 'Obstetrics.' *Lancet* 148 (3805): 343–344.

———. (1901). 'Edinburgh Obstetrical Society: Psychoses Following Pelvi-Abdominal Operations.' *Lancet* 157 (4044): 630–631.

Cullen, William. (1778). *First Lines of the Practice of Physic*, Vol. 4. Edinburgh: C. Elliot, T. Kay, & Co.

Cullingworth, Charles. (1887). 'A Tabular Statement of Sixty-Four Abdominal Sections; Including Forty-Five Completed Ovariotomies with Remarks.' *Lancet* 130 (3335): 205–209.

Cushing, Harvey. (1940). *The Life of Sir William Osler: Vol. 1*. London, New York and Toronto: Oxford University Press.

Delaporte, Jean. (1753). 'Hydropsie Enkistée de l'Ovarie Attaquée Par Incision.' *Mémoires de l'Académie Royale de Chirurgie* 2: 455.

Denman, Thomas. (1794). *An Introduction to the Practice of Midwifery*, Vol. 1. London: J. Johnson.

Dent, C.T. (1889). 'Insanity Following Surgical Operations.' *British Journal of Psychiatry* 35 (149): 1–14.

De Styrap, Jukes. (1878). *A Code of Medical Ethics*. London: J. & A. Churchill.

———. (1890). *The Medico-Chirurgical Tariffs (Prepared for the Late Shropshire Ethical Branch of the British Medical Association)*. London: H. K. Lewis.

Dickens, Charles. (1994). *The Pickwick Papers*. London: Penguin.

Dolan, Thomas M. (1889). 'Gynaecological Specialism and General Practice.' *British Gynaecological Journal* 5 (19): 284–304.

Doran, Alban. (1887). *Handbook of Gynaecological Operations*. Philadelphia: P. Blakiston & Son.

———. (1888). 'The Details of Ovariotomy.' *Annals of Surgery* 7: 321–328.

Dorr, James. A. (1847). 'Are Improvements in Medicine and Surgery Proper Subjects of Patents?' *Lancet* 49 (1237): 523–524.

Douglas, John. (1720). *Lithotomia Douglassiana*. London: Thomas Woodward.

Dudley, A Palmer. (1903). 'The Trend of Gynecologic Work To-Day.' *Journal of the American Medical Association* 41 (25): 1527–1532.

Duncan, James Matthews. (1857). 'Is Ovariotomy Justifiable?' *Lancet* 69 (1748): 212–214.

Eliot, George. (2007). *Middlemarch: A Study of Provincial Life*. London: Vintage.

Epps, Richard. (1875). *On Ovarian Dropsy and Ascites: Their Diagnosis and Treatment. Also on Prolapsus of the Uterus*. London and Edinburgh: Simpkin, Marshall & Co.

Erichsen, John. (1874). 'Impressions of American Surgery.' *Lancet* 104 (2673): 717–720.

———. (1886). 'An Address Delivered at the Opening of the Section of Surgery.' *British Medical Journal* 2 (1337): 314–316.

Fergusson, William. (1867). *Lectures on the Progress of Anatomy and Surgery During the Present Century*. London: John Churchill.

Fisher, S.S. (1871). *Reports of Cases Arising Upon Letters Patent for Inventions Determined in the Circuit Courts of the United States*, Vol. 2. Cincinnati: Robert Clarke & Co.

Fothergill, John. (1772). 'On the Use of Tapping Early in Dropsies.' *Medical Observations and Inquiries* 4: 115.

'F.R.C.S.' (1886). 'Nomenclature for Operations Upon the Ovary.' *British Medical Journal* 2 (1334): 187–188.

Gaillard, Theodore. (1880). *A Practical Treatise on the Diseases of Women*. London: Henry Kimpton.

Gamgee, Arthur. (1886). 'An Address on the Employment of Compressed and Rarefied Air in the Treatment of Cases of Chronic Bronchitis, Emphysema, and Spasmodic Asthma.' *British Medical Journal* 2 (1355): 1205–1207.

Gamgee, Sampson. (1867a). 'The Present State of Surgery in Paris.' *Lancet* 90 (2296): 273–274.

———. (1867b). 'The Present State of Surgery in Paris.' *Lancet* 90 (2313): 799–802.

———. (1871). *A Lecture on Ovariotomy*, 2nd ed. London: Churchill.

Gant, Frederick. (1872). 'Abstract of an Oration on Modern Surgery as a Science and an Art.' *Lancet* 100 (2560): 401–404.

Giles, Arthur E. (1910). *Study of the After-Results of Abdominal Operations on the Pelvic Organs: Based on a Series of 1000 Consecutive Cases*. London: Baillière, Tindall and Cox.

———. (1912). 'Address in Surgery.' *Canadian Medical Association Journal* 2 (9): 751–763.

———. (1914). 'Meditation on 1000 Consecutive Abdominal Operations at the Prince of Wales's General Hospital, Tottenham.' *Lancet* 184 (4740): 8–16.

Godlee, Rickman John. (1917). *Lord Lister*. London: Macmillan.

Godson, Clement. (1884). 'Porro's Operation.' *British Medical Journal* 1 (1204): 142–159.

Gooch, Benjamin. (1773). *Medical and Chirurgical Observations, as an Appendix to a Former Publication*. London and Norwich: G. Robinson and R. Beatniffe.

Goodell, William. (1873). *Lessons in Gynecology*. Philadelphia: D. & G. Brinton.

Gorham, John. (1839a). 'Excision in Ovarian Dropsy.' *Lancet* 33 (852): 506–507.

———. (1839b). 'Observations on the Propriety of Extirpating the Cyst in Some Cases of Ovarian Dropsy.' *Lancet* 33 (843): 155–161.

———. (1874), 'On the Revival of Ovariotomy.' *Lancet* 103 (2639): 440–441.

Gould, Alfred Pearce. (1906). *The Influence of Surgical Operations upon the Expectation of Life: Lecture for the Life Assurance Medical Officer's Association*. London: C.E. Gray.

Granville, Augustus. (1826). 'Case in Which an Attempt Was Made to Extirpate Ovarian Tumors.' *London Medical and Physical Journal* 56 (330): 141–143.

Granville, Augustus. (1874). *Autobiography of A. B. Granville.* Edited by P. Granville. London: Henry S. King & Co.

Gregory, John. (1770). *Observations on the Duties and Offices of a Physician, and on the Method of Prosecuting Enquiries in Philosophy.* London: W. Strahan and T. Cadell.

Hall-Williams, Mary J. (1899). *Ovariotomy Averted.* Plymouth.

Halton, John. (1843). 'On the Average Number of Deaths in Capital Operations.' *London Medical Gazette* 33: 390–400.

Hegar, Alfred, Robert Battey, and Thomas Spencer Wells. (1886). 'Castration for Nervous and Mental Diseases: A Symposium.' *American Journal of Medical Sciences* 184: 455–490.

H.E.M. (1940). 'Medical Nomenclature.' *Canadian Medical Association Journal* 43 (6): 597–598.

Herman, George E. (1903). *Diseases of Women: A Clinical Guide to Their Diagnosis and Treatment.* London and New York: Cassell.

Holt, B.W. (1841). 'Case of Extensive Scrofulous Disease of the Knee-Joint. Amputation-Recovery.' *Lancet* 37 (944): 30–31.

Hopfer. (1829). 'On Extirpation of Diseased Ovaria.' *London Medical Gazette* 3: 401–405.

Houstoun, Robert. (1724). 'An Account of a Dropsy in the Left Ovary of a Woman, Aged 58. Cured by a Large Incision Made in the Side of the Abdomen.' *Philosophical Transactions of the Royal Society* 33: 8–15.

Hunter, John. (1787). 'An Experiment to Determine the Effect of Extirpating One Ovarium Upon the Number of Young Produced.' *Philosophical Transactions of the Royal Society* 77: 233–239.

Hunter, William. (1758). 'The History of Emphysema.' *Medical Observations and Inquiries* 2: 17–70.

Hunter, William. (2008). *Correspondence of Dr. William Hunter—Vol. 1.* Edited by C. Helen Brock. London: Pickering and Chatto.

Jeaffreson, William. (1837). 'A Case of Ovarian Tumour Successfully Removed.' *Transactions of the Provincial Medical and Surgical Association* 5: 239–245.

———. (1839). 'Ovarian Cysts.' *Lancet* 33 (846): 287.

———. (1843). 'Mr Jeaffreson's Operation for Ovarian Dropsy.' *Lancet* 41 (1055): 217.

Jennings, Charles. (1886). 'Nomenclature for Operations Upon the Ovaries.' *British Medical Journal* 2 (1331): 187.

Jesse, George. (1882). *Correspondence of George Jesse with T.S. Wells and Other Medical Men on Ovariotomy.* London: Pickering & Co.

Joubert, C.H. (1892). 'The History of Ovariotomy in Bengal.' *Indian Medical Gazette* 27 (2): 52–54.

Keith, Thomas. (1867). 'Fifty-One Cases of Ovariotomy.' *Lancet* 90 (2297): 290–291.

———. (1878). 'Results of Ovariotomy Before and After Antiseptics.' *British Medical Journal* 2 (929): 590–593.

———. (1885). 'Thirteen Cases of Hysterectomy, with Remarks on Carbolic Acid Spray in Abdominal Surgery.' *British Medical Journal* 1 (1257): 214–215.

Kelly, Howard A. (1896). 'Conservatism in Ovariotomy.' *Journal of the American Medical Association* 26 (2): 249–251.

King, Robert. (1837). 'New Operations for the Removal of Abdominal Tumours.' *Lancet* 27 (699): 586–590.

L'Aumonier, Jean-Baptiste. (1787). 'Observations Sur Un Dêpot de La Trompe et Sur L'extirpation Des Ovaires.' *Histoire de La Société Royale de Médecine* 5: 296–300.

Lane, James R. (1884). 'The Revival of Ovariotomy.' *British Medical Journal* 2 (1250): 1212.

Lawrence, William. (1829a). 'A Lecture Introductory to a Course of Surgery.' *Lancet* 11 (285): 612–618.

———. (1829b). 'Lectures on Surgery, Medical and Operative. Lecture 1: Introduction.' *Lancet* 13 (318): 33–42.

———. (1829c). 'Lectures on Surgery, Medical and Operative. Lecture 2: On the Nature and Seat of Diseases.' *Lancet* 13 (319): 65–71.

———. (1830). 'Lectures on Surgery: Lecture LXXV.' *London Medical Gazette* 6: 822–828.

Laycock, Thomas. (1840). *A Treatise on the Nervous Diseases of Women*. London: Longman, Orme, Brown, Green, and Longmans.

Leake, John. (1777). *Medical Instructions Towards the Prevention and Cure of Chronic or Slow Diseases Peculiar to Women*. London: R. Baldwin.

Le Dran, Henri. (1749). *The Operations in Surgery of Monsieur Le Dran*. Translated by Thomas Gataker. London: C. Hitch & R. Dodsley.

———. (1753). 'Hydropsie Enkistée Attaquée Par Une Opération Dont Il Resta Fistule' in 'Plusieurs Mémoires et Observations Sur l'Enkistée et Le Skirre Des Ovaires.' *Memoires de l'Academie Royale de Chirurgie* 2: 431–442.

———. (1766). *Consultation on Most of the Disorders That Require the Assistance of Surgery*. London: Robert Horsfield.

Lee, Robert. (1853). *Clinical Reports of Ovarian and Uterine Diseases*. London: John Churchill.

Lettsom, John Coakley. (1797). *Hints Designed to Promote Beneficence, Temperance and Medical Science*, Vol. I. London: H. Fry.

Lindsay, James A. (1899). 'An Inaugural Address on Our Position and Outlook.' *Lancet* 154 (3983): 1797–1800.

Liston, Robert. (1835). *Elements of Surgery*. London: Longman.

————. (1837). *Practical Surgery*. London: John Churchill.

————. (1845). 'Practical Surgery: A Course of Lectures on the Operations of Surgery and Diseases and Accidents Requiring Operations.' *Lancet* 45 (1119): 145–148.

Lizars, John. (1825). *Observations on Extraction of Diseased Ovaria*. Edinburgh: Daniel Lizars.

Lockhart-Mummery, J.P. (1903). *The After-Treatment of Operations: A Manual for Practitioners and House Surgeons*. London: Baillière, Tindall and Cox.

Logie, H.B. (1934). 'Medical Nomenclature.' *American Speech* 9 (1): 17–25.

Lückes, Eva. (1884). *Lectures on General Nursing*. London: Kegan Paul.

Luxmoore, William. (1766). *An Address to Hydropic Patients*. London: W. Wilson.

MacCormac, William. (1880). *Antiseptic Surgery*. London: Smith, Elder.

————. (1881). *Transactions of the International Medical Congress*, Vol. 2. London: J.W. Kolckmann.

Mackenzie, Morell. (1885). 'Medical Specialism.' *Fortnightly Review* 38 (224): 272–276.

Madden, Thomas More. (1886). 'On the So-Called Laparotomy Epidemic.' *Dublin Journal of Medical Science* 82 (1): 1–9.

Manchester Medico-Ethical Association. (1879). *Tariff of Medical Fees Issued by the Manchester Medico-Ethical Association*. Manchester: J. & E. Cornish.

————. (1893). *Tariff of Medical Fees Issued by the Manchester Medico-Ethical Association*. Manchester: J. & E. Cornish.

Manning, Henry. (1771). *A Treatise on Female Diseases*. London: R. Baldwin.

Martin, Christopher. (1898). 'On the Conservative Surgery of the Ovary.' *British Medical Journal* 2 (1968): 791–792.

————. (1921). 'Reminiscences of Lawson Tait.' *British Journal of Obstetrics and Gynaecology* 28 (1): 117–123.

Martineau, Philip Meadows, and John Hunter. (1784). 'An Extraordinary Case of a Dropsy of the Ovarium.' *Philosophical Transactions of the Royal Society* 74: 471–476.

McDowell, Ephraim. (1817). 'Three Cases of Extirpation of Diseased Ovaria.' *Eclectic Repertory and Analytical Review* 7: 242–245.

————. (1819). 'Observations on Diseased Ovaria.' *Eclectic Repertory and Analytical Review* 9: 546–552.

Michener, Ezra. (1818). 'Case of Diseased Ovarium.' *Eclectic Repertory and Analytical Review* 8: 111–115.

Monro, Donald. (1756). *An Essay on the Dropsy and Its Different Species*. London: D. Wilson & T. Durham.

Morand, Sauveur-François. (1753). 'Remarques sur le Observations précédentes, avec un précis de quelques autres, sur le meme sujet' in 'Plusieurs Mémoires et Observations sur l'Enkistée et le Skirre des Ovaires.' *Memoires de l'Academie Royale de Chirurgie* 2: 455–460.

Morison, Rutherford. (1916). *Surgical Contributions from 1881–1916. Vol. II: Abdominal Surgery.* Bristol: John Wright and Sons.

Moss, B.N. Henry, and F. Curtis Dohan. (1958). 'Surgical Convalescence: When Does It End?' *Annals of the New York Academy of Sciences* 73: 455–464.

Moynihan, Berkeley. (1910). *The Pathology of the Living and Other Essays.* Philadelphia and London: W.B. Saunders.

———. (1927). 'Lister as Surgeon.' *Lancet* 209 (5406): 746–748.

Needham, Joseph. (1959). *A History of Embryology.* Cambridge: Cambridge University Press.

Newman, David. (1901). 'History of Renal Surgery (Part 4).' *Lancet* 157 (4049): 1033–1035.

O'Flanagan, James. (1877). *Contradiction! Or English Medical Men and Manners of the Nineteenth Century.* London: Baillière, Tindall and Cox.

Paget, James. (1862). 'The Address in Surgery.' *British Medical Journal* 2 (155): 155–162.

Peaslee, Edmund R. (1867). 'Ovariotomy, When and How to Operate; After-Treatment.' *Southern Journal of the Medical Sciences* 2: 546–552.

———. (1872). *Ovarian Tumors: Their Pathology, Diagnosis and Treatment, Especially by Ovariotomy.* New York: D. Appleton.

'Pen Oliver' (Henry Thompson). (1885). *Charley Kingston's Aunt.* London: Macmillan.

Phillips, Benjamin. (1840). 'Extraction of an Ovarian Cyst.' *London Medical Gazette* 27: 83–88.

———. (1844). 'Observations on the Recorded Cases of Operations for the Extraction of Ovarian Tumours.' *Medico-Chirurgical Transactions* 27: 468–492.

Pott, Percivall. (1775). *Chirurgical Observations.* London: T. J. Carnegy.

Potter, Jonathan. (1873). 'The History of Ovariotomy.' *British Medical Journal* 2 (678): 770–771.

Rabagliati, Andrea. (1886). 'Notes on Abdominal Section for Ovariotomy, Oophorectomy, and Hysterectomy.' *Medical Press and Circular* 41 (2455): 444–445.

Ridenbaugh, Mary Young. (1890). *The Biography of Ephraim McDowell: The "Father" of Ovariotomy.* New York: Charles L. Webster.

Rivington, Walter. (1888). *The Medical Profession of the United Kingdom.* Dublin: Fannin & Co.

Robson, Arthur Mayo. (1895). 'An Address on the Surgery of To-Day as Compared with That of Twenty-Five Years Ago: Illustrated by the Work in the General Infirmary at Leeds.' *Lancet* 146 (3766): 1094–1096.

———. (1902). 'An Introductory Address on the Advance in Surgery During 30 Years.' *Lancet* 160 (4127): 912–916.

———. (1903). 'Address in Surgery: Observations on the Evolution of Abdominal Surgery from Personal Reminiscences Extending Over a Third of a Century and the Performance of 2000 Operations,' *Lancet* 162 (4170): 292–297.

———. (1904). 'The Bradshaw Lecture on the Treatment of Cancer.' *British Medical Journal* 2 (2292): 1501–1506.

Rogers, David. (1829). 'Extirpation of an Enlarged Ovary.' *London Medical Gazette* 5: 271–272.

Routh, Charles H. F. (1894a). 'On Castration in Females: Its Frequent Inexpediency and the Signal Advantages of Conservative Surgery in These Cases—Part II.' *Medical Press and Circular* 108 (18): 457–459.

———. (1894b). 'The Conservative Treatment of Disease of the Uterine Appendages.' *British Gynaecological Journal* 10: 51–87.

Rowlette, Robert J. (1939). *The Medical Press and Circular, 1839–1939*. London: MPC.

Royal College of Physicians of London. (1906). *The Nomenclature of Diseases*. London: Printed for His Majesty's Stationery Office by Darling and Son.

Sampson, Henry. (1677). 'Anatomical Observations in the Body of a Woman, About 50 Years Old, Who Died Hydropical in the Left Testicle.' *Philosophical Transactions of the Royal Society* 12: 1001.

Schachner, August. (1921). *Ephraim McDowell: "Father of Ovariotomy" and Founder of Abdominal Surgery*. Philadelphia and London: J. B Lippincott.

Seymour, Edward. (1830). *Illustrations of Some of the Principal Diseases of the Ovaria*. London: Longman, Rees, Orme, Brown and Green.

Shaw, George Bernard. (1909). 'The Socialist Criticism of the Medical Profession.' *Transactions of the Medico-Legal Society* 6: 202–228.

———. (1957). *The Doctor's Dilemma*. London: Penguin.

Short, Thomas. (1728). *A Discourse Concerning the Causes and Effects of Corpulency*. London: J. Roberts.

Simpson, Alexander Russell. (1879). 'History of a Case of Double Oophorectomy, or Battey's Operation: With Remarks.' *British Medical Journal* 1 (960): 763–766.

Sims, James Marion. (1869). 'Ovariotomy: Pedicle Secured by Silver-Wire Ligatures: Cure.' *British Medical Journal* 1 (432): 326.

———. (1877). 'Remarks on Battey's Operation.' *British Medical Journal* 2 (877): 916–918.

———. (1884). *The Story of My Life*. New York: D. Appleton.

Skene, Alex. (1896). 'Thomas Keith.' *Brooklyn Medical Journal* 10 (2): 73–80.

Smiles, Samuel. (2008). *Self-Help: With Illustrations of Conduct and Perseverance*. Rockville: Serenity.

Smith, Alban. (1826). 'Account of a Case in Which an Ovarium Was Successfully Extirpated.' *North American Medical and Surgical Journal* 1: 30–38.

Smith, Heywood. (1879). 'Successful Case of Battey's Operation or Oöphorectomy.' *British Medical Journal* 2 (967): 41–45.

———. (1893). 'The Early History of Ovariotomy.' *Lancet* 142 (3658): 898.

Smith, James Greig. (1888). *Abdominal Surgery.* London and Bristol: J. & A. Churchill and J. W. Arrowsmith.

———. (1894). 'The Art of the Surgeon, and How We Train Men to Practise It.' *Lancet* 144 (3701): 245–249.

Smith, Nathan. (1822). 'Case of Ovarian Dropsy Successfully Removed by a Surgical Operation.' *Edinburgh Medical and Surgical Journal* 18: 532–534.

Smollett, Tobias. (1966). *The Expedition of Humphry Clinker.* London: Oxford University Press.

Solly, Samuel. (1846). 'Clinical Lecture on Ovariotomy.' *London Medical Gazette* 38: 51–58.

Southam, George. (1845). 'Ovariotomy: Removal of an Encysted Tumour of the Left Uterine Appendages.' *The Provincial Medical and Surgical Journal* 9 (37): 561–565.

Southwood Smith, Thomas. (1832). *A Lecture Delivered Over the Remains of Jeremy Bentham.* London: Effingham Wilson.

Spencer, Herbert R. (1933). 'A Review of 658 Ovariotomies.' *Proceedings of the Royal Society of Medicine* 26 (11): 1435–1444.

Sprigge, Samuel Squire. (1897). *The Life and Times of Thomas Wakley.* London: Longmans, Green and Co.

Stafford, Ezra Hurlbert. (1901). *Medicine, Surgery and Hygiene in the Nineteenth Century.* London, Toronto and Philadelphia: Linscott Publishing.

Stephenson, W. (1903). 'The British Association Meeting at Swansea: Obstetrics and Gynaecology.' *Lancet* 162 (4170): 350–352.

Stoker, Bram. (1994). *Dracula.* London: Penguin.

Stokes, W. (1886). 'An Address on Finality in Surgery.' *Lancet* 128 (3299): 959–962.

Swain, William P. (1866). 'Transaction of Branches: On Recent Improvements in Surgery.' *British Medical Journal* 2 (298): 303–305.

Syme, J. (1832). *The Principles of Surgery.* Edinburgh: MacLachlan and Stewart.

Tait, Robert Lawson. (1882). 'Removal of the Uterine Appendages.' *British Medical Journal* 2 (1125): 153.

———. (1884a). 'Recent Advances in Pelvic Surgery.' *Medical Press and Circular* 37: 321–323.

———. (1884b). 'The Revival of Ovariotomy.' *British Medical Journal* 2 (1249): 1165.

———. (1885). 'Abstract of an Address on One Thousand Abdominal Sections.' *British Medical Journal* 1 (1257): 218–219.

———. (1886). 'Removal of the Uterine Appendages.' *Medical Press and Circular* 42: 202–203.

———. (1886). 'Casey vs Imlach.' *Lancet* 128 (3286): 375–376.

———. (1888). 'Menstruation and the Ovaries.' *Lancet* 132 (3404): 1044–1045.

———. (1889). *Diseases of Women and Abdominal Surgery*, Vol. 1. Philadelphia: Lea Bros.

———. (1891). 'Address on the Principle of Exploratory and Confirmatory Incisions.' *Lancet* 137 (3519): 292–296.

———. (1896). 'The Evolution of the Surgical Treatment of the Broad Ligament Pedicle.' *Lancet* 147 (3794): 1334–1338.

Taylor, William, Fountain Elwin and William Dalrymple (1831). *A Memoir of the Late Philip Meadows Martineau, Surgeon*. Norwich: Bacon and Kinnerbrook.

Thomson, St. Clair. (1927). 'Memories of a House Surgeon.' *Lancet* 209 (5406): 775–780.

Thomson, William. (1885). 'Three Cases of Ovariotomy.' *Transactions of the Royal Academy of Medicine in Ireland* 3 (1): 121–130.

Thorne, May. (1899). 'After-Effects of Abdominal Section.' *British Medical Journal*, 1, 1988: 264–265.

Thornton, John Knowsley. (1886). 'Ovariotomy.' In *Dictionary of Practical Surgery*, Vol. 2, ed. Christopher Heath, 151–159. London: Smith, Elder & Co.

Tilt, Edward. (1882). *The Change of Life in Health and Disease*. Philadelphia: P. Blakiston, Son & Co.

———. (1885). *On Diseases of Menstruation and Ovarian Inflammation, in Connexion with Sterility, Pelvic Tumours, and Affections of the Womb*. London: J. & A. Churchill.

Treves, Frederick. (1900). 'Address in Surgery: The Surgeon in the Nineteenth Century.' *Lancet* 4014: 156.

Trombley, Stephen. (1989). *Sir Frederick Treves*. London and New York: Routledge.

Tyson, Edward. (1680). *Phocaena, or the Anatomy of a Porpess*. London: Benjamin Tooke.

Walne, D. Henry. (1843). *Cases of Dropsical Ovaria Removed by the Large Abdominal Section*. London: Longman, Brown, Green, and Longmans.

Walsham, William Johnson. (1897). *Surgery: Its Theory and Practice*, 6th ed. London: J. & A. Churchill.

Warren, John Collins. (1906). *The Influence of Anaesthesia on the Surgery of the Nineteenth Century, Being the Address of the President Before the American Surgical Association*. Boston: Privately Printed.

Weatherly, Lionel. (1898). 'Remarks on Medical Progress.' *Lancet* 152 (3918): 851–854.

Wells, Thomas Spencer. (1863). 'On the History and Progress of Ovariotomy in Great Britain.' *The Medico-Chirurgical Transactions* 46: 33–55.

———. (1865). *Diseases of the Ovaries: their Diagnosis and Treatment.* London: John Churchill.

———. (1865). 'Results of Ovariotomy.' *Lancet* 85 (2167): 272.

———. (1866). 'Clinical Remarks on Different Modes of Dealing with the Pedicle in Ovariotomy.' *British Medical Journal* 2 (301): 377–379.

———. (1877). 'The Address in Surgery.' *Lancet* 110 (2815): 189–194.

———. (1884a). 'An Inaugural Address on the Revival of Ovariotomy, and Its Influences on Modern Surgery.' *Lancet* 124 (3193): 811–814.

———. (1884b). 'An Inaugural Address on the Revival of Ovariotomy, and Its Influences on Modern Surgery.' *Lancet* 124 (3194): 857–860.

———. (1891). *Modern Abdominal Surgery: The Bradshaw Lecture Delivered at the Royal College of Surgeons of England December 18th, 1890 with an Appendix on the Castration of Women.* London: J. & A. Churchill.

West, William J. (1837). 'Successful Operation for the Removal of an Ovarian Tumour.' *Lancet* 29 (743): 307–308.

Whitehead, James. (1842). 'Case of Caesarean Section.' *London Medical Gazette* 28: 939–947.

Wilkes, Richard. (1781). *An Historical Essay on the Dropsy.* London: Law & Ray.

Williams, Roger W. (1900). 'Some Reasons for Believing That Oophorectomy Tends to Favour Rather Than to Prevent the Development of Cancer.' *British Medical Journal* 2 (2081): 1471–1472.

———. (1902). 'Correspondence.' *British Medical Journal* 1 (2141): 111–112.

Withering, William. (1785). *An Account of the Foxglove and Some of Its Medical Uses.* Birmingham: Swinney.

Wynter, Andrew. (1872). 'Review Essay.' *Edinburgh Review, or Critical Journal* 136 (278): 488–515.

Yonge, James. (1706). 'An Account of Balls of Hair Taken from the Uterus and Ovaria of Several Women; By Mr. James Yonge, F.R.S. Communicated to Dr. Hans Sloane, R.S. Secr.' *Philosophical Transactions of the Royal Society* 25 (309): 2387–2392.

Zola, Émile. (1957). *Fécondité.* Paris: Fasquelle Éditeurs.

Secondary Literature

Absolon, Karel B. (1979). *Theodor Billroth—Vol. 1.* Lawrence: Coronado Press.

Adams, Annmarie, and Thomas Schlich. (2006). 'Design for Control: Surgery, Science, and Space at the Royal Victoria Hospital, Montreal, 1893–1956.' *Medical History* 50 (3): 303–324.

Adams, James Eli. (1995). *Dandies and Desert Saints: Styles of Victorian Manhood.* Ithaca: Cornell University Press.

Alderson, D., and J. J. Earnshaw. (2013). 'A Century at the Cutting Edge.' *The British Journal of Surgery* 100 (2): 169.

Allender, Tim. (2016). *Learning Femininity in Colonial India, 1820–1932*. Manchester: Manchester University Press.

Angelos, Peter. (2010). 'The Art of Medicine: The Ethical Challenges of Surgical Innovation for Patient Care.' *Lancet* 376 (9746): 1046–1047.

Anger, Suzy. (2001). 'Introduction: Knowing the Victorians.' In *Knowing the Past: Victorian Literature and Culture*, ed. Suzy Anger, 1–24. Ithaca and London: Cornell University Press.

———. (2005). *Victorian Interpretation*. Ithaca and London: Cornell University Press.

Anonymous. (1997). 'Sir William Watson Cheyne.' In *Plarr's Lives of the Fellows*, Vol. 3, ed. D'Arcy Power, 143–146. London: Royal College of Surgeons of England. https://livesonline.rcseng.ac.uk/biogs/E000222b.htm.

———. (2000). 'McDowell, Ephraim.' *American National Biography*. Online. http://www.anb.org/articles/12/12-00598.html.

———. (2007). 'Russell Claude Brock, Lord Brock of Wimbledon (1903–1980).' In *Plarr's Lives of the Fellows Online*. London: Royal College of Surgeons of England. http://livesonline.rcseng.ac.uk/biogs/E000235b.htm.

Armitage, David. (2012). 'What's the Big Idea? Intellectual History and the Longue Durée.' *History of European Ideas* 38 (4): 493–507.

Bailey, Joanne. (2008). 'Is the Rise of Gender History "Hiding" Women from History Once Again?' *History in Focus*, 7–20. http://www.history.ac.uk/ihr/Focus/Gender/articles2.html.

Bartrip, Peter. (1990). *Mirrors of Medicine: A History of the BMJ*. Oxford: Oxford University Press.

———. (1996). *Themselves Writ Large: The British Medical Association 1832–1966*. London: BMA Publishing Group.

Baston, K. Grudzien. (2004). 'Bell, John (1763–1820).' *Oxford Dictionary of National Biography*. Oxford University Press. http://www.oxforddnb.com/view/article/2013.

Batty Shaw, A. (1970). 'The Norwich School of Lithotomy.' *Medical History* 14 (3): 221–259.

Beaumont, Matthew. (2009). *Utopia Ltd: Ideologies of Social Dreaming in England 1870–1900*. Chicago: Haymarket Books.

Beck, Ulrich. (1992). *Risk Society: Towards a New Modernity*. London: Sage.

Benedict, Barbara M. (2000). 'Making a Monster: Socializing Sexuality and the Monster of 1790.' In *"Defects": Engendering the Modern Body*, eds. Helen Deutsch and Felicity Nussbaum, 127–153. Ann Arbor: University of Michigan Press.

Beninghaus, Christina. (2012). 'Beyond Constructivism? Gender, Medicine and the Early History of Sperm Analysis, Germany 1870–1900.' *Gender and History* 24 (3): 647–676.

Berkowitz, Carin. (2011). 'The Beauty of Anatomy: Visual Displays and Surgical Education in Early-Nineteenth-Century London.' *Bulletin of the History of Medicine* 85 (2): 248–278.

Bland, Lucy. (2002). *Banishing the Beast: Feminism, Sex and Morality.* London and New York: I.B. Tauris.

Bowler, Peter J. (1989). *The Invention of Progress: The Victorians and the Past.* Oxford: Basil Blackwell.

Bowra, Jean. (2005). 'Making a Man a Great Man: Ephraim McDowell, Ovariotomy and History.' Paper Presented to the Social Change in the 21st Century Conference, Centre for Social Change Research, Queensland University of Technology. http://eprints.qut.edu.au/3454/1/3454.pdf.

Brieger, Gert. H. (1992). 'From Conservative to Radical Surgery in Late Nineteenth-Century America.' In *Medical Theory, Surgical Practice: Studies in the History of Surgery*, ed. Christopher Lawrence, 216–231. London and New York: Routledge.

Brock, Claire. (2011). 'Surgical Controversy at the New Hospital for Women, 1872–1892.' *Social History of Medicine* 24 (3): 1–16.

———. (2013). 'Risk, Responsibility and Surgery in the 1890s and Early 1900s.' *Medical History* 57 (3): 317–337.

———. (2017). *British Women Surgeons and Their Patients, 1860–1918.* Cambridge: Cambridge University Press.

Brock, R. (1962). 'A Philosophy of Surgery.' *Canadian Medical Association Journal* 86: 370–372.

Brockliss, Laurence, and Colin Jones. (1997). *The Medical World of Early Modern France.* Oxford: Clarendon Press.

Brockwell, Holly. (2015). 'Why Can't I Get Sterilised in My 20s?' *The Guardian.* http://www.theguardian.com/commentisfree/2015/jan/28/why-wont-nhs-let-me-be-sterilised#comment-46773414. Accessed 11 December 2017.

Brown, Michael. (2011). *Performing Medicine: Medical Culture and Identity in Provincial England*, c. 1760–1850. Manchester and New York: Manchester University Press.

———. (2017). 'Redeeming Mr. Sawbone: Compassion and Care in the Cultures of Nineteenth-Century Surgery.' *Journal of Compassionate Healthcare* 4 (13).

Buckley, Jerome Hamilton. (1967). *The Triumph of Time: A Study of the Victorian Concepts of Time, History, Progress, and Decadence.* Cambridge, MA: The Belknap Press of Harvard University Press.

Buklijas, Tatjana. (2008). 'Surgery and National Identity in Late Nineteenth-century Vienna.' *Studies in History and Philosophy of Biological and Biomedical Sciences* 38 (4): 756–774.

Burney, Ian. (2003). 'Medicine in the Age of Reform.' In *Rethinking the Age of Reform: Britain 1780–1850*, 163–181. Cambridge: Cambridge University Press.

———. (2006). 'Anaesthetic Death and the Evaluation of Risk in Nineteenth-Century English Surgery.' In *The Risks of Medical Innovation*, eds. Thomas Schlich and Ulrich Tröhler, 38–52. Abingdon: Routledge.

Burnham, John. (1992). 'The British Medical Journal in America.' In *Medical Journals and Medical Knowledge: Historical Essays*, eds. William F. Bynum, Stephen Lock, and Roy Porter, 165–187. London and New York: Routledge.

Butterfield, Herbert. (1965). *The Whig Interpretation of History*. London and New York: The Norton Library.

Bynum, William F. (1985). 'Physicians, Hospital and Career Structures in Eighteenth-Century London.' In *William Hunter and the Eighteenth-Century Medical World*, eds. William F. Bynum and Roy Porter, 105–128. Cambridge: Cambridge University Press.

———. (1994). *Science and the Practice of Medicine in the Nineteenth Century*. Cambridge: Cambridge University Press.

———. (2001). 'Hunter, John.' In *Encyclopaedia of Life Sciences*. https://doi.org/10.1038/npg.els.0002437.

Bynum, William F., and Janice C. Wilson. (1992). 'Periodical Knowledge: Medical Journals and Their Editors in Nineteenth-Century Britain.' In *Medical Journals and Medical Knowledge: Historical Essays*, eds. William F. Bynum, et al., 29–48. London and New York: Routledge.

Carlson, Bob. (2010). 'Surprise District Court Ruling Invalidates Myriad Genetics' BRCA Patents, but Appeal Is Pending.' *Biotechnology Healthcare* 7 (2): 8–9.

Carr, Eloise et al. (2006). 'Patterns and Frequency of Anxiety in Women Undergoing Gynaecological Surgery.' *Journal of Clinical Nursing* 15 (3): 341–352.

Chakrabarti, B. and N. Mondal. (2009). 'O160 Adolescent Ovarian Malignancy.' *International Journal of Gynecology & Obstetrics* 107: S138–S138.

Chaney, Sarah. (2011). '"A Hideous Torture on Himself": Madness and Self-Mutilation in Victorian Literature.' *Journal of Medical Humanities* 32 (4): 279–289.

Chapman, Raymond. (1986). *The Sense of the Past in Victorian Literature*. London and Sydney: Croom Helm.

Churchill, Wendy D. (2005). 'The Medical Practice of the Sexed Body: Women, Men, and Disease in Britain, c. 1600–1740.' *Social History of Medicine* 18 (1): 3–22.

———. (2012). *Female Patients in Early Modern Britain: Gender Diagnosis and Treatment*. Farnham: Ashgate.

Cody, Lisa Forman. (2005). *Birthing the Nation: Sex, Science and the Conception of Eighteenth-Century Britons.* Oxford: Oxford University Press.

Condrau, Florin. (2007). 'The Patient's View Meets the Clinical Gaze.' *Social History of Medicine* 20 (3): 525–540.

Cooke, A.M. (1982). 'Queen Victoria's Medical Household.' *Medical History* 26 (3): 307–320.

Cooper Owens, Deirdre. (2017). *On Medical Bondage: Race, Gender and the Origins of American Gynecology.* Athens: University of Georgia Press.

Cooter, Roger. (1993). *Surgery and Society in Peace and War.* Basingstoke: Macmillan.

———. (1995). 'Review Article: The Resistible Rise of Medical Ethics.' *Social History of Medicine* 8 (2): 257–270.

———. (2004). '"Framing" the End of the Social History of Medicine.' In *Locating Medical History: The Stories and Their Meanings*, eds. Frank Huisman and John Harley Warner, 309–337. Baltimore and London: The Johns Hopkins University Press.

Corley, T.A.B. (1987). *Interactions Between the British and American Patent Medicine Industries, 1708–1914* (Pamphlet Reprint from Business and Economic History, Series 2).

Crenner, Christopher. (2005). *Private Practice: In the Early Twentieth-Century Medical Office of Dr. Richard Cabot.* Baltimore and London: The Johns Hopkins University Press.

Cronon, William. (2012). 'Two Cheers for the Whig Interpretation of History.' *Perspectives on History* 50 (6). http://www.historians.org/perspectives/issues/2012/1209/Two-Cheers-for-the-Whig-Interpretation-of-History.cfm.

Crowther, M. Anne, and Marguerite W. Dupree. (2007). *Medical Lives in the Age of the Surgical Revolution.* Cambridge: Cambridge University Press.

Culler, A. Dwight. (1985). *The Victorian Mirror of History.* New Haven and London: Yale University Press.

Cunningham, Andrew. (2010). *The Anatomist Anatomis'd.* Farnham and Burlington: Ashgate.

Curran, Andrew. (2004). 'Afterword: Anatomical Readings in the Early Modern Era.' In *Monstrous Bodies/Political Monstrosities in Early Modern Europe*, eds. Laura Lunger Knoppers and Joan B. Landes, 227–246. Ithaca and London: Cornell University Press.

Dally, Ann. (1991). *Women Under the Knife: A History of Surgery.* London: Hutchinson Radius.

Darby Robert. (2005). *A Surgical Temptation: The Demonization of the Foreskin and the Rise of Circumcision in Britain.* Chicago: University of Chicago Press.

———. (2007). 'The Benefits of Psychological Surgery: John Scoffern's Satire on Isaac Baker Brown.' *Medical History* 51 (4): 527–544.

Daston, Lorraine, and Katharine Park. (2001). *Wonders and the Order of Nature.* New York: Zone Books.

Daunton, Martin. (2005). 'Introduction,' In *The Organisation of Knowledge in Victorian Britain,* ed. Martin Daunton, 1–28. Oxford: Oxford University Press.

De Costa, Caroline, and Francesca Miller. (2006). 'Portrait of a Ladies' Man: Dr. Samuel-Jean Pozzi.' *History Today* 56 (3): 10–17.

———. (2010). *The Diva and Doctor God: Letters from Sarah Bernhardt to Doctor Samuel Pozzi.* Bloomington: XLibris.

Degeling, Chris. (2009). 'Fractured Hips: Surgical Authority, Futility and Innovation in Nineteenth Century Medicine.' *Endeavour* 33 (4): 129–134.

De Graaf, Regnier (Translated by H. D. Jocelyn, and B. P. Setchell). (1972). *Regnier de Graaf on the Human Reproductive Organs.* Oxford: Blackwell.

Desmond, Adrian. (1989). *The Politics of Evolution: Morphology, Medicine and Reform in Radical London.* Chicago: University of Chicago Press.

Devlin, Hanna, and Nicola Davis. (2017, November 27). 'Vaginal Mesh Operations for Prolapse Should Be Banned, Watchdog to Say.' *The Guardian.* https://www.theguardian.com/society/2017/nov/27/vaginal-mesh-opera-tions-should-be-banned-health-watchdog-to-say. Accessed 5 December 2017.

DeVries, Jacqueline. (2015). 'A Moralist and Modernizer: Mary Scharlieb and the Creation of Gynecological Knowledge, c. 1880–1914.' *Social Politics* 22 (3): 298–318.

Digby, Anne. (1994). *Making a Medical Living: Doctors and Patients in the English Market for Medicine, 1720–1911.* Cambridge: Cambridge University Press.

Digby, Anne, and Nick Bosanquet. (1988). 'Doctors and Patients in an Era of National Health Insurance and Private Practice, 1913–1938.' *The Economic History Review* 41 (1): 74–94.

Dixon, Thomas. (2008). *The Invention of Altruism: Making Moral Meanings in Victorian Britain.* Oxford and New York: British Academy and Oxford University Press.

Duden, Barabara. (1991). *The Woman Beneath the Skin: A Doctor's Patients in Eighteenth-Century Germany.* Cambridge, MA and London: Harvard University Press.

Duffin, Lorna. (1978). 'The Conspicuous Consumptive: Woman as an Invalid.' In *The Nineteenth-Century Woman,* eds. Sara Delamont and Lorna Duffin, 26–56. London: Croom Helm Ltd.

Dupree, Marguerite W. (1997). 'Other Than Healing: Medical Practitioners and the Business of Life Assurance During the Nineteenth and the Early Twentieth Centuries.' *Social History of Medicine* 10 (1): 79–103.

————. (2013). 'From Mourning to Scientific Legacy: Commemorating Lister in London and Scotland.' *Notes and Records of the Royal Society* 67 (3): 261–280.

Dutton, H. I. (1984). *The Patent System and Inventive Activity during the Industrial Revolution, 1750–1852*. Manchester: Manchester University Press.

Dzelzainis, Ella. (2012). 'Introduction: Production and Consumption in Victorian Literature and Culture.' *Victorian Network* 4 (1): 1–7.

Eaton, Margaret L., and Donald Kennedy. (2007). *Innovation in Medical Technology*. Baltimore: The Johns Hopkins University Press.

Edgerton, David. (2006). *The Shock of the Old: Technology and Global History Since 1900*. London: Profile.

Ehrenreich, Barbara, and Deirdre English. (1979). *For Her Own Good: 150 Years of the Experts' Advice to Women*. London: Pluto Press.

Elston, Mary Ann. (1990). 'Women and Anti-vivisection in Victorian England, 1870–1900.' In *Vivisection in Historical Perspective*, ed. Nicolaas A. Rupke, 259–294. London and New York: Routledge.

Evenden, Doreen. (2000). *The Midwives of Seventeenth-Century London*. Cambridge: Cambridge University Press.

Fee, Elizabeth, and Theodore M. Brown. (2004). 'Using Medical History to Shape a Profession: The Ideals of William Osler and Henry E Sigerist.' In *Locating Medical History: The Stories and Their Meanings*, eds. Frank Huisman and John Harley Warner. Baltimore and London: The Johns Hopkins University Press.

Fissell, Mary E. (1991). 'The Disappearance of the Patient's Narrative and the Invention of Hospital Medicine.' In *British Medicine in the Age of Reform*, eds. Roger French and Andrew Wear, 92–109. London and New York: Routledge.

————. (1995). 'Gender and Generation: Representing Reproduction in Early Modern England.' *Gender & History* 7 (3): 433–456.

————. (2004). *Vernacular Bodies: The Politics of Reproduction in Early Modern England*. Oxford: Oxford University Press.

Forster, F.M. (1965). 'A Case of Ovariotomy Instruments Sent by Thomas Spencer Wells to Richard Thomas Tracy.' *The Journal of Obstetrics and Gynaecology of the British Commonwealth* 72 (5): 810–815.

Fort, John M.T. (2003). 'William John West (1794–1848): Abdominal Surgeon and Distraught Father.' *Journal of Medical Biography* 11: 107–113.

Foucault, Michel (Translated by A. M. Sheridan). (2003). *The Birth of the Clinic: An Archaeology of Medical Perception*. London: Routledge.

Frampton, Sally. (2008). '*Applause and Amazement*': Social Identity and the London Surgical Elite, 1880–1905. Unpublished MA thesis, University College London.

———. (2016). '"Honour and Subsistence": Invention, Credit and Surgery in the Nineteenth Century.' *British Journal of the History of Science* 49 (4): 561–576.

Frampton, Sally, and Roger Kneebone. (2017). 'John Wickham's New Surgery: "Minimally Invasive Therapy", Innovation, and Approaches to Medical Practice in Twentieth-Century Britain.' *Social History of Medicine* 30 (3): 544–566.

Gabriel, Joseph M. (2009). 'A Thing Patented Is a Thing Divulged: Francis E. Stewart, George S. Davis, and the Legitimization of Intellectual Property Rights in Pharmaceutical Manufacturing, 1879–1911.' *Journal of the History of Medicine and Allied Sciences* 64 (2): 135–172.

Gelfand, Toby. (1972). 'The "Paris Manner" of Dissection: Student Anatomical Dissection in Early Eighteenth-Century Paris.' *Bulletin of the History of Medicine* 2: 99–130.

———. (1980). *Professionalizing Modern Medicine*. Westport and London: Greenwood.

Georgopoulos, Dimitris-Solon G. (2004). 'In Pursuit of an Eponym.' *Texas Heart Institute Journal / from the Texas Heart Institute of St. Luke's Episcopal Hospital, Texas Children's Hospital* 31 (3): 335.

Gilman, Sander. (2011). 'Representing Health and Illness: Thoughts for the Twenty-First Century.' *Medical History* 55 (3): 295–300.

Godin, Benoît. 'Social Innovation: Utopias of Innovation from c. 1830 to the Present.' Project on the Intellectual History of Innovation, Working Paper No. 11 (Montreal: INRS, 2012). http://www.csiic.ca/PDF/SocialInnovation_2012.pdf.

Gooday, Graeme. (2000). 'Lies, Damned Lies and Declinism: Lyon Playfair, the Paris 1867 Exhibition and Contested Rhetorics of Scientific Education and Industrial Performance.' In *The Golden Age: Essays in British Social and Economic History, 1850–1870*, eds. Ian Inkster et al., 105–120. Aldershot: Ashgate.

Gooding, Richard. (2008). '"A Complication of Disorders": Bodily Health, Masculinity, and the Discourse of Gout and Dropsy in Henry Fielding's the Journal of a Voyage to Lisbon.' *Literature and Medicine* 26 (2): 386–407.

Gradmann, Christoph (Translated by Elborg Forster). (2009). *Laboratory Disease: Robert Koch's Medical Bacteriology*. Baltimore: John Hopkins University Press.

Granshaw, Lindsay. (1989). '"Fame and Fortune by Means of Bricks and Mortar": The Medical Profession and Specialist Hospitals in Britain 1800–1948.' In *The Hospital in History*, eds. Lindsay Granshaw and Roy Porter, 199–220. London and New York: Routledge.

Green, Monica H. (2008). *Making Women's Medicine Masculine: The Rise of Male Authority in Pre-Modern Gynaecology*. Oxford: Oxford University Press.

Greenwood, Anna. (1998). 'Lawson Tait and Opposition to Germ Theory: Defining Science in Surgical Practice.' *Journal of the History of Medicine and Allied Sciences* 53 (2): 99–131.

Guerrini, A. (2004). 'Anatomists and Entrepreneurs in Early Eighteenth-Century London.' *Journal of the History of Medicine and Allied Sciences* 59 (2): 219–239.

Hacking, Ian. (1990). *The Taming of Chance.* Cambridge: Cambridge University Press.

Hagner, Michael. (1999). 'Enlightened Monsters.' In *The Sciences in Enlightened Europe,* eds. William Clark et al., 175–217. Chicago and London: University of Chicago Press.

Hall, Stuart. (1997). 'The Work of Representation.' In *Representation: Cultural Representations and Signifying Practices,* eds. Stuart Hall et al. 13–74. Milton Keynes: Open University.

Handley, R.S. (1971). 'Gordon-Taylor, Breast Cancer and the Middlesex Hospital.' *Annals of the Royal College of Surgeons of England* 49 (3): 151–164.

Hannaway, Caroline C. (1972). 'The Société Royale de Médecine and Epidemics in the Ancien Régime.' *Bulletin of the History of Medicine* 46 (3): 257–273.

Harley, C.K. (2004). 'Trade, 1870–1939: From Globalisation to Fragmentation.' In *Cambridge Economic History of Modern Britain, Vol. 11: Economic Maturity, 1860–1939,* eds. Roderick Floud and Paul Johnson, 161–189. Cambridge: Cambridge University Press.

Harvey, Karen. (2002). 'The Substance of Sexual Difference: Change and Persistence in Representations of the Body in Eighteenth-Century England.' *Gender and History* 14 (2): 202–223.

Heaman, E.A. (2003). *St. Mary's: The History of a London Teaching Hospital.* Montreal: McGill-Queen's University Press.

Herbert, Christopher. (2002). 'Filthy Lucre: Victorian Ideas of Money.' *Victorian Studies* 44 (2): 185–213.

Hewitt, Martin. (1996). *The Emergence of Stability in the Industrial City: Manchester, 1832–1867.* Aldershot: Scolar.

———. (2006). 'Why the Notion of Victorian Britain Does Make Sense.' *Victorian Studies* 48 (3): 395–438.

Hirschauer, Stefan. (1998). 'Performing Sexes and Genders in Medical Practices.' In *Differences in Medicine: Unraveling Practices, Techniques and Bodies,* eds. Marc Berg and Annemarie Mol, 13–27. Durham, NC and London: Duke University Press.

Hollender, L.F. (2001). 'Eugène Koeberlé (1828–1915): Père de La Chirurgie Moderne.' *Annales de Chirurgie* 126 (6): 572–581.

Horrocks, Thomas A. (2000). 'James, Thomas C.' *American National Biography.* Online. http://www.anb.org/articles/12/12-00450.html.

———. (2000, February). 'Physick, Philip Syng.' *American National Biography*. Online. http://www.anb.org/articles/12/12-00722.html.

Huff, Joyce L. (2001). 'A "Horror of Corpulence": Interrogating Bantingism and Mid-Nineteenth Century Fat-Phobia.' In *Bodies out of Bounds: Fatness and Transgression*, eds. Jana Evans Braziel and Kathleen LeBesco, 39–59. Berkeley: University of California Press.

Hughes, Thomas P. (2012). 'The Evolution of Large Technological Systems.' In *The Social Construction of Technological Systems: New Directions in the Sociology and History of Technology*, eds. Wiebe E. Bijker et al., 51–82. Cambridge, MA: MIT Press.

Huisman, Frank, and John Harley Warner. (2004). 'Medical Histories.' In *Locating Medical History: The Stories and Their Meanings*, eds. Frank Huisman and John Harley Warner, 1–30. Baltimore and London: The Johns Hopkins University Press.

Hurwitz, Brian. (2006). 'Form and Representation in Clinical Case Reports.' *Literature and Medicine* 25 (2): 216–240.

Inkster, Ian. (2000a). 'Introduction: A Lustrous Age?' In *The Golden Age: Essays in British Social and Economic History, 1850–1870*, ed. Ian Inkster, 1–8. Aldershot: Ashgate.

———. (2000b). 'Machinofacture and Technical Change: The Patent Evidence.' In *The Golden Age: Essays in British Social and Economic History, 1850–1870*, ed. Ian Inkster. 121–142. Aldershot: Ashgate.

Jackson, Holbrook. (1976). *The Eighteen Nineties: A Review of Art and Ideas at the Close of the Century*. Brighton: The Harvester Press.

Jackson, R.V. (1987). 'The Structure of Pay in Nineteenth-Century Britain.' *Economic History Review* 40 (4): 561–570.

Jacyna, Stephen. (1992). 'Physiological Principles in the Surgical Writings of John Hunter.' In *Medical Theory, Surgical Practice: Studies in the History of Surgery*, ed. Christopher Lawrence, 135–152. London: Routledge.

———. (1994). *Philosophic Whigs: Medicine, Science and Citizenship in Edinburgh, 1789–1848*. London: Routledge.

———. (2004). 'Lawrence, Sir William, First Baronet (1783–1867).' In *Oxford Dictionary of National Biography*. Oxford University Press. http://www.oxforddnb.com/view/article/16191.

Jasen, Patricia. (2002). 'Breast Cancer and the Language of Risk, 1750–1950.' *Social History of Medicine* 15 (1): 17–43.

———. (2009). 'From the "Silent Killer" to the Whispering Disease: Ovarian Cancer and the Uses of Metaphor.' *Medical History* 5 (4): 489–512.

Jenner, Mark, and Patrick Wallis. (2007). 'The Medical Marketplace.' In *Medicine and the Market in England and Its Colonies* c. 1450–1850, eds. Mark Jenner and Patrick Wallis, 1–23. Basingstoke: Palgrave Macmillan.

Johnson, Jane, and Wendy Rogers. (2012). 'Innovative Surgery: The Ethical Challenges.' *Journal of Medical Ethics* 38 (1): 9–12.

Jones, Claire L. (2012). '(Re-)Reading Medical Trade Catalogs: The Uses of Professional Advertising in British Medical Practice, 1870–1914.' *Bulletin of the History of Medicine* 86 (3): 361–393.

Jones, David S. (2000). 'Visions of a Cure: Visualization, Clinical Trials, and Controversies in Cardiac Therapeutics, 1968–1998.' *Isis* 91 (3): 504–541.

Jones, Greta. (2010). '"Strike Out Boldly for the Prizes That Are Available to You": Medical Emigration from Ireland 1860–1905.' *Medical History* 54 (1): 55–74.

Jordanova, Ludmilla. (1989). *Sexual Visions: Images of Gender in Science and Medicine Between the Eighteenth and Twentieth Centuries.* Hemel Hempstead: Harvester Wheatsheaf.

Joyce, Simon. (2004). 'On or About 1901: The Bloomsbury Group Looks Back at the Victorians.' *Victorian Studies* 46 (4): 631–654.

———. (2007). *The Victorians in the Rearview Mirror.* Athens: Ohio University Press.

Kargon, Robert H. (1977). *Science in Victorian Medicine: Enterprise and Expertise.* Manchester: Manchester University Press.

Keating, Peter, and Alberto Cambrosio. (2006). 'Risk on Trial: The Interaction of Innovation and Risk in Cancer Clinical Trials.' In *The Risks of Medical Innovation: Risk Perception and Assessment in Historical Context,* eds. Thomas Schlich and Ulrich Tröhler, 225–241. Abingdon and New York: Routledge.

Kennedy, Meegan. (2010). *Revising the Clinic: Vision and Representation in Victorian Medical Narrative and the Novel.* Columbus: Ohio State University Press.

Keynes, Geoffrey. (1966). *The Life of William Harvey.* Oxford: Oxford University Press.

King, Helen. (2007). *Midwifery, Obstetrics and the Rise of Gynaecology.* Aldershot and Burlington: Ashgate.

Koselleck, Reinhart. (2004). *Futures Past: On the Semantics of Historical Time.* New York: Columbia University Press.

La Berge, Ann, and Mordechai Feingold. (1994). *French Medical Culture in the Nineteenth Century.* Amsterdam: Rodopi.

Laqueur, Thomas. (1990). *Making Sex: Body and Gender from the Greeks to Freud.* Cambridge, MA and London, England: Harvard University Press.

Lawrence, Cera. (2008). 'Spermism.' *The Embryo Project Encyclopedia.* Arizona State University. http://embryo.asu.edu/pages/spermism.

Lawrence, Christopher. (1992). 'Democratic, Divine and Heroic: The History and Historiography of Surgery.' In *Medical Theory, Surgical Practice: Studies in the History of Surgery,* ed. Christopher Lawrence, 1–47. London: Routledge.

————. (1998). 'Medical Minds, Surgical Bodies.' In *Science Incarnate: Historical Embodiments of Natural Knowledge*, eds. Christopher Lawrence and Steven Shapin, 156–201. Chicago and London: University of Chicago Press.

Lawrence, Christopher, and Michael Brown. (2016). 'Quintessentially Modern Heroes: Surgeons, Explorers and Empire, c. 1840–1914.' *Journal of Social History* 50 (1): 148–178.

Lawrence, Christopher, and Richard Dixey. (1992). 'Practising on Principle: Joseph Lister and the Germ Theories of Disease.' In *Medical Theory, Surgical Practice: Studies in the History of Surgery*, ed. Christopher Lawrence, 153–215. London and New York: Routledge.

Lawrence, Susan C. (1985). '"Desirous of Improvements in Medicine": Pupils and Practitioners in the Medical Societies at Guy's and St. Bartholomew's Hospitals, 1795–1815.' *Bulletin of the History of Medicine* 59: 89–104.

Levine, George. (2002). *Dying to Know: Scientific Epistemology and Narrative in Victorian England*. Chicago: Chicago University Press.

Levine-Clarke, Marjorie. (2004). *Beyond the Reproductive Body: The Politics of Women's Health in Early Victorian England*. Columbus: Ohio State University Press.

Linker, Beth. (2017). 'Prosthetic Imaginaries: Spinal Surgery and Innovation from the Patient's Perspective.' In *Technological Change in Modern Surgery*, eds. Thomas Schlich and Christopher Crenner, 100–128. Rochester: University of Rochester Press.

Livingstone, David N. (2003). *Putting Science in Its Place: Geographies of Scientific Knowledge*. Chicago: The University of Chicago Press.

Loeb, Lori. (2001). 'Doctors and Patent Medicines in Modern Britain: Professionalism and Consumerism.' *Albion: A Quarterly Journal of British Studies* 33 (3): 404–425.

Longo, Lawrence D. (1979). 'The Rise and Fall of Battey's Operation: A Fashion in Surgery.' *Bulletin of the History of Medicine* 53 (2): 244–267.

Loudon, Irvine. (1986). *Medical Care and the General Practitioner, 1750–1850*. Oxford: Clarendon Press.

Löwy, Ilana. (1993). 'Introduction: Medicine and Change.' In *Medicine and Change: Historical and Sociological Studies of Medical Innovation*, ed. Ilana Löwy, 1–22. Montrouge: John Libbey Eurotext.

————. (2010). *Preventive Strikes: Women, Precancer, and Prophylactic Surgery*. Baltimore: Johns Hopkins University Press.

————. (2011). '"Because of Their Praiseworthy Modesty, They Consult Too Late": Regime of Hope and Cancer of the Womb.' *Bulletin of the History of Medicine* 85 (3): 356–383.

Lyon, John, and Philip R. Sloan. (1981). 'Introduction.' In *From Natural History to the History of Nature: Readings from Buffon and His Critics*, eds. John Lyon and Philip R. Sloan, 1–32. Notre Dame: University of Notre Dame Press.

MacDonald, Helen. (2010). *Possessing the Dead.* Melbourne: Melbourne University Press.

MacLeod, Christine. (1991). 'The Paradoxes of Patenting: Invention and Its Diffusion in 18th- and 19th-Century Britain, France and North America.' *Technology and Culture* 32 (4): 885–910.

———. (2007). *Heroes of Invention.* Cambridge: Cambridge University Press.

MacLeod, Christine, and Gregory Radick. (2013). 'Claiming Ownership in the Technosciences: Patents, Priority and Productivity.' *Studies in History and Philosophy of Science Part A* 44 (2): 188–201.

Magee, Reginald. (2000). 'Surgery in the Pre-Anaesthetic Era: The Life and Work of Robert Liston.' *Health and History* 2 (1): 121–133.

Marx, Paul. (1985). 'Un Conflit Médical à l'Hôtel-Dieu de Rouen en 1790.' *Histoire des Sciences Médicales* 19 (4): 382.

———. (1992). 'Un Conflit Médical à l'Hôtel-Dieu de Rouen en 1790.' *Échanges Magazine* 19: 33.

Mays, Kelly J. (2011). 'Looking Backward, Looking Forward: The Victorians in the Rearview Mirror of Future History.' *Victorian Studies* 53 (3): 445–456.

McClive, Cathy. (2002). 'The Hidden Truths of the Belly: The Uncertainties of Pregnancy in Early Modern Europe.' *Social History of Medicine* 15 (2): 209–227.

McCray Beier, Linda. (1987). *Sufferers and Healers: The Experience of Illness in Seventeenth-Century England.* London and New York: Routledge and Kegan Paul.

McKinlay, J.B. (1981). 'From "Promising Report" to "Standard Procedure": Seven Stages in the Career of a Medical Innovation.' *The Milbank Memorial Fund Quarterly. Health and Society* 59 (3): 374–411.

Merton, Robert K. (1973). *The Sociology of Science.* Chicago: University of Chicago Press.

Miller, Ian. (2009). 'Necessary Torture? Vivisection, Suffragette Force-feeding, and Responses to Scientific Medicine in Britain c. 1870–1920.' *Journal of the History of Medicine and Allied Sciences* 64 (3): 333–372.

Mohr, Peter D. (2004). 'Clay, Charles (1801–1893).' *Oxford Dictionary of National Biography.* Oxford University Press. http://www.oxforddnb.com/view/article/5558.

Moore, Wendy. (2005). *The Knife Man: Blood, Bodysnatching and the Birth of Modern Surgery.* London: Bantam Press.

Morantz-Sanchez, Regina. (1999). *Conduct Unbecoming a Woman: Medicine on Trial in Turn-of-the-Century Brooklyn.* Oxford: Oxford University Press.

———. (2000). 'Negotiating Power at the Bedside: Historical Perspectives on Nineteenth-Century Patients and Their Gynecologists.' *Feminist Studies* 26 (2): 287–309.

Moscucci, Ornella. (1990). *The Science of Woman: Gynaecology and Gender in England 1800–1929*. Cambridge: Cambridge University Press.

———. (2005). 'Gender and Cancer in Britain, 1860–1910: The Emergence of Cancer as a Public Health Concern.' *American Journal of Public Health* 95 (8): 1312–1321.

———. (2007). 'The "Ineffable Freemasonry of Sex": Feminist Surgeons and the Establishment of Radiotherapy in Early Twentieth-Century Britain.' *Bulletin of the History of Medicine* 81 (1): 139–163.

———. (2010). 'The British Fight Against Cancer: Publicity and Education, 1900–1948.' *Social History of Medicine* 23 (2): 356–373.

———. (2017). *Gender and Cancer in England, 1860–1948*. Basingstoke: Palgrave Macmillan.

Munslow, Alan. (2003). *The New History*. Harlow: Pearson.

Murphy, T.D. (1981). 'Medical Knowledge and Statistical Methods in Early Nineteenth-Century France.' *Medical History* 25 (3): 301–319.

Nathoo, Ayesha. (2009). *Hearts Exposed: Transplants and the Media in 1960s Britain*. Basingstoke: Palgrave Macmillan.

Nicolson, Malcolm. (2004). 'Lizars, John (1791/2–1860).' *Oxford Dictionary of National Biography*. Oxford University Press. http://www.oxforddnb.com/view/article/16814.

Nolte, K. (2008). 'Carcinoma Uteri and "Sexual Debauchery"—Morality, Cancer and Gender in the Nineteenth Century.' *Social History of Medicine* 21 (1): 31–46.

Nowell-Smith, Harriet. (1995). 'Nineteenth-Century Narrative Case Histories: An Inquiry into Stylistics and History.' *Canadian Bulletin of Medical History/ Bulletin Canadien D'histoire de La Médecine* 12 (1): 47–67.

Nussbaum, Felicity A. (1995). *Torrid Zones: Maternity, Sexuality, and Empire in Eighteenth-Century Narratives*. Baltimore and London: Johns Hopkins University Press.

O'Connor, Erin. (2000). *Raw Material: Producing Pathology in Victorian Culture*. Durham: Duke University Press.

Olson, James S. (2002). *Bathsheba's Breast: Women, Cancer and History*. Baltimore: Johns Hopkins University Press.

Parker, Sarah. (2016). 'Subtle Bodies: The Limits of Categories in Girolamo Cardano's De Subtilitate.' In *Anatomy and the Organization of Knowledge, 1500–1850*, eds. Matthew Landors and Brian Muñoz, 71–84. London and New York: Routledge.

Patterson, James T. (1987). *The Dread Disease: Cancer and Modern American Culture*. Cambridge and London: Harvard University Press.

Payne, Lynda. (2007). *With Words and Knives: Learning Medical Dispassion in Early Modern England*. Aldershot and Burlington: Ashgate.

Peitzman, Steven J. (1992). 'From Bright's Disease to End-Stage Renal Disease.' In *Framing Disease: Studies in Cultural History*, eds. Charles Rosenberg and Janet Golden, 3–32. New Brunswick: Rutgers University Press.

Pernick, Martin S. (1985). *A Calculus of Suffering: Pain, Professionalism, and Anesthesia in Nineteenth-Century America*. New York: Columbia University Press.

Pettitt, Clare. (2004). *Patent Inventions: Intellectual Property and the Victorian Novel*. Oxford and New York: Oxford University Press.

Pickering, Andrew. (1995). *The Mangle of Practice: Time, Agency and Science*. Chicago: University of Chicago Press.

Pickstone, John V. (1992). 'Introduction.' In *Medical Innovations in Historical Perspective*, ed. John V. Pickstone, 1–16. Basingstoke: Macmillan.

———. (2005). 'Review Article: "Medical History as a Way of Life."' *Social History of Medicine* 18 (2): 307–323.

Pies, N.J, and C.W. Beardsmore. (2003). 'West & West Syndrome—A Historical Sketch About the Eponymous Doctor, His Work and His Family.' *Brain and Development* 25: 84–101.

Pinto-Correia, Clara. (1997). *The Ovary of Eve: Egg and Sperm and Preformation*. Chicago: University of Chicago Press.

Poovey, Mary. (1986). '"Scenes of an Indelicate Character": The Medical "Treatment" of Victorian Women.' *Representations* 14: 137–168.

———. (2008). *Genres of the Credit Economy: Mediating Value in Eighteenth and Nineteenth-Century Britain*. Chicago and London: University of Chicago Press.

Porter, Roy. (1989). *Health for Sale: Quackery in England 1660–1850*. Manchester and New York: Manchester University Press.

Powderly, Kathleen E. (2000). 'Patient Consent and Negotiation in the Brooklyn Gynecological Practice of Alexander J.C. Skene: 1863–1900.' *Journal of Medicine and Philosophy* 25 (1): 12–27.

Power, D'Arcy. (2004). 'Liston, Robert (1794–1847).' *Oxford Dictionary of National Biography*. Oxford University Press. http://www.oxforddnb.com/view/article/16772.

Putnam, Constance E. (2008). 'Smith, Nathan.' *American National Biography*. Online. http://www.anb.org/articles/12/12-00858.html.

Rice, Gillian. (1987). 'The Bell-Magendie-Walker Controversy.' *Medical History* 31 (2): 190–200.

Richards, Thomas. (1990). *The Commodity Culture of Victorian England: Advertising and Spectacle, 1851–1914*. Stanford: Stanford University Press.

Richardson, Ruth. (1987). *Death, Dissection and the Destitute*. London: Routledge and Kegan Paul.

———. (2008). *The Making of Mr. Gray's Anatomy*. Oxford: Oxford University Press.

Riches, E. (1968). 'The History of Lithotomy and Lithotrity.' *Annals of the Royal College of Surgeons of England* 43 (4): 185–199.

Riskin, Daniel J. et al. (2006). 'Innovation in Surgery: A Historical Perspective.' *Annals of Surgery* 244 (5): 686–963.

Risse, Guenter B. (1999). *Mending Bodies, Saving Souls: A History of Hospitals.* Oxford: Oxford University Press.

Rivlin, J.J. (2000). 'Francis Imlach (1851–1920) and the Liverpool Medical Establishment.' *Medical Historian* 42–50, 1999.

Roberts, M.J.D. (2009). 'The Politics of Professionalization: MPs, Medical Men, and the 1858 Medical Act.' *Medical History* 52 (1): 37–56.

Roberts, Mary Louise. (1998). 'Gender, Consumption and Commodity Culture.' *American Historical Review* 103 (3): 817–844.

Roe, Shirley A. (1981). *Matter, Life and Generation: Eighteenth-Century Embryology and the Haller-Wolff Debate.* Cambridge: Cambridge University Press.

Romano, Terrie M. (2000). 'Halsted, William Stewart.' *American National Biography.* Online. http://www.anb.org/articles/12/12-00365.html.

Rosenberg Charles W., and Janet Golden. (1992). *Framing Disease: Studies in Cultural History.* New Brunswick: Rutgers University Press.

Schiebinger, Londa. (1989). *The Mind Has No Sex? Women in the Origins of Modern Science.* Cambridge, MA and London: Harvard University Press.

Schlich, Thomas. (2002). *Surgery, Science and Industry: A Revolution in Fracture Care, 1950s–1980s.* Basingstoke: Palgrave Macmillan.

———. (2004). 'The Emergence of Modern Surgery.' In *Medicine Transformed: Health, Disease and Society in Europe: 1800–1930*, ed. Deborah Brunton, 61–91. Manchester: Manchester University Press.

———. (2006). 'Risk and Medical Innovation: A Historical Perspective.' In *The Risks of Medical Innovation*, eds. Thomas Schlich and Ulrich Tröhler, 1–19. Abingdon and New York: Routledge.

———. (2007). 'Surgery, Science and Modernity: Operating Rooms and Laboratories as Spaces of Control.' *History of Science* 45: 231–256.

———. (2010). *The Origins of Organ Transplantation: Surgery and Laboratory Science 1880–1930.* Rochester and Woodbridge: University of Rochester Press.

———. (2012). 'Asepsis and Bacteriology: A Realignment of Surgery and Laboratory Science.' *Medical History* 56 (3): 308–334.

———. (2015). '"The Days of Brilliancy Are Past": Skill, Styles and the Changing Rules of Surgical Performance, c. 1820–1920.' *Medical History* 59 (3): 379–403.

Schlich, Thomas, and Christopher Crenner. (2017). 'Technological Change in Surgery: An Introductory Essay.' In *Technological Change in Modern Surgery*, eds. Thomas Schlich and Christopher Crenner, 1–20. Rochester: University of Rochester Press.

Scull, Andrew. (2005). *Madhouse: A Tragic Tale of Megalomania and Modern Medicine*. New Haven and London: Yale University Press.

———. (2006). *The Insanity of Place/The Place of Insanity*. London: Routledge.

Searle, G.R. (1998). *Morality and the Market in Victorian Britain*. Oxford: Clarendon Press.

Secord, James A. (2000). *Victorian Sensation: The Extraordinary Publication, Reception, and Secret Authorship of Vestiges of the Natural History of Creation*. Chicago: University of Chicago Press.

Sengoopta, Chandak. (2000). 'The Modern Ovary: Constructions, Meanings, Uses.' *History of Science* 38 (122) Pt 4: 425–88.

Sewell, Jane Eliot. (1990). *Bountiful Bodies: Spencer Wells, Lawson Tait and the Birth of British Gynaecology*. Unpublished PhD thesis, Johns Hopkins University.

———. (2004). 'Wells, Sir Thomas Spencer, First Baronet (1818–1897).' *Oxford Dictionary of National Biography*. Oxford University Press. http://www.oxforddnb.com/view/article/29018.

Shapin, Steven. (1979). 'The Politics of Observation: Cerebral Anatomy and Social Interests in the Edinburgh Phrenology Disputes.' In *On the Margins of Science: The Social Construction of Rejected Knowledge*, ed. Roy Wallis, 139–178. Staffordshire: University of Keele.

Shapin, Steven. (1994). *A Social History of Truth: Civility and Science in Seventeenth-Century England*. Chicago: University of Chicago Press.

Shapin, Steven, and Simon Schaffer. (2011). *Leviathan and the Air-Pump: Hobbes, Boyle, and the Experimental Life*. Princeton: Princeton University Press.

Shaw, George Bernard. (1909). 'The Socialist Criticism of the Medical Profession.' *Transactions of the Medico-Legal Society* 6: 202–228.

Sheldon, Peter. (2004). *The Life and Times of William Withering: His Work, His Legacy*. Studley: Brewin Books.

Shepherd, John A. (1965a). 'William Jeaffreson (1790–1865): Surgical Pioneer.' *British Medical Journal* 2 (5470): 1119–1120.

———. (1965b). *Spencer Wells: The Life and Work of a Victorian Surgeon*. Edinburgh and London: E. & S. Livingstone Ltd.

Shonfield, Zuzanna. (1987). *The Precariously Privileged: A Medical Man's Family in Victorian London*. Oxford and New York: Oxford University Press.

Shortt, S.E.D. (1983). 'Physicians, Science and Status: Issues in the Professionalization of Anglo-American Medicine in the Nineteenth Century.' *Medical History* 27 (1): 51–68.

Showalter, Elaine. (1987). *The Female Malady: Women, Madness and English Culture, 1830–1980*. London: Virago.

Smith, Dale C. (1996). 'Appendicitis, Appendectomy, and the Surgeon.' *Bulletin of the History of Medicine* 70 (3): 414–441.

Smith, Lisa W. (2010). 'Imagining Women's Fertility Before Technology.' *The Journal of Medical Humanities* 31 (1): 69–79.

Smith-Rosenberg, Carroll, and Charles Rosenberg. (1973). 'The Female Animal: Medical and Biological Views of Woman and Her Role in Nineteenth-Century America.' *Journal of American History* 60 (2): 332–356.

Sparks, Tabitha. (2009). *The Doctor in the Victorian Novel: Family Practices*. Farnham and Burlington: Ashgate.

Srirangam, Shalom J., et al. (2009). 'Nephroptosis: Seriously Misunderstood?' *BJU International* 103 (3): 296–300.

Stanley, Peter. (2003). *For Fear of Pain: British Surgery, 1790–1850*. Amsterdam and New York: Rodopi.

Stark, James F. (2016). 'Introduction: Plurality in Patenting: Medical Technology and Cultures of Protection.' *British Journal of the History of Science* 49 (4): 533–540.

Stinson, Daniel T.T. (1969). *The Role of William Lawrence in 19th Century Surgery*. Zurich: Jurie-Verlag.

Studd, John. (2006). 'Ovariotomy for Menstrual Madness and Premenstrual Syndrome—19th Century History and Lessons for Current Practice.' *Gynecological Endocrinology : The Official Journal of the International Society of Gynecological Endocrinology* 22 (8): 411–415.

Sturdy, Steve. (2011). 'Looking for Trouble: Medical Science and Clinical Practice in the Historiography of Modern Medicine.' *Social History of Medicine* 24 (3): 739–757.

Sturdy, Steve, and Roger Cooter. (1998). 'Science, Scientific Management, and the Transformation of Medicine in Britain c.1870–1950.' *History of Science* 36: 421–466.

Swazey, Judith P., and Renée C. Fox. (1988). 'The Clinical Moratorium.' In *Essays in Medical Sociology: Journeys into the Fields*, ed. Renée C. Fox, 325–365. New York: Transaction Publishers.

Takahiro, Ueyama. (2010). *Health in the Marketplace: Professionalism, Therapeutic Desires, and Medical Commodification in Late-Victorian London*. Palo Alto: The Society for the Promotion of Science and Scholarship.

Tames, Richard. (1972). *Economy and Society in Nineteenth Century Britain*. London: George Allen & Unwin.

Tang Cynthia L., and Thomas Schlich. (2017). 'Surgical Innovation and the Multiple Meanings of Randomized Controlled Trials: The First RCT on Minimally Invasive Cholecystectomy (1980–2000).' *Journal of the History of Medicine and Allied Sciences*, 72 (2): 117–141.

Temkin, Oswei. (1977). *The Double Face of Janus and Other Essays in the History of Medicine*. Baltimore: Johns Hopkins University Press.

Thiery, Michel. (1998). 'Battey's Operation : An Exercise in Surgical Frustration.' *European Journal of Obstetrics & Gynecology and Reproductive Biology* 81: 243–246.

Thomas, David Wayne. (2000). 'Replicas and Originality: Picturing Agency in Dante Gabriel Rossetti and Victorian Manchester.' *Victorian Studies* 43 (1): 67–102.

Timmermans, Stefan, and Marc Berg. (2003). *The Gold Standard: The Challenge of Evidence-Based Medicine and Standardization in Health Care*. Philadelphia: Temple University Press.

Todd, Dennis. (1995). *Imagining Monsters: Miscreations of the Self in Eighteenth-Century England*. Chicago and London: University of Chicago Press.

Tröhler, Ulrich. (1978). *Quantification in British Medicine and Surgery 1750–1830, With Special Reference to Its Introduction into Therapeutics*. Unpublished PhD thesis, University College London.

———. (2005). 'Quantifying Experience and Beating Biases: A New Culture in Eighteenth-Century British Clinical Medicine.' In *Body Counts: Medical Quantification in Historical and Sociological Perspective*, eds. Gérard Jorland et al., 19–50. Montreal: McGill-Queen's University Press.

———. (2006). 'To Assess and Improve: Practitioners Approaches to Doubts Linked with Medical Innovations 1720–1920.' In *The Risks of Medical Innovation*, eds. Thomas Schlich and Ulrich Tröhler, 20–37. Abingdon: Routledge.

Vila, Anna C. (1998). *Enlightenment and Pathology: Sensibility in the Literature and Medicine of Eighteenth-Century France*. Baltimore: The Johns Hopkins University Press.

Waddington, Keir. (2003). *Medical Education at St. Bartholomew's Hospital*. Woodbridge: Boydell Press.

———. (2012). 'Dying Scientifically: Gothic Romance and London's Teaching Hospitals.' Paper presented at the 2012 Conference for the British Society for Literature and Science, Oxford, April 13, 2012. http://www.academia.edu/1721140/Dying_Scientifically_Gothic_romance_and_Londons_Teaching_Hospitals.

Wagner, Daniel. (2011). 'Visualisations of the Womb Through Tropes, Dissection and Illustration (circa 1660–1774).' In *Book Illustration in the Long Eighteenth Century: Reconfiguring the Visual Periphery of the Text*, ed. Christina Ionescu, 541–572. Newcastle: Cambridge Scholars.

Walker, Katherine A. (2015). 'Pain and Surgery in England, circa 1620–circa 1740.' *Medical History* 59 (2): 255–274.

Walkowitz, Judith. (1992). *City of Dreadful Delight: Narratives of Sexual Danger in Late Victorian London*. Chicago: University of Chicago Press.

Wall, L. Lewis. (2006). 'The Medical Ethics of Dr J. Marion Sims: a Fresh Look at the Historical Record.' *Journal of Medical Ethics* 32 (6): 346–350.

Wangensteen, Owen H., and Sarah D. Wangensteen. (1978). *The Rise of Surgery: From Empiric Craft to Scientific Discipline*. Minneapolis: University of Minnesota Press.

Warner, John Harley. (1998). *Against the Spirit of the System*. Princeton: Princeton University Press.

Washington, Deleso Alford. (2009). 'Critical Race Feminist Bioethics: Telling Stories in Law School and Medical School in Pursuit of "Cultural Competency".' *Albany Law Review* 72 (4): 961–998.

Wear, Andrew, Johanna Geyer-Kordesch, and Roger French. (1993). 'Introduction.' In *Doctors and Ethics: The Earlier Historical Setting of Professional Ethics*, eds. Andrew Wear et al., 1–9. Amsterdam: Rodopi.

Weatherall, M.W. (1996). 'Making Medicine Scientific: Empiricism, Rationality, and Quackery in mid-Victorian Britain.' *Social History of Medicine* 9 (2): 175–194.

Webster, Charles. (2002). *The National Health Service: A Political History*. Oxford: Oxford University Press.

Weisz, George. (1995). *The Medical Mandarins: The French Academy of Medicine in the Nineteenth and Early Twentieth Centuries*. Oxford: Oxford University Press.

———. (2003). 'The Emergence of Medical Specialization in the Nineteenth Century.' *Bulletin of the History of Medicine* 77 (3): 536–574.

Wellman, Kathleen Anne. (2002). 'Physicians and Philosophes: Physiology and Sexual Morality in the French Enlightenment.' *Eighteenth-Century Studies* 35 (2): 267–277.

Wilde, Sally. (2009). 'Truth, Trust, and Confidence in Surgery, 1890–1910: Patient Autonomy, Communication, and Consent.' *Bulletin of the History of Medicine* 83 (2): 302–330.

———. (2010). *The History of Surgery: Trust, Patient Autonomy, Medical Dominance and Australian Surgery, 1890–1940*. Byron Bay: Finesse Press.

Wilde, Sally, and Geoffrey Hirst. (2009). 'Learning from Mistakes: Early Twentieth-Century Surgical Practice.' *Journal of the History of Medicine and Allied Sciences* 64 (1): 38–77.

Wilson, Adrian. (1985). 'William Hunter and the Varieties of Man-midwifery.' In *William Hunter and the Eighteenth-Century Medical World*, eds. William F. Bynum and Roy Porter, 343–369. Cambridge: Cambridge University Press.

———. (1995). *The Making of Man-Midwifery: Childbirth in England 1660–1770*. London: UCL Press.

Wilson, Philip K. (2002). 'Eighteenth-Century "Monsters" and Nineteenth-Century "Freaks": Reading the Maternally Marked Child.' *Literature and Medicine* 21 (1): 1–25.

Winau, Rolf. (1983). 'The Role of Medical History in the History of Medicine in Germany.' In *Functions and Uses of Disciplinary Histories*, eds. Loren Graham et al., 105–118. Dordrecht: D. Reidel Press.

Winter, Alison. (1991). 'Ethereal Epidemic: Mesmerism and the Introduction of Inhalation Anaesthesia to Early Victorian London.' *Social History of Medicine* 4 (1): 1–27.

Wood, Anthony. (1982). *Nineteenth-Century Britain 1814–1914.* Harlow: Longman House.

Worboys, Michael. (2001). 'British Medicine and its Past at Queen Victoria's Jubilees and the 1900 Centennial.' *Medical History* 45 (4): 461–482.

Xin Zhao et al. (2005). 'Ovariotomy and Persistent Pain Affect Long-Term Fos Expression in Spinal Cord.' *Neuroscience Letters* 375 (3): 165–169.

Young, J.H. (1964). 'James Blundell (1790–1878) Physiologist and Obstetrician.' *Medical History* 8 (2): 159–169.

Permissions

The contributors of this book come from diverse backgrounds, making this book a truly international effort. This book will bring forth new frontiers with its revolutionizing research information and detailed analysis of the nascent developments around the world.

We would like to thank all the contributing authors for lending their expertise to make the book truly unique. They have played a crucial role in the development of this book. Without their invaluable contributions this book wouldn't have been possible. They have made vital efforts to compile up to date information on the varied aspects of this subject to make this book a valuable addition to the collection of many professionals and students.

This book was conceptualized with the vision of imparting up-to-date information and advanced data in this field. To ensure the same, a matchless editorial board was set up. Every individual on the board went through rigorous rounds of assessment to prove their worth. After which they invested a large part of their time researching and compiling the most relevant data for our readers.

The editorial board has been involved in producing this book since its inception. They have spent rigorous hours researching and exploring the diverse topics which have resulted in the successful publishing of this book. They have passed on their knowledge of decades through this book. To expedite this challenging task, the publisher supported the team at every step. A small team of assistant editors was also appointed to further simplify the editing procedure and attain best results for the readers.

Apart from the editorial board, the designing team has also invested a significant amount of their time in understanding the subject and creating the most relevant covers. They scrutinized every image to scout for the most suitable representation of the subject and create an appropriate cover for the book.

The publishing team has been an ardent support to the editorial, designing and production team. Their endless efforts to recruit the best for this project, has resulted in the accomplishment of this book. They are a veteran in the field of academics and their pool of knowledge is as vast as their experience in printing. Their expertise and guidance has proved useful at every step. Their uncompromising quality standards have made this book an exceptional effort. Their encouragement from time to time has been an inspiration for everyone.

The publisher and the editorial board hope that this book will prove to be a valuable piece of knowledge for researchers, students, practitioners and scholars across the globe.

Index

CPSIA information can be obtained
at www.ICGtesting.com
Printed in the USA
BVHW062117290822
645775BV00003B/206

9 781639 894024